The Clozapine Handbook

T0177164

The Clozapine Handbook

Stahl's Handbooks

Jonathan M. Meyer

University of California, San Diego

Stephen M. Stahl

University of California, San Diego

With illustrations by

Nancy Muntner

Neuroscience Education Institute

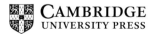

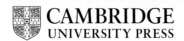

Shaftesbury Road, Cambridge CB2 8EA, United Kingdom

One Liberty Plaza, 20th Floor, New York, NY 10006, USA

477 Williamstown Road, Port Melbourne, VIC 3207, Australia

314–321, 3rd Floor, Plot 3, Splendor Forum, Jasola District Centre, New Delhi – 110025, India

103 Penang Road, #05–06/07, Visioncrest Commercial, Singapore 238467

Cambridge University Press is part of Cambridge University Press & Assessment,
a department of the University of Cambridge.

We share the University's mission to contribute to society through the pursuit of
education, learning and research at the highest international levels of excellence.

www.cambridge.org
Information on this title: www.cambridge.org/9781108447461

DOI: 10.1017/9781108553575

First published 2020 (version 3, July 2024)

Printed in Mexico by Litográfica Ingramex, S.A. de C.V., July 2024

A catalogue record for this publication is available from the British Library.

Library of Congress Cataloging-in-Publication data
Names: Meyer, Jonathan M., 1962– author. | Stahl, Stephen M., 1951– author. |
Title: The clozapine handbook / Jonathan M. Meyer, Stephen M. Stahl.
Other titles: Stahl's handbooks.
Description: Cambridge ; New York, NY : Cambridge University Press, 2019. | Series: Stahl's
handbooks | Includes bibliographical references and index.
Identifiers: LCCN 2018054843 | ISBN 9781108447461 (paperback : alk. paper)
Subjects: | MESH: Clozapine – administration & dosage | Clozapine – therapeutic use |
Clozapine – adverse effects | Antipsychotic Agents | Schizophrenia – drug therapy
Classification: LCC RM333.5 | NLM QV 77.9 | DDC 615.7/882–dc23
LC record available at https://lccn.loc.gov/2018054843

ISBN 978-1-108-44746-1 Paperback

Jonathan M. Meyer, M.D. is a Clinical Professor of Psychiatry at the University of California San Diego, and a Psychopharmacology Consultant to the California Department of State Hospitals. Over the past 36 months Dr. Meyer reports having served as a **consultant** to Acadia Pharmaceuticals, Alkermes, Allergan, Intra-Cellular Therapies, Merck, Neurocrine and Teva Pharmaceutical Industries; he has served on the **speakers bureaus** for Acadia Pharmaceuticals, Alkermes, Allergan, Intra-Cellular Therapies, Merck, Neurocrine, Otsuka America, Inc., Sunovion Pharmaceuticals and Teva Pharmaceutical Industries.

Stephen M. Stahl, M.D., PhD, Dsc (Hon.) is an Adjunct Professor of Psychiatry at the University of California San Diego, Honorary Visiting Senior Fellow at the University of Cambridge, UK and Director of Psychopharmacology for California Department of State Hospitals. Over the past 36 months (January 2016 – December 2018) Dr. Stahl has served as a **consultant** to Acadia, Adamas, Alkermes, Allergan, Arbor Pharmaceutcials, AstraZeneca, Avanir, Axovant, Axsome, Biogen, Biomarin, Biopharma, Celgene, Concert, ClearView, DepoMed, Dey, EnVivo, EMD Serono, Ferring, Forest, Forum, Genomind, Innovative Science Solutions, Intra-Cellular Therapies, Janssen, Jazz, Lilly, Lundbeck, Merck, Neos, Novartis, Noveida, Orexigen, Otsuka, PamLabs, Perrigo, Pfizer, Pierre Fabre, Reviva, Servier, Shire, Sprout, Sunovion, Taisho, Takeda, Taliaz, Teva, Tonix, Trius, Vanda, Vertex and Viforpharma; he has been a **board member** of RCT Logic and Genomind; he has served on **speakers bureaus** for Acadia, Astra Zeneca, Dey Pharma, EnVivo, Eli Lilly, Forum, Genentech, Janssen, Lundbeck, Merck, Otsuka, PamLabs, Pfizer Israel, Servier, Sunovion and Takeda and he has received **research and/or grant support** from Acadia, Alkermes, AssureX, Astra Zeneca, Arbor Pharmaceuticals, Avanir, Axovant, Biogen, Braeburn Pharmaceuticals, BristolMyer Squibb, Celgene, CeNeRx, Cephalon, Dey, Eli Lilly, EnVivo, Forest, Forum, GenOmind, Glaxo Smith Kline, Intra-Cellular Therapies, ISSWSH, Janssen, JayMac, Jazz, Lundbeck, Merck, Mylan, Neurocrine, Neuronetics, Novartis, Otsuka, PamLabs, Pfizer, Reviva, Roche, Sepracor, Servier, Shire, Sprout, Sunovion, TMS NeuroHealth Centers, Takeda, Teva, Tonix, Vanda, Valeant and Wyeth

All illustrations by Nancy Muntner provided by permission of Neuroscience Education Institute.

Contents

Foreword

It is 30 years since the Clozaril Collaborative Study Group published the pivotal trial results in September 1988 that established clozapine's efficacy in treatment-resistant schizophrenia, with subsequent research noting clozapine's unique benefit for suicidal and persistently aggressive schizophrenia patients [1–3]. Over the ensuing decades no other medication has proven effective for this multiplicity of uses, yet many candidate patients throughout the world are deprived of a clozapine trial. That clozapine is underutilized has been lamented in numerous publications, and remains a source of consternation for the psychiatric profession as treatment-resistant patients are repeatedly exposed to ineffective medications with little likelihood of response.

Yet, there is hope in reversing the long-standing problem of mental health clinicians refusing to prescribe a potentially effective and in some instances life-saving/life-changing medication. The past half decade has the seen the rise of initiatives to increase clozapine use in certain parts of Europe and the United States, efforts that are informed by a body of literature documenting the benefits accrued to the individual, as well as to a society at large that bears the economic and social burdens of managing treatment-resistant schizophrenia. In 2015 the United States Food and Drug Administration (FDA) modernized and streamlined its clozapine prescribing guidelines, and in doing so created an evidenced-based model that can be emulated throughout the world. There have also been advances in our understanding of effective strategies to manage common adverse effects such as sialorrhea and constipation, and data-driven approaches to more vexing problems such as fever occurring during the initial 6–8 weeks of clozapine treatment.

Despite overwhelming international support in favor of increased clozapine access, one stumbling block is the need to support and nurture relevant clinicians, many of whom cite lack of education regarding clozapine's nuances as a primary reason to avoid prescribing this medication [4,5]. The present volume thus appears at an opportune time, and, in a comprehensive manner, covers the latest information and updated guidelines in a practical and easily accessible format. Nowhere is this breadth of information and clinical insights about clozapine use provided within a single volume; moreover, of great benefit to clinicians is the manner in which Dr. Meyer and Dr. Stahl walk the reader through common issues in clozapine management and present a rationale for the next steps.

The time has come to turn the tide on the regrettable practice patterns that lead to clozapine underutilization. It is hoped that clinicians and health-care systems will take advantage of this valuable handbook to increase patient access to clozapine.

John M. Kane MD

Professor and Chairman, Department of Psychiatry, The Donald and Barbara Zucker School of Medicine at Hofstra/Northwell

Senior Vice President, Behavioral Health Services, Northwell Health

References

1. Kane, J., Honigfeld, G., Singer, J., et al. (1988). Clozapine for the treatment-resistant schizophrenic. A double-blind comparison with chlorpromazine. *Archives of General Psychiatry*, 45, 789–796.

2. Meltzer, H. Y., Alphs, L., Green, A. I., et al. (2003). Clozapine treatment for suicidality in schizophrenia: International Suicide Prevention Trial (InterSePT). *Archives of General Psychiatry*, 60, 82–91.

3. Krakowski, M. I., Czobor, P., Citrome, L., et al. (2006). Atypical antipsychotic agents in the treatment of violent patients with schizophrenia and schizoaffective disorder. *Archives of General Psychiatry*, 63, 622–629.

4. Nielsen, J., Dahm, M., Lublin, H., et al. (2010). Psychiatrists' attitude towards and knowledge of clozapine treatment. *Journal of Psychopharmacology*, 24, 965–971.

5. Cohen, D. (2014). Prescribers fear as a major side-effect of clozapine. *Acta Psychiatrica Scandinavica*, 130, 154–155.

Introduction

The year 2018 marked the 60th anniversary of clozapine's synthesis, and the 30th anniversary of the September 1988 *Archives of General Psychiatry* paper by Kane and colleagues documenting clozapine's superior efficacy in treatment-resistant schizophrenia [1]. The peer view literature since 1988 demonstrates ongoing interest in clozapine, with 350–450 papers per year listed in PubMed (see Figure 1). The ensuing decades have also seen other evidence-based uses for clozapine (e.g. schizophrenia patients with suicidality or aggression, Parkinson's disease psychosis, treatment-resistant mania), but treatment-resistant schizophrenia spectrum disorders remain the most common indication. Lamentably, clozapine remains significantly underutilized for treatment-resistant schizophrenia despite compelling evidence of efficacy in this population, and the enormous individual and societal benefits that can accrue from effective management of treatment-resistant patients [2].

To fully appreciate the economic impact of treatment-resistant schizophrenia, one must understand the enormity of the disease burden exacted by schizophrenia. Schizophrenia prevalence remains low, with the global estimate of 0.28% remaining unchanged from 1990 to 2016. The 2016 age distribution of disease also mirrored that in 1990, but the total number of cases rose nearly 60% due to population increases (see Figure 2 and Table 1). There are now close to 21 million persons worldwide with schizophrenia, most of whom require extensive supportive resources. A 2012 meta-analysis indicated that only 13.5% of schizophrenia patients meet criteria for functional recovery; moreover, in addition to lengthy periods of disability, schizophrenia patients suffer premature mortality due to natural and unnatural causes [3]. The World Health Organization (WHO) quantifies the dual impact of disorders using the outcome of disability-adjusted life year, a measure that sums the years lived with disability and those lost due to early mortality. Schizophrenia ranked twelfth overall among 310 conditions (i.e. diseases or injuries) studied in the WHO Global Burden of Disease Study 2016, and acute schizophrenia carried the highest disability weight

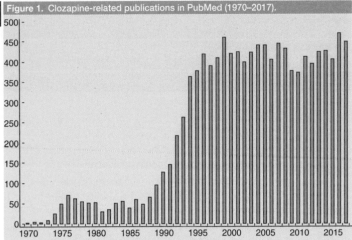

Figure 1. Clozapine-related publications in PubMed (1970–2017).

among all disorders [3,4]. Despite its low global prevalence of 0.28%, schizophrenia contributed 13.4 million years of life lost due to disability in 2016. This represented 1.7% of the total in the 2016 WHO study, a value sixfold greater than the prevalence of schizophrenia. For the United States (US) alone, the combination of direct health care costs, direct nonhealth-care costs (law enforcement, homeless shelters, health-care training and research) and indirect costs (productivity loss from disability, premature mortality, caregiving) was estimated at $155.7 billion for 2013 [5]. The largest components were excess costs associated with unemployment (38%), productivity loss due to caregiving (34%) and direct health-care costs (24%).

Treatment-resistant schizophrenia patients are but a fraction of the schizophrenia population, yet they exert an outsized influence on the costs associated with this disorder. While there is active debate about the definition of treatment resistance for clinical and research purposes, an estimated 20–30% of schizophrenia patients fail to adequately respond to two or more documented antipsychotic trials of sufficient dosage and duration [6,7]. A 2014 review on the social and economic burden of treatment-resistant schizophrenia found 65 papers published from 1996 to 2012 to provide data for relative cost estimates [6]. Based on this extensive literature review, annual costs for patients with schizophrenia in the US were three- to 11-fold higher for those who were treatment-resistant, with hospitalization costs and total health-resource utilization 10-fold higher among this cohort than for schizophrenia patients in general (see Figure 3). The authors concluded that treatment-resistant schizophrenia

Figure 2. Mean schizophrenia prevalence by age in 2016.

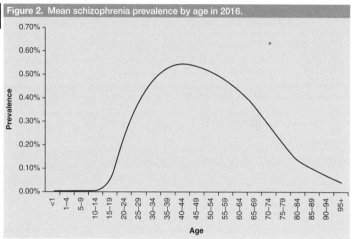

(Adapted from: Charlson, F. J., Ferrari, A. J., Santomauro, D. F., et al. (2018). Global epidemiology and burden of schizophrenia: findings from the Global Burden of Disease Study 2016. *Schizophrenia Bulletin* 44, 1195–1203.)

Table 1 Age-standardized schizophrenia prevalence in 1990 and 2016 [3].

Region	Total number of cases (in 1000s)		Prevalence (%)	
	1990	2016	1990	2016
Southeast Asia, East Asia, and Oceania	5869.3	9109.4	0.38	0.38
Central Europe, Eastern Europe, and Central Asia	865.9	987.0	0.20	0.21
South Asia	2112.1	3986.1	0.25	0.25
Australasia	71.5	105.9	0.33	0.33
Western Europe	1029.4	1242.9	0.24	0.25
High-income North America	884.6	1214.7	0.30	0.30
Latin America and Caribbean	635.0	1186.5	0.20	0.20
North Africa and Middle East	443.9	1014.7	0.18	0.19
Sub-Saharan Africa	619.0	1314.1	0.19	0.19
Global	13,122.1	20,883.0	0.28	0.28

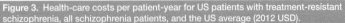

Figure 3. Health-care costs per patient-year for US patients with treatment-resistant schizophrenia, all schizophrenia patients, and the US average (2012 USD).

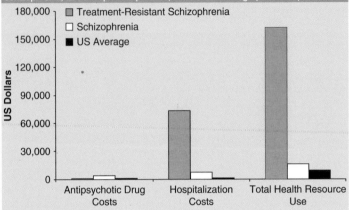

(Adapted from: Kennedy, J. L., Altar, C. A., Taylor, D. L., et al. (2014). The social and economic burden of treatment-resistant schizophrenia: a systematic literature review. *International Clinical Psychopharmacology*, 29, 63–76 [6].)

conservatively adds more than $34 billion in annual direct medical costs in the US [6]. On a personal level, quality of life for schizophrenia patients who are unresponsive or intolerant to treatment is 20% lower than that of patients who achieve more robust symptomatic improvement [6].

Clinicians are often more focused on alleviating individual suffering than the societal impact of disease burden, but despite widespread availability and compelling efficacy data clozapine remains underutilized for treatment-resistant schizophrenia [2]. Although 20–30% of schizophrenia patients are treatment-resistant, only six of 50 states in the US report that more than 10% of schizophrenia patients have received a prescription for clozapine; moreover, many clozapine candidates are subjected to years of multiple, ineffective antipsychotic trials. Systemic issues are one disincentive to clozapine use for outpatients, with one workgroup noting that most mental health-care systems lack "a centralized infrastructure for coordinating the array of services required by persons receiving clozapine" [2]. While one might assume that more densely populated urban areas would have the resources to support new clozapine treatment, a 2014 analysis of US clozapine prescribing in 2002–2005 noted that, on a county level, there was no significant effect of population density or measures of poverty or income on clozapine initiation, though a higher density of psychiatrists (≥ 15 per 100,000 population) was associated with a greater likelihood of commencing clozapine [8]. Certain factors, such as age, gender, race, substance use and medical comorbidity all played roles in clozapine usage, but geographic location emerged as a significant overriding predictor, suggesting that local culture in certain areas reinforces evidence-based practice, while that in other areas tolerates the notion that "We don't prescribe clozapine in this area" as an acceptable response to managing treatment-resistant schizophrenia (see Figure 4). Bolstering this argument are data from that 2014 analysis which indicate that patients residing in US counties that had historically

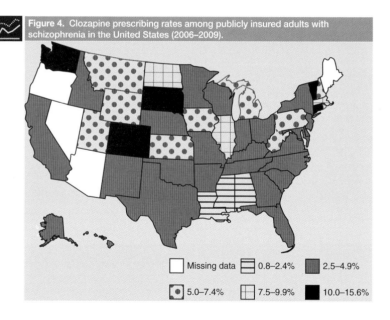

Figure 4. Clozapine prescribing rates among publicly insured adults with schizophrenia in the United States (2006–2009).

Missing data   0.8–2.4%   2.5–4.9%   5.0–7.4%   7.5–9.9%   10.0–15.6%

(Adapted from: Olfson, M., Gerhard, T., Crystal, S., et al. (2016). Clozapine for schizophrenia: state variation in evidence-based practice. *Psychiatric Services*, 67, 152 [16].)

high clozapine usage were nearly twice as likely to start clozapine as patients residing in historically low-use counties [8]. This problem is not unique to the US, as 2002 prescribing data from the United Kingdom (UK) found a 34-fold variation in clozapine use across National Health Service (NHS) trusts [9]. One practical obstacle to clozapine treatment among patients of African descent has been benign ethnic neutropenia (BEN), but revisions of absolute neutrophil count (ANC) thresholds for BEN individuals in many countries has markedly reduced the impact of this benign variant [10].

 PRESCRIBER FEAR

While recent US changes to ANC thresholds for all patients (including new BEN thresholds) have enlarged the pool of individuals who can start clozapine, there is one barrier that no regulatory authority can overcome, and that is clinician fear of prescribing clozapine [10,11]. Despite the overwhelming evidence that patients on clozapine have lower mortality from natural and unnatural causes, enhanced quality of life due to reduced symptom burden, and that no other antipsychotic is robustly effective for treatment-resistant schizophrenia, numerous papers document overestimation of safety concerns combined at times with a misunderstanding of the tremendous efficacy difference between clozapine and other antipsychotics for treatment-resistant schizophrenia. In an article entitled "Prescribers Fear as a Major Side-Effect of Clozapine", Professor Dan Cohen (Mental Health Organization North-Holland North, Heerhugowaard, The Netherlands) comments:

> This unscientific and irrational fear is a clinically relevant phenomenon as it causes psychiatrists to withhold their patients an effective, evidence-based treatment, thereby unnecessarily prolonging their patients' suffering. [11]

The net result is that many psychiatrists either refuse to prescribe clozapine, or do so in a limited manner, a finding seen in studies across the globe including the US, Denmark, India and the UK [12–15]. Given the enormous social and economic impact of clozapine use, large health-care systems have taken note of this gap between evidence-based practice and the routine underuse of clozapine for treatment-resistant schizophrenia, and have commenced initiatives to promote clozapine prescribing. In the UK, variation in clozapine use across NHS trusts was reduced from 34-fold in 2002 to 5-fold by 2006 in part due to the publication of national guidelines recommending clozapine after inadequate response to two antipsychotics [9]. In other places, more intensive, coordinated efforts have been devised employing some or all of the principles outlined in Box 1.

Box 1 Strategies for Increasing Clozapine Utilization [11,15]

1. Establishment of national or regional (e.g. state-wide) clozapine expertise centers tasked with performing three essential functions:

   a. Real-time consultation without a fee on treatment indications, clozapine initiation, drug–drug interactions, prevention or management of adverse effects.

   b. Provide educational outreach to mental health professionals through lectures, publications, and written summaries of important clinical points (e.g. constipation management).

   c. Modernizing local clozapine prescribing guidelines (as recently performed in the US) to reduce initiation and treatment burdens, remove unnecessary monitoring requirements (e.g. total white blood cell count), lower absolute neutrophil count (ANC) thresholds for all patients, establish appropriate lower ANC thresholds for those with benign ethnic neutropenia, and other evidence-based changes as indicated by developments in the literature.

2. Development of a national or regional (e.g. state-wide) pharmacy surveillance system to identify all schizophrenia patients that are prescribed a third antipsychotic other than clozapine. When this occurs, the prescriber must provide documentation justifying this choice in lieu of clozapine. Such documentation must include the fact that the patient has been informed of the specific benefits of clozapine (e.g. symptom reduction, mortality reduction, lower suicide rate), and include the patient's signature (and that of a caregiver or guardian if the patient lacks capacity) noting the date of the discussion.

3. Incentivizing clinic systems to promote clozapine prescribing through financial methods (e.g. money for training or technical assistance).

4. Publication of regional clozapine usage rates for clinic systems (per 100 schizophrenia spectrum patients) on an annual basis to clearly identify persistent areas of underutilization. Detailed action plans will be demanded from centers with low levels of clozapine use.

5. Creation of internet-based education programs geared towards consumers and family members. One model is the New York State Office of Mental Health web-based module "Considering Clozapine" that provides information about clozapine (including benefits and risks), and includes a series of testimonials from consumers who describe personal benefits from clozapine along with its challenges.

Elements of these programs include support and education of clinicians to enhance their ability to manage clozapine-treated patients, and ongoing system-wide surveillance of clozapine usage rates to reinforce the new cultural norm that underuse of clozapine is a mark of substandard psychiatric practice. The engendered fear of using clozapine is often simply a byproduct of inadequate education and not clinician indifference to the patient's condition, but providing information to clinicians, patients and families about clozapine's benefits is not enough. The creation of a clozapine resource center was an important aspect of programs established in the Netherlands and in New York State. These centers were typically staffed by knowledgeable senior psychiatrists and thereby allowed clinicians immediate answers to pressing questions during working hours. The value of the personal connection and the immediacy of the response cannot be underestimated. In the Netherlands prescriptions for all antipsychotics rose 8.2% from 2008 and 2012, but through the efforts of the Dutch Clozapine Collaboration Group (www.clozapinepluswerkgrocp.nl) clozapine use in this same interval rose by 20% [11]. Across the state of New York the proportion of new clozapine starts increased by 40% from 2009 to 2013 following commencement of their "Best Practices Initiative – Clozapine" in 2010 [15]. Importantly, the quarterly percentage change in rate of clozapine initiation among state run facilities was threefold higher than in other settings, illustrating the concept that local changes in culture with respect to clozapine prescribing are self-reinforcing. As more clinicians in a practice setting develop comfort with and expertise in clozapine prescribing, those who fail to meet the new expectations of competence will increasingly be viewed in a negative light by their colleagues.

 CONCLUSIONS

There is a worldwide effort to increase clozapine use, but many clinicians lack access to expert consultation services or other centralized resources of information about clozapine. It is hoped that this volume will serve as a unified guide for those clinicians who strive to provide optimal, evidence-based care for their patients in need of clozapine. The focus of this handbook is on the practical management of clozapine initiation and adverse effects, with the idea that each chapter will present a self-contained discussion of a particular topic for the busy clinician. As the reader will discover, there is a paucity of double-blind, placebo-controlled trials governing most aspects of clozapine side-effect management, but patients must be treated with the best tools available, and this handbook uses the extant literature to guide clinicians through various options. The net goal is to demystify the use of clozapine, and empower mental health providers everywhere to provide their patients with this effective, and at times life-saving, medication.

References

1. Kane, J., Honigfeld, G., Singer, J., et al. (1988). Clozapine for the treatment-resistant schizophrenic. A double-blind comparison with chlorpromazine. *Archives of General Psychiatry*, 45, 789–796.

2. Kelly, D. L., Freudenreich, O., Sayer, M. A., et al. (2018). Addressing barriers to clozapine underutilization: a national effort. *Psychiatric Services*, 69, 224–227.

3. Charlson, F. J., Ferrari, A. J., Santomauro, D. F., et al. (2018). Global epidemiology and burden of schizophrenia: findings from the Global Burden of Disease Study 2016. *Schizophrenia Bulletin*, 44, 1195–1203.

4. Vos, T., Abajobir, A. A., Abbafati, C., et al. (2017). Global, regional, and national incidence, prevalence, and years lived with disability for 328 diseases and injuries for 195 countries, 1990–2016: A systematic analysis for the Global Burden of Disease Study 2016. *Lancet*, 390, 1211–1259.

5. Cloutier, M., Aigbogun, M. S., Guerin, A., et al. (2016). The economic burden of schizophrenia in the United States in 2013. *Journal of Clinical Psychiatry*, 77, 764–771.

6. Kennedy, J. L., Altar, C. A., Taylor, D. L., et al. (2014). The social and economic burden of treatment-resistant schizophrenia: A systematic literature review. *International Clinical Psychopharmacology*, 29, 63–76.

7. Howes, O. D., McCutcheon, R., Agid, O., et al. (2017). Treatment-resistant schizophrenia: Treatment Response and Resistance in Psychosis (TRRIP) Working Group consensus guidelines on diagnosis and terminology. *American Journal of Psychiatry*, 174, 216–229.

8. Stroup, T. S., Gerhard, T., Crystal, S., et al. (2014). Geographic and clinical variation in clozapine use in the United States. *Psychiatric Services*, 65, 186–192.

9. Downs, J. and Zinkler, M. (2007). Clozapine: National review of postcode prescribing. *Psychiatric Bulletin*, 31, 384–387.

10. Sultan, R. S., Olfson, M., Correll, C. U., et al. (2017). Evaluating the effect of the changes in FDA guidelines for clozapine monitoring. *Journal of Clinical Psychiatry*, 78, e933–e939.

11. Cohen, D. (2014). Prescribers fear as a major side-effect of clozapine. *Acta Psychiatrica Scandinavica*, 130, 154–155.

12. Nielsen, J., Dahm, M., Lublin, H., et al. (2010). Psychiatrists' attitude towards and knowledge of clozapine treatment. *Journal of Psychopharmacology*, 24, 965–971.

13. Grover, S., Balachander, S., Chakarabarti, S., et al. (2015). Prescription practices and attitude of psychiatrists towards clozapine: A survey of psychiatrists from India. *Asian Journal of Psychiatry*, 18, 57–65.

14. Tungaraza, T. E. and Farooq, S. (2015). Clozapine prescribing in the UK: Views and experience of consultant psychiatrists. *Therapeutic Advances in Psychopharmacology*, 5, 88–96.

15. Carruthers, J., Radigan, M., Erlich, M. D., et al. (2016). An initiative to improve clozapine prescribing in New York State. *Psychiatric Services*, 67(4), 369–371.

16. Olfson, M., Gerhard, T., Crystal, S., et al. (2016). Clozapine for schizophrenia: state variation in evidence-based practice. *Psychiatric Services*, 67, 152.

1

The Efficacy Story: Treatment-Resistant Schizophrenia, Psychogenic Polydipsia, Treatment-Intolerant Schizophrenia, Suicidality, Violence, Mania and Parkinson's Disease Psychosis

QUICK CHECK

INTRODUCTION

The 60th anniversary of clozapine's synthesis by Schmutz and Eichenberger at Wander Pharmaceuticals was celebrated in 2018, although the chemists involved hoped that their tricyclic compound HF-1854 would possess antidepressant effects [1]. In January 1961, the first pharmacological report on HF-1854 described an agent with sedative and antiadrenergic properties that resembled chlorpromazine, but which did not induce catalepsy [1]. Further animal testing reported in December 1961 established a range of activities comparable to chlorpromazine but without the catalepsy induction seen with haloperidol. In 1962 the first open clinical trial of HF-1854 found limited efficacy at the dose of 160 mg TID ($n = 19$), but later that year Gross and Langer in Vienna found good results in 21 of 28 patients at similar dosing, again without neurological adverse effects [2]. Further trial reports to Wander

- Clozapine is the only effective antipsychotic for treatment-resistant schizophrenia. When treatment resistance is rigorously defined using all three Kane criteria, the response rate to most antipsychotics is < 5%, and for olanzapine 7%.

- Delaying clozapine initiation beyond 3 years after treatment resistance is identified reduces the likelihood of response.

- Compared to other antipsychotics, real-world data indicate that clozapine-treated patients have lower rehospitalization rates, and decreased mortality from all causes (natural and unnatural).

- Clozapine is uniquely effective in schizophrenia patients with psychogenic polydipsia.

- Clozapine is effective for schizophrenia patients with suicidality on the basis of a large clinical trial vs. olanzapine. Clozapine has an approved indication for this purpose in the US.

- Clozapine's impact on suicidality and aggression is independent of the antipsychotic effect.

- Clozapine has proven efficacy in treatment-resistant mania when used adjunctively with mood-stabilizing medications, and is effective in nonpsychotic bipolar patients.

- Prior to the development of pimavanserin, clozapine was the antipsychotic with the strongest evidence for efficacy and tolerability in Parkinson's disease psychosis.

Pharmaceuticals in 1966 by Hippius in Berlin and Engelmeier in Vienna indicated that this was an effective but sedating antipsychotic that appeared free of neurological side effects. Wander completed further toxicological assays in 1967 and embarked on multiple clinical trials resulting in product registration in 1971, and marketing the following year under the trade name Leponex [1]. A spate of severe neutropenia cases from Finland in 1975 led to clozapine's withdrawal from the market in most countries, although it was available under humanitarian programs with hematological monitoring [3].

Three double-blind studies comparing clozapine to other antipsychotics were published in the 1970s and 1980s based on perceived benefit in those who did not respond to other agents, or improved tolerability in patients with a history of severe intolerance to D_2 antagonism (i.e. akathisia, parkinsonism, tardive dyskinesia (TD) or neuroleptic malignant syndrome (NMS)). While clozapine was clearly better tolerated and more effective than chlorpromazine among those with a history of D_2 sensitivity [4], the two large efficacy trials used modest dosages of the comparator antipsychotics (chlorpromazine 360 mg/day, haloperidol 7.6 mg/day), raising doubts about clozapine's greater effectiveness [5]. The latter question was definitively settled with publication of the pivotal clozapine trial for treatment-resistant schizophrenia in 1988, using criteria elaborated by Dr. John Kane for this purpose [6]. A crucial element of the trial design was the third criterion for treatment resistance: demonstrating in a prospective manner failure to respond to high levels of D_2 antagonism. Fewer than 2% of patients met response criteria in the prospective haloperidol arm of the Kane study (mean dose 61 mg/day), while 80% were nonresponders and 18% intolerant of high-dose haloperidol. Using only those schizophrenia patients who met all three of the treatment-resistance criteria ($n = 268$), response rates in the short (6-week) double-blind, randomized trial were 4% for the chlorpromazine arm vs. 30% for the clozapine group [6]. Additional experience over the next decade combined with insights regarding therapeutic plasma levels has increased the expected clozapine response rate to at least 40% in longer-term studies, with values up to 60% reported [7]. Clozapine has also demonstrated efficacy in schizophrenia patients with psychogenic polydipsia, an effect seen with doses as low as 300 mg/day [8].

Box 1.1 Essential Components of the Kane Definition of Treatment-Resistant Schizophrenia for Patients Enrolled in the Pivotal Clozapine Trial

1. At least three periods of treatment in the preceding 5 years with antipsychotics (from at least two different chemical classes) at dosages equivalent to or greater than 1000 mg/day of chlorpromazine for a period of 6 weeks, each without significant symptomatic relief.
2. No period of good functioning within the preceding 5 years.
3. Failure to respond to a prospective high-dose trial of a typical antipsychotic (haloperidol at doses up to 60 mg/day or higher administered with benztropine 6 mg/day). Response was defined as a 20% decrease in the Brief Psychiatric Rating Scale (BPRS) total score plus either a post-treatment Clinical Global Impression (CGI) severity rating of mildly ill (≤ 3) or a post-treatment BPRS score ≤ 35.

The unique benefits of clozapine extend beyond treatment-resistant schizophrenia and include a number of other uses, many of which are supported by rigorous double-blind, placebo or active comparator trials. In some instances, the value of clozapine lies in its low affinity for D_2 receptors, thus permitting treatment of schizophrenia patients intolerant of D_2 antagonism, or Parkinson's disease psychosis (PDP) patients. For other applications, the underlying mechanism for clozapine's effectiveness is unknown, but it appears independent of the antipsychotic effect when employed for treatment-resistant mania, in schizophrenia patients with persistent aggression, and in schizophrenia patients with a history of suicidality. By mastering the details of hematologic monitoring and management of adverse effects, clinicians have a range of evidence-based uses for clozapine in difficult-to-treat patient groups.

A Treatment-Resistant Schizophrenia

While inconvenient, criterion 3 of the Kane 1988 criteria is central to a research definition of treatment resistance. Studies using "modified Kane criteria" that lack this crucial element report unrealistically high response rates for atypical antipsychotics other than clozapine. The enormous impact of criterion 3 can be seen in the three double-blind studies of olanzapine for treatment-resistant schizophrenia (Table 1.1). Response rates to olanzapine at doses up to 50 mg/day were 0% and 7% in the two studies that included criterion 3 [9,10], but response to olanzapine was 50% when this step was omitted [11].

Unfortunately the literature is littered with numerous papers in which patients with varying degrees of treatment resistance and intolerance are grouped together, leading the unwary reader to question clozapine's benefit in treatment-resistant patients. Adding to the confusion was a 2016 meta-analysis that included literally any definition of treatment resistance in its examination of the literature, and reviewed studies that also enrolled treatment-intolerant patients [12]. Although that meta-analysis did not change perceptions regarding clozapine's efficacy for treatment-resistant schizophrenia, it reinforced the concept that one must take a jaundiced view of studies for treatment-resistant schizophrenia that do not subject patients to a prospective antipsychotic trial and rely solely on historical records of prior antipsychotic treatment. Aside from treatment resistance, there are many reasons that patients may fail to respond adequately to an antipsychotic, with nonadherence, underdosing and kinetic issues playing significant roles. To further emphasize this point, in a recent outpatient

Table 1.1 Double-blind olanzapine trials using strict criteria for treatment-resistant schizophrenia.

Reference	Population included	% Responders
Conley et al., 1998 [9]	Treatment-resistant schizophrenia, defined by Kane criteria: • Inpatients with poor function for ≥ 5 years • Historical failure with two typical antipsychotics for at least 6 weeks on daily doses > 1000 mg/day chlorpromazine equivalents • **Failure of a prospective 6-week haloperidol trial at daily doses of 10–40 mg** **Study method:** 8-week fixed-dose trial of olanzapine 25 mg/day vs. chlorpromazine 1200 mg/day (n = 84). Response defined as ≥ 20% improvement in the total BPRS score, endpoint BPRS score ≤ 35, and a CGI severity score ≤ 3.	Olanzapine 7%[1] Chlorpromazine 0%
Conley et al., 2003 [10]	Treatment-resistant schizophrenia, defined by Kane criteria: • Inpatients with poor function for ≥ 5 years • Historical failure with two typical antipsychotics for at least 6 weeks on daily doses > 1000 mg/d chlorpromazine equivalents • **Failure of a prospective 6-week haloperidol trial at daily doses of 10–40 mg** **Study method:** Double-blind, randomized crossover study of olanzapine 50 mg/day vs. clozapine 450 mg/day (with option for reduction to 30 mg/day olanzapine or 300 mg/day clozapine for tolerability) (n = 23). Patients received 8 weeks on olanzapine or clozapine including a 2-week titration to the target dose. At the end of 8 weeks subjects were switched to the other medication. Response was defined as ≥ 20% improvement in total BPRS score, and a final BPRS score ≤ 35 or a 1 point improvement on the CGI severity score.	Olanzapine 0% Clozapine 20%
Meltzer et al., 2008 [11]	Treatment-resistant schizophrenia, defined as historical failure of two or more trials of typical or atypical antipsychotics "with usually adequate doses" for at least 6 weeks. **Study method:** 1-year double-blind study of olanzapine up to 45 mg/day and clozapine up to 900 mg/day (n = 40). Response was defined as ≥ 20% improvement in total PANSS score at 6 months, or at 6 weeks if drop out was due to reasons other than lack of efficacy.	Olanzapine 50%[2] Clozapine 60%

Comments
1. Twenty-seven olanzapine-treated subjects who failed to respond in this study were titrated on open-label clozapine and followed for 8 weeks. Using the same response definition as the prior trial, 41% met response criteria on clozapine [71].
2. No prospective trial of high-dose typical antipsychotic (Kane criterion 3).

study of 99 schizophrenia patients deemed treatment-resistant, 35% had plasma antipsychotic levels that were subtherapeutic [13].

One positive outcome of the confusing 2016 meta-analysis was a sharpening of the debate regarding the need to define treatment resistance in research and clinical settings [14]. There is little question that, when rigorously defined using all three Kane criteria, the anticipated response rate to antipsychotics other than clozapine is < 5%, compared to rates ≥ 40% for clozapine. Because implementing criterion 3 is often impractical for routine clinical care, a consensus panel published guidelines in 2017 to help clinicians ascertain when patients are treatment-resistant. Included in this recommendation is that the term "refractory" no longer be used (Table 1.2).

Table 1.2 Consensus criteria for defining an adequate antipsychotic trial in resistant schizophrenia patients [14].

	Minimum requirement	Optimum requirement
Duration	• ≥ 6 weeks at a therapeutic dosage • Record minimum and mean (SD) duration for each treatment episode	• ≥ 6 weeks at a therapeutic dosage • Record minimum and mean (SD) duration for each treatment episode
Dosage	• Equivalent to ≥ 600 mg of chlorpromazine per day • Record minimum and mean (SD) dosage for each drug	• Equivalent to ≥ 600 mg of chlorpromazine per day • Record minimum and mean (SD) dosage for each drug
Number of antipsychotics	• ≥ Two past adequate treatment episodes with different antipsychotic drugs • Specify median number of failed antipsychotic trials	• ≥ Two past adequate treatment episodes with different antipsychotic drugs, and at least one utilizing a long-acting injectable antipsychotic (for at least 4 months) • Specify median number of failed antipsychotic trials
Current adherence	• ≥ 80% of prescribed doses taken • Adherence should be assessed using at least two sources (pill counts, dispensing chart reviews, and patient/caregiver report) • Antipsychotic plasma levels monitored on at least one occasion • Specify methods used to establish adherence	• Same as the minimum criteria, with the addition of trough antipsychotic serum levels measured on at least two occasions separated by at least 2 weeks (without prior notification of patient)

These criteria emphasize that clinicians must be mindful of high nonadherence rates in schizophrenia patients before concluding that prior antipsychotic trials were failures. When prior trials lacked plasma levels, or had features associated with antipsychotic nonadherence (e.g. missed refills, homelessness, substance use, no documented adverse effects), it is not unreasonable to conduct a trial with a long-acting injectable and plasma level monitoring to confirm adequate antipsychotic exposure. If prior trials employed relatively weaker D_2 antagonists (e.g. quetiapine) or a D_2 partial agonist (e.g. aripiprazole, brexpiprazole, cariprazine), and there is no history of unusual D_2 sensitivity at routine doses, one should consider use of a stronger D_2 antagonist for the depot formulation. Clinicians can be guided by the literature in cases where exploring higher antipsychotic plasma levels appears feasible in a nonresponding and adherent patient (by plasma levels) who is not exhibiting dose-limiting adverse effects [15]. Nonetheless, despite a clinician's best efforts, at least 20–30% of schizophrenia patients will be inadequate responders to nonclozapine antipsychotics.

Outside of the academic sphere, there are large data sets that substantiate clozapine's effectiveness in 'real-world' circumstances. Table 1.3 summarizes the latest and best-designed of these studies. Two of these studies examined enormous samples of schizophrenia patients (18,869 and 29,823) for up to 8 years [16,17], while another looked at two matched cohorts of 3123 schizophrenia patients who met clinically defined criteria for treatment resistance [18].

By selecting those patients who would be deemed treatment-resistant by routine clinical standards, the latter study emphasizes the benefits of clozapine compared to other antipsychotics for that population [18]. As opposed to the outcomes found in an inpatient research unit or highly supervised research clinic, these naturalistic data sets provide a compelling picture of clozapine's effectiveness in the hands of clinicians working with a challenging population with varying degrees of motivation, adherence and illness severity. Regardless of the treatment setting, clozapine remains the option with best chance of success for the treatment-resistant schizophrenia patient.

● Impact of Delays in Commencing Clozapine

One important variable in maximizing the chance of clozapine response involves minimizing the time to initiation once the patient meets clinical criteria for treatment resistance. Given the reluctance of many clinicians to prescribe clozapine, it is not surprising that the literature documents unnecessary delays in commencing

Table 1.3 Summary of large real-world effectiveness studies in schizophrenia 2016–2017.

Reference	Comments
Vanasse et al., 2016 [16]	**Sample:** Retrospective analysis of outcomes for 18,869 adult schizophrenia patients living in Quebec, Canada and starting an antipsychotic between January 1998 and December 2005. **Outcomes of interest:** Any mental health event (suicide, hospitalization or emergency visit for mental disorders), and any physical health event (death other than suicide, hospitalization or emergency visit for physical disorders). **Results:** Compared to FGAs, patients on quetiapine at the time of the event was associated with increased risk of mental health events (HR = 1.38, 95% CI 1.24–1.54, $p < 0.0001$) and also of physical health events (HR = 1.24, 95% CI 1.12–1.37, $p < 0.0001$). Patients not using any antipsychotic were also at an increased risk of mental health events (HR = 1.54, 95% CI 1.44–1.65, $p < 0.0001$), and physical health events (HR = 1.24, 95% CI 1.17–1.32, $p < 0.0001$). Clozapine was associated with slightly lower risk of mental or physical health events than FGAs, and was associated with markedly lower rates of discontinuation or antipsychotic switching compared to FGA and other SGAs.
Stroup et al., 2016 [18]	**Sample:** Retrospective examination of outcomes for 3123 adult schizophrenia patients extracted from US national Medicaid data 2001–2009 with clinical evidence of treatment resistance that required clozapine. This cohort was matched with a similar cohort of 3123 patients with clinical evidence of treatment resistance that initiated a standard antipsychotic. **Outcomes of interest:** Hospital admission for a mental disorder. Secondary efficacy outcomes included discontinuation of the antipsychotic, and use of an additional antipsychotic. **Results:** Initiation of clozapine was associated with a significantly lower rate of psychiatric hospital admission (HR = 0.78, 95% CI 0.69–0.88). Clozapine was also associated with lower rates of antipsychotic discontinuation (HR = 0.60, 95% CI 0.55–0.65), and the need for an additional antipsychotic (HR = 0.76, 95% CI 0.70–0.82).
Tiihonen et al., 2017 [17]	**Sample:** Retrospective examination of outcomes for 29,823 patients in Sweden with a schizophrenia diagnosis who were 16–64 years of age in 2006. Psychiatric outcomes were analyzed for July 1, 2006, to December 31, 2013. **Outcomes of interest:** Risk of rehospitalization and treatment failure (defined as psychiatric rehospitalization, suicide attempt, discontinuation or switch to other medication, or death). **Results:** Risk of psychiatric rehospitalization was the lowest during monotherapy with once-monthly long-acting injectable paliperidone (HR = 0.51; 95% CI 0.41–0.64), long-acting injectable zuclopenthixol (HR = 0.53, 95% CI 0.48–0.57), clozapine (HR = 0.53, 95% CI 0.48–0.58), long-acting injectable perphenazine (HR = 0.58, 95% CI 0.52–0.65), and long-acting injectable olanzapine (HR = 0.58, 95% CI 0.44–0.77) compared with no use of antipsychotic medication. Oral flupentixol (HR = 0.92, 95% CI 0.74–1.14), quetiapine (HR = 0.91; 95% CI 0.83–1.00), and oral perphenazine (HR = 0.86, 95% CI 0.77–0.97) were associated with the highest risk of rehospitalization.

FGA, first-generation antipsychotic; SGA, second-generation antipsychotic; HR, hazard ratio.

clozapine treatment. A clinical review of all 149 patients started on clozapine at the South London and Maudsley NHS Foundation Trust from 2006 to 2010 found that the mean delay in initiating clozapine was 47.7 months, with 36% of patients receiving antipsychotic polypharmacy and 34% receiving high-dose antipsychotic therapy during the delay [19]. A subsequent paper covering 162 clozapine starts at the Istanbul Faculty of Medicine, Department of Psychiatry noted a mean delay of 29 months after fulfilling treatment-resistance criteria [20]. While those who responded to clozapine tended to be younger, have shorter illness duration and fewer numbers of adequate antipsychotic trials before clozapine, the extent of delay in starting clozapine was an independent contributor to the odds of clozapine response [20]. The mean delay in initiating clozapine in the good response group was 21 months, compared to 47 months in those with minimal or no improvement ($p = 0.04$). Utilizing the concept that the biological onset of treatment resistance was not when the patient was finally deemed to have failed their second antipsychotic but when that period of exacerbation commenced, a group from a tertiary care inpatient hospital in Okayama, Japan analyzed data in 90 new clozapine starts who remained on treatment for at least 3 months (see Figure 1.1) [21]. Using this definition, they found that a delay in clozapine initiation of 2.8 years best predicted those who would benefit from clozapine treatment. In patients with a delay ≤ 2.8 years the response rate was 81.6%, while it fell to 30.8% in those with a delay > 2.8 years. Consistent with the Turkish data, older age and longer duration of illness were associated with lower response rates.

● Clozapine and Mortality

Symptomatic exacerbation and rehospitalization are inherent to schizophrenia, but so is increased risk of mortality from all causes, natural and unnatural (i.e. accidents, suicide) [22]. Increasingly sophisticated database studies indicate that clozapine is associated with lower mortality rates than other antipsychotics, that clozapine reduces mortality from both natural and unnatural causes, and that the mortality reduction is not solely due to increased clinical monitoring or other treatment factors (Table 1.4). The impact of clozapine on mortality is only present if the patient continues on clozapine. A 2018 meta-analysis of 24 long-term mortality studies found mortality rate ratios were 44% lower in patients continuously treated with clozapine (compared to other antipsychotics), but were not significant lower in those who ever used clozapine [23]. The loss of clozapine's protective effect on mortality emerges soon after

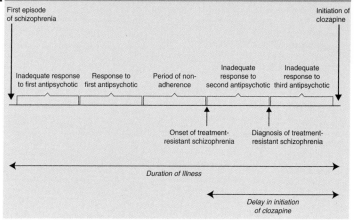

Figure 1.1. Delaying the time to starting clozapine reduces likelihood of response in resistant schizophrenia.

(Adapted from: Yoshimura, B., Yada, Y., So, R., et al. (2017). The critical treatment window of clozapine in treatment-resistant schizophrenia: Secondary analysis of an observational study. *Psychiatry Research*, 250, 65–70 [21].)

treatment stoppage, with Danish data showing that mortality was highest in periods after clozapine discontinuation (HR: 2.65, 95% CI 1.47–4.78) [22].

What is interesting about this literature is that the Quebec study (Table 1.3) showed that clozapine lowered the odds of all physical health events despite subanalayses showing that current clozapine use was associated with higher risk for serious physical health events (i.e. hospitalization or death from nonpsychiatric medical causes) [16]. As noted in Chapters 7 and 9, use of clozapine is associated with constipation and sialorrhea that in some cases can result in ileus or aspiration pneumonia. As clinicians become more adept at managing those two adverse effects of clozapine, it will be interesting to note whether the mortality gap between clozapine and other antipsychotics further widens in favor of clozapine for treatment-resistant schizophrenia patients. Antipsychotic treatment is the foundation upon which patients can build skills to achieve functional goals, but such goals can only be attained if the patient remains alive. Even with clozapine's burden of somatic adverse effects, the

Table 1.4 Summary of recent large antipsychotic mortality studies in schizophrenia.

Reference	Comments
Tiihonen et al., 2009 [32]	**Sample:** Nationwide registers in Finland were used to examine mortality in 66,881 outpatients with schizophrenia between 1996 and 2006, and to link these data with the use of antipsychotic drugs. Perphenazine was used as the comparison medication.
	Outcomes of interest: All-cause mortality using Cox regression models for the period. Secondary outcomes included mortality due to suicide and ischemic heart disease.
	Results: Compared with current use of perphenazine, the highest risk for overall mortality was recorded for quetiapine (adjusted HR = 1.41, 95% CI 1.09–1.82), and the lowest risk for clozapine (HR = 0.74, 95% CI 0.60–0.91). Use of clozapine significantly decreased risk of death by suicide (HR = 0.34, 95% CI 0.20–0.57), and did not increase risk of death due to ischemic heart disease.
Hayes et al., 2015 [72]	**Sample:** The South London and Maudsley National Health Service Foundation Trust case register linked to a national (UK) mortality database was used to identify 14,754 individuals with serious mental illnesses including schizophrenia, schizoaffective and bipolar disorders aged ≥ 15 years.
	Outcomes of interest: The effect of clozapine on mortality over a 5-year period (2007–2011) using Cox regression models for the period.
	Results: There was a significant association between being prescribed clozapine and lower mortality after controlling for numerous potential confounders including clinical monitoring associated with clozapine use and markers of disease severity (adjusted HR = 0.4, 95% CI 0.2–0.7; p = 0.001). For natural causes of death the adjusted HR = 0.5 (95% CI 0.2–0.9). For unnatural causes of death the adjusted HR = 0.2 (95% CI 0.05–0.9).
Wimberley et al., 2017 [22]	**Sample:** The Danish National Prescription Registry and clinical databases were used to identify a cohort of 2370 individuals with treatment-resistant schizophrenia after January 1, 1996. The cohort was followed until death, first episode of self-harm, emigration, or June 1, 2013.
	Outcomes of interest: Time to all-cause death and time to first episode of self-harm were analyzed in Cox regression models for the period.
	Results: The absence of clozapine treatment was associated with an elevated all-cause mortality (HR = 1.88, 95% CI 1.16–3.05) in adjusted models. Estimates were substantially higher for no antipsychotic treatment (HR = 2.50, 95% CI 1.50–4.17) and nonclozapine antipsychotic treatment (HR = 1.45, 95% CI 0.86–2.45*). Mortality was highest in periods after clozapine discontinuation (HR = 2.65, 95% CI 1.47–4.78). When compared with clozapine, nonclozapine antipsychotics were associated with an elevated rate of self-harm (HR = 1.36, 95% CI 1.04–1.78).
Vermeulen et al., 2019 [23]	**Sample:** Meta-analysis of 24 mortality studies in adults diagnosed with schizophrenia spectrum disorders who had received clozapine treatment with > 52 weeks of follow-up.
	Outcome of interest: Comparative mortality rates between clozapine and other antipsychotics.

continued overleaf

Table 1.4 continued

Reference	Comments
Vermeulen et al., 2019 [23] cont'd	**Results:** For clozapine-treated patients, 1327 deaths were recorded during 217,691 patient-years of follow-up. Mortality rate ratios (mRR) were significantly lower in patients continuously treated with clozapine compared to other antipsychotics (mRR = 0.56, 95% CI 0.36–0.85). The mRR of studies including patients who ever used clozapine during follow-up compared to other antipsychotics was not significant (mRR = 0.74, 95% CI 0.38–1.45).

HR, hazard ratio.
*Not statistically significant.

published literature indicates that clozapine lowers the risk of premature mortality compared to other options for resistant schizophrenia.

● Psychogenic Polydipsia

Primary polydipsia is a scenario of increased water intake occurring in the absence of impairment in water excretion. This can be distinguished from the secondary polydipsia seen with lithium-treated patients who increase water intake due to obligatory losses from nephrogenic diabetes insipidus. Both groups may have low urine osmolality, but the latter group maintains normal serum osmolality and serum sodium levels, while the primary polydipsia patient will suffer from severe hyponatremia and low serum osmolality during water binges [24]. The association of water intoxication and schizophrenia was reported in the pre-antipsychotic era, with a 1923 paper correlating increased water excretion with greater psychosis severity. By 1936 it was noted that excessive water intake occurred in approximately 25% of patients and was the most common metabolic abnormality in the severely mentally ill; moreover, it could be associated with life-threatening hyponatremia [24]. Modern prevalence data obtained over 5 years in a state hospital (1996–200) confirm that polydipsia continues to be present in at least 20% of chronic psychiatric inpatients [25]. The excessive drinking in primary polydipsia is not due to excessive thirst, but is motivated instead by delusions or psychic discomfort that is relieved by water binges [24].

Shortly after clozapine's approval in 1989, cases emerged in which water intoxication associated with schizophrenia was not addressed by typical antipsychotics, but which responded to clozapine. A 1996 case series of five state hospital patients with polydipsia who met Kane criteria reported that all were successfully discharged on clozapine and had no recurrence of polydipsia over 17 months of outpatient follow-up [26]. A subsequent 24-week open-label study was performed in eight male schizophrenia patients with polydipsia to document longitudinal changes in urine and serum osmolality after starting clozapine [8]. The protocol involved 6 weeks with a typical antipsychotic (per Kane criterion 3), followed by sequential 6-week periods of clozapine at 300, 600 and then 900 mg/day (if tolerated). During treatment with typical antipsychotics both serum and urine osmolality remained grossly abnormal; however, on clozapine the mean plasma osmolality normalized, and rose on average by 15.2 mosm/kg (95% CI 5.5–25.0); moreover, this effect was evident at the dose of 300 mg/day of clozapine (see Figures 1.2 and 1.3) [8]. With ongoing clozapine titration, urine osmolality also normalized. No other prospective clozapine studies have emerged for polydipsia, but the

Figure 1.2. Mean plasma osmolality during 6 weeks of typical antipsychotic treatment followed by 6 weeks each of clozapine at 300, 600 and then 900 mg/day in schizophrenia patients with polydipsia.

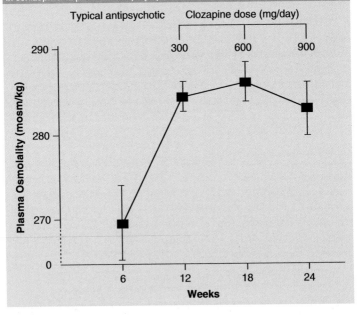

(Adapted from: Canuso, C. M. and Goldman, M. B. (1999). Clozapine restores water balance in schizophrenic patients with polydipsia–hyponatremia syndrome. *Journal of Neuropsychiatry and Clinical Neuroscience*, 11, 86–90 [8].)

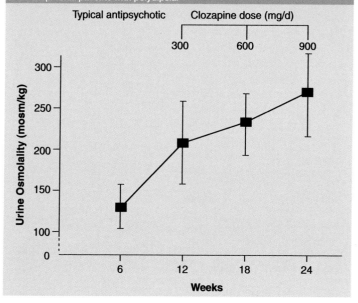

Figure 1.3. Mean urine osmolality during 6 weeks of typical antipsychotic treatment followed by 6 weeks each of clozapine at 300, 600 and then 900 mg/day in schizophrenia patients with polydipsia.

(Adapted from: Canuso, C. M. and Goldman, M. B. (1999). Clozapine restores water balance in schizophrenic patients with polydipsia–hyponatremia syndrome. *Journal of Neuropsychiatry and Clinical Neuroscience*, 11, 86–90 [8].)

accumulated literature is substantial enough that a 2010 comprehensive review of water imbalance issues in psychosis patients concluded that primary polydipsia generally appears resistant to antipsychotics except clozapine. Evidence-based treatment options for preventing water intoxication includes targeted fluid restriction, clozapine therapy, and removal of agents that may be causing hyponatremia (e.g. carbamazepine, valproate, sodium-wasting diuretics). The titration and therapeutic plasma levels for schizophrenia spectrum polydipsia patients are consistent with the use of clozapine for treatment-resistant schizophrenia.

Treatment-Intolerant Schizophrenia

Early in its clinical development, clozapine's extremely low rate of neurological adverse became apparent, leading to small trials in patients with tardive dyskinesia (TD), and for patients intolerant of D_2 antagonism due to akathisia, parkinsonism, acute dystonia or neuroleptic malignant syndrome (NMS) [27]. While use in TD patients was a focus of several studies, evidence for benefit in D_2 antagonist-intolerant patients is based on experience reported in case series where these patients were often included along with treatment-resistant individuals [28]. The conclusions from this case-based literature is that clozapine is unlikely to induce acute movement disorders, although there are a handful of NMS cases reported [29]. With respect to TD, both the efficacy outcomes and quality of prior studies led the American Academy of Neurology to state that the data were insufficient to support or refute use of clozapine for tardive syndromes [30]. Despite the abundance of case data, only three prospective studies involving a switch to clozapine for TD management were of sufficient quality to be reviewed: two were positive, one was not. A subsequent 2018 review found no further data to indicate that antipsychotic switching is an evidence-based practice for management of TD [31].

Since clozapine's reintroduction in 1989 the psychopharmacology landscape has changed in two ways: there are numerous options to high-potency typical antipsychotics, and there are three vesicular monoamine transporter type 2 (VMAT2) inhibitors available for TD treatment. The expanded group of atypical antipsychotics (including the D_2 partial agonists) provides a range of options for those with significant sensitivity to D_2 antagonism. Quetiapine has very low D_2 affinity and consequentially low rates of acute movement disorders, but enthusiasm for its use as a schizophrenia treatment has waned based on real-world effectiveness data associating quetiapine with higher rates of overall mortality [32], rehospitalization[17], any mental health event (suicide, hospitalization or emergency visit) or physical health event (death other than suicide, hospitalization or emergency visit for physical disorders) [16]. Although the pool of treatment-intolerant patients is smaller than when first-generation antipsychotics were the only available choices, these individuals do exist and should be offered clozapine. For stable TD patients who require ongoing antipsychotic therapy, the addition of a VMAT2 inhibitor is preferable to antipsychotic switching as the combination is well tolerated in severely mentally ill individuals on antipsychotic therapy (see Chapter 13). Clozapine should be considered if there are other ongoing sources of treatment intolerance (e.g. akathisia), or the patient meets clinical criteria for treatment resistance.

Suicidality

Conceptually, suicide and violence are separate domains of schizophrenia spectrum disorders that are not necessarily driven by psychotic thought processes, and thus respond incompletely to traditional antipsychotic therapy [33]. A review of suicidal acts among 10,118 schizophrenia patients participating in placebo-controlled clinical trials found that rates of suicide and attempted suicide did not differ significantly between the placebo-treated and drug-treated groups despite greater symptom reduction for the latter [34]. Patients with schizophrenia spectrum disorders have ninefold higher rates of unnatural causes of death (suicide, violent accidents) compared to the general population, with suicide risk especially prominent in the first 5 years after diagnosis [35,36]. Death from suicide comprises 30% of all causes of mortality in studies of new-onset schizophrenia patients, but wanes over ensuing decades. The estimated lifetime risk of death from suicide is 4.9% in patients with schizophrenia [36].

The impact of clozapine on suicidality was first noticed in treatment-resistant schizophrenia patients, but the antisuicide effects were later seen in those without treatment resistance, and in bipolar disorder patients [37–39]. From these observations the foundation was laid for a large international trial to examine clozapine's comparative efficacy vs. olanzapine in a nonresistant schizophrenia population. The International Suicide Prevention Trial (InterSePT) enrolled 980 patients at high risk for suicide due to prior attempts or current symptoms, with 24 months of follow-up (see Figure 1.4) [40]. In this cohort of schizophrenia patients who were not treatment-resistant, clozapine's superior impact on suicidality was clearly independent of the reduction in psychotic symptoms, as both clozapine and olanzapine had comparable improvements in total Positive and Negative Syndrome Scale (PANSS) scores. This principle will be echoed in data supporting clozapine's effect on aggression: *the reduction in suicidality and violence is independent of clozapine's antipsychotic effect.* The InterSePT study resulted in an indication for reducing risk of recurrent suicidal behavior in patients with schizophrenia or schizoaffective disorder "who are judged to be at chronic risk for re-experiencing suicidal behavior, based on history and recent clinical state" [41]. Naturalistic data summarized in Table 1.4 substantiate the findings from InterSePT: clozapine treatment is associated with a reduction of 66–80% in deaths by suicide or other unnatural causes, and a 36% lower rate of self-harm compared with nonclozapine antipsychotics.

Figure 1.4. Time to suicidal events in the InterSePT study.

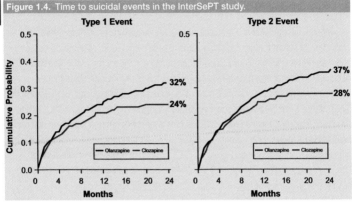

HR, hazard ratio. Type 1 Event: Significant suicide attempt or hospitalization due to imminent suicide risk. Type 2 Event: Worsening suicidality.
(Adapted from: Meltzer, H. Y., Alphs, L., Green, A. I., et al. (2003). Clozapine treatment for suicidality in schizophrenia: International Suicide Prevention Trial (InterSePT). *Archives of General Psychiatry*, 60, 82–91 [40].)

Box 1.2 Important Conclusions from the 24-Month Prospective, Randomized International Suicide Prevention Trial (InterSePT) [40]

1. In this group of 980 schizophrenia patients who were not treatment-resistant but at high risk for suicide, clozapine and olanzapine had comparable reductions in symptom ratings (PANSS total score).

2. Despite equivalent reduction in psychosis symptoms, clozapine was superior to olanzapine for overall suicidal behavior (HR = 0.76; 95% CI 0.58–0.97). Specifically, *fewer clozapine-treated patients*:

   – attempted suicide

   – required hospitalizations or needed rescue interventions to prevent suicide

   – required concomitant treatment with antidepressants or anxiolytics/hypnotics

3. Clozapine delayed the time to occurrence of suicidal events compared to olanzapine treatment, and this effect was increasingly more significant over time for both Type 1 and Type 2 events as defined below:

Type 1 Event: Significant suicide attempt or hospitalization due to imminent suicide risk

Type 2 Event: Worsening suicidality (as indicated by a rating of "much worse" or "very much worse" from baseline on the Clinical Global Impression Severity of Suicidality scale)

D Violence and Aggression

The association between psychosis and violence has been noted for over a century, but only in recent decades have there been systematic attempts to understand the intrinsic neurobiological factors and extrinsic factors (e.g. substance use) that moderate this risk. Quantifying this risk has been challenging because violence or aggression can include a spectrum of behaviors from verbal threats to physical violence or murder. The lack of consensus definitions for the term "violence" in research papers leads to a range of reported rates [42]. Despite these limitations, a comprehensive 2009 review noted that violence risk is increased for both male and female schizophrenia patients, and that substance use further increases risk of violence 3.7- to 4.2-fold in this population compared to psychosis patients without substance use (see Figure 1.5) [43,44].

Aggression in undermedicated or untreated schizophrenia patients is approached with standard pharmacological interventions including antipsychotics alone or with mood stabilizers (if there is a bipolar diathesis) [33]. The more problematic clinical scenario revolves around the type of schizophrenia patient encountered

Figure 1.5. Risk estimates for violence in schizophrenia and other psychoses for male samples, female samples and mixed gender samples.

		OR (95%CI)
Males		3.98 (2.98, 5.31)
Mixed Genders		5.02 (3.41, 7.39)
Females		7.85 (4.00, 15.40)

.5 1 2 4 8 16 32
Odds Ratio

OR, Odds Ratio; CI, Confidence Interval.
(Adapted from: Fazel, S., Gulati, G., Linsell, L., et al. (2009). Schizophrenia and violence: Systematic review and meta-analysis. *PLoS Medicine*, 6, e1000120 [43].)

in psychiatric inpatient and forensic settings who remains persistently aggressive despite antipsychotic treatment. In addressing the persistently violent schizophrenia spectrum patient, one must first categorize the nature of the aggression. The most robust and empirically validated classification method was developed within the New York State Hospital system based on reviewed videotaped assaults supplemented with assailant and victim interviews to determine the motivation for each violent act. These detailed assessments led the authors to conclude that three categories could be used to define aggressive acts: psychotic, impulsive, and predatory (also called organized or instrumental) [33]. The latter group comprises intentional acts for secondary gain (e.g. theft, intimidation), and requires a custodial solution, not pharmacotherapy. Psychotic violence is due to persistent delusions or hallucinations that drive behaviors, while impulsive acts involve inappropriate responses to real-world stimuli. A classic example of impulsive violence is a patient who assaults a peer after being gently bumped in a line despite the innocuous nature of the contact and the fact that the assault will have repercussions for

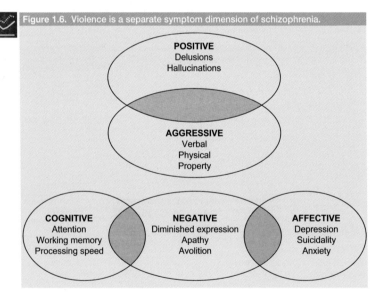

Figure 1.6. Violence is a separate symptom dimension of schizophrenia.

POSITIVE
Delusions
Hallucinations

AGGRESSIVE
Verbal
Physical
Property

COGNITIVE
Attention
Working memory
Processing speed

NEGATIVE
Diminished expression
Apathy
Avolition

AFFECTIVE
Depression
Suicidality
Anxiety

the assailant (e.g. legal, loss of privileges, etc.). Utilizing this classification, there are two core concepts that underlie treatment of ongoing violence in medicated schizophrenia patients:

a. Among persistently aggressive forensic schizophrenia inpatients the most common type of assault is impulsive (54%), followed by organized (29%) and psychotic (17%) [45].

b. Impulsive violence/aggression is a separate symptom dimension of schizophrenia that may not respond to nonclozapine antipsychotics (see Figure 1.6) [33].

The initial approach to any violent patient requires the clinician to classify the nature of the violence. That motivated by delusions or hallucinations involves optimization of antipsychotic treatment, and use of clozapine in those who are treatment-resistant. For those who are impulsive, further antipsychotic titration is appropriate if there are no dose-limiting adverse effects (e.g. akathisia, parkinsonism). In schizophrenia patients who continue to be impulsively violent despite maximal use of nonclozapine antipsychotics, clozapine is the preferred agent, and its anti-aggressive property in these individuals is independent of its impact on psychotic symptoms. Evidence for this assertion comes from studies summarized in Table 1.5 [46]. The most rigorous study design was a randomized, double-blind, parallel-group, 12-week trial specifically for physically assaultive New York State Hospital patients with schizophrenia or schizoaffective disorder [47]. At study end there were nonsignificant numerical changes in PANSS total scores across all three drug groups, but clozapine significantly reduced verbal, physical and total aggression scores compared to haloperidol or olanzapine. Clozapine's effect was more pronounced in those with cognitive dysfunction, despite the fact that poor executive function at study baseline predicted higher levels of aggression (see Figure 1.7) [48].

Further evidence that clozapine's anti-aggression effect is independent of its antipsychotic properties includes a small case series of clozapine therapy for impulsive aggression among nonpsychotic patients with antisocial personality disorders. Not only did clozapine significantly decrease rates of impulsive aggression and violence in this cohort, it did so at a mean plasma level of 171 ng/ml, well below the 350 ng/ml threshold used to manage treatment-resistant schizophrenia [49]. A 2018 review outlines the challenges to prescribing clozapine in forensic settings,

Table 1.5 Summary of randomized studies of clozapine for aggression in schizophrenia.

Reference	Comments
Niskanen et al., 1974 [73]	**Sample:** Randomized, double-blind, 40-day trial of clozapine vs. chlorpromazine in 48 patients with chronic schizophrenia, 75% of whom were experiencing acute symptoms or exacerbation of chronic symptoms. **Outcomes of interest:** Change in BPRS score. **Results:** Improvements in tension, hostility and excitement were seen in the clozapine group compared to baseline, with no between-group differences in BPRS scores.
Chow et al., 1996 [74]	**Sample:** Open-label, 14-week randomized trial in aggressive inpatients with schizophrenia ($n = 12$), schizoaffective disorder ($n = 2$) or dementia with psychotic features ($n = 1$). Subjects were randomized to clozapine or remaining on their current antipsychotic. **Outcomes of interest:** Change in total score on the MOAS. Secondary outcome was change in PANSS total score. **Results:** Aggression scores improved in the clozapine group at week 10 and at week 14 compared to baseline. PANSS total scores did not improve for either group.
Citrome et al., 2001 [75] Volavka et al., 2002 [76] Volavka et al., 2004 [77]	**Sample:** Randomized, double-blind, 14-week trial of clozapine, olanzapine, risperidone or haloperidol in 157 adult inpatients (ages 18–60) with total PANSS ≥ 60, suboptimal response to treatment and poor functioning over the prior 2 years. **Outcome of interest:** Change in PANSS total score, and total aggression severity score. **Results:** Atypical antipsychotics were superior to haloperidol for symptom reduction, and clozapine was superior to haloperidol in reducing the number and severity of aggressive incidents. Risperidone and olanzapine had less antipsychotic efficacy in aggressive patients; the opposite was true for clozapine.
Krakowski et al., 2006 [47]	**Sample:** Randomized, double-blind, parallel-group, 12-week trial. Subjects were physically assaultive inpatients with schizophrenia or schizoaffective disorder in New York State psychiatric facilities randomly assigned to clozapine ($n = 37$), olanzapine ($n = 37$) or haloperidol ($n = 36$). **Outcome of interest:** Changes in total score on the MOAS-30, and the three MOAS-30 subscales (physical aggression against other people, verbal aggression, and physical aggression against objects). Nursing staff reported all behaviors on a monitoring form with 30- to 60-minute intervals. Research personnel interviewed the nursing staff after each event. **Results:** There were no significant between-group differences for mean change in PANSS total score. Clozapine was superior to olanzapine for change in MOAS-30, for physical aggression against other people, and for verbal aggression. Clozapine was superior to haloperidol for MOAS-30 total score, and for physical aggression against other people, verbal aggression, and physical aggression against objects.

BPRS, Brief Psychiatric Rating Scale; MOAS, Modified Overt Aggression Scale; PANSS, Positive and Negative Syndrome Scale

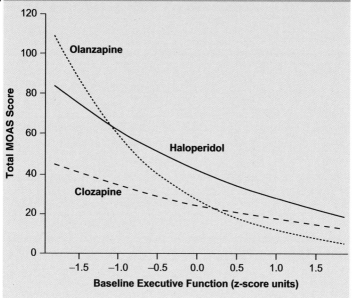

Figure 1.7. Clozapine's superiority for aggression compared to olanzapine and haloperidol among schizophrenia patients with cognitive dysfunction.

MOAS, Modified Overt Aggression Scale.
(Adapted from: Krakowski, M. I. and Czobor, P. (2012). Executive function predicts response to antiaggression treatment in schizophrenia: A randomized controlled trial. *Journal of Clinical Psychiatry*, 73, 74–80 [48].)

including the lack of an intramuscular formulation in most countries, and the greater attention required for management of adverse effects. Nonetheless, the authors note the cost-effectiveness of clozapine treatment as an important part of any strategy to manage aggressive, severely mentally ill patients in health-care and criminal justice systems [50].

 Treatment-Resistant Mania

The value of clozapine for treatment-resistant mania was noted in case reports as early as 1977 [51], but not until 1994 was a trial conducted in patients who met a standardized definition of treatment resistance: documented response failure or

31

intolerance to lithium, an anticonvulsant, and at least two typical antipsychotics. All subjects ($n = 25$) in that 13-week open-label trial met DSM-IIIR criteria for the manic phase of bipolar disorder or schizoaffective disorder, bipolar type [52]. At study endpoint, 72% of patients demonstrated at least 50% decrease in the Young Mania Rating Scale (YMRS) score. A subsequent 1-year trial with 38 treatment-resistant patients meeting DSM-IV criteria for the manic phase of schizoaffective or bipolar disorder randomly assigned subjects to adjunctive open-label clozapine ($n = 19$) or treatment as usual (TAU) ($n = 19$), with monthly ratings of mood and psychosis symptoms [53]. Significant between-group differences were found in scores on all rating scales except the Hamilton Depression scale, and medication use decreased significantly in the clozapine group. Importantly, patients with nonpsychotic bipolar I disorder randomized to clozapine exhibited similar improvement in mania symptoms as did the entire clozapine-treated group, providing evidence that clozapine's antimanic effect is independent of the antipsychotic effect [53]. There were differences in mean clozapine doses between those with schizophrenia spectrum disorders (623 mg/day) and nonpsychotic bipolar I patients (234 mg/day). A subsequent 12-week trial of 22 bipolar I patients with mania and psychotic features noted a mean dose among completers of 334 mg/day [54]. Double-blind, placebo controlled adjunctive studies do not exist, but there are case series for use in rapid cycling bipolar disorder [55].

Real-world data support the conclusions of open-label studies that clozapine is effective for treatment-resistant mania in bipolar I patients. Using the Denmark national database for the years 1996–2007, investigators examined outcomes in bipolar disorder patients started on clozapine ($n = 326$) specifically excluding those with a schizophrenia spectrum disorder. The study used a mirror image design to look at comparative hospital days, number of psychiatric admissions, and medication usage for the 2 years before and 2 years after starting clozapine [56]. After a mean follow-up of 544 ± 280 days, the number of hospital bed days decreased by 80% from 178 to 35 ($p < 0.001$), and the mean number of admissions decreased by 37.5% from 3.2 to 2.0 ($p < 0.001$). Overall, 74% had reduced bed days and 40% were not admitted at all while on clozapine. Using defined daily doses (DDD), the number of psychotropic medications decreased by 13% from 4.5 to 3.9 DDD ($p = 0.045$). Nonpsychiatric hospital visits for intentional self-harm or medication overdose also decreased significantly from 8.3% to 3.1% ($p = 0.004$). The mean clozapine dose at the end of follow-up was 307.4 mg/day. After 1 year of clozapine exposure, use of medications to manage nonpsychiatric medical conditions did not increase. As noted in schizophrenia, clozapine is only effective for mania when patients adhere to treatment. Bipolar patients deemed "irregular" clozapine users in a Taiwan analysis by virtue of low medication possession ratios had twofold higher adjusted risk for emergency room visits, and 2.5 times greater risk for hospitalizations compared to more adherent clozapine patients [57].

Box 1.3 Essential Facts about Use of Clozapine For Treatment-Resistant Mania

1. Adjunctive clozapine is equally effective in treatment-resistant nonpsychotic bipolar patients and those with a diagnosis of schizoaffective disorder, bipolar type.

2. Use of clozapine is associated with reduced hospital admissions, number of hospital days, hospital visits for self-harm or intentional overdose, and total psychotropic medication use.

3. Mean endpoint doses for bipolar I patients in long-term studies of 1 year or more range from 234 to 305 mg/day [53,56]. Higher doses (and plasma levels) typical of schizophrenia spectrum disorders are usually needed for schizoaffective disorder, bipolar type patients. There is one study of rapid clozapine titration among treatment-resistant bipolar disorder inpatients, but this reduced time to discharge readiness by less than 4 days. In a forced titration study that advanced clozapine by 25 mg/day to a target dose of 550 mg/day (if tolerated), only 14 of 22 manic bipolar I patients managed to complete the 12-week trial [54].

 Parkinson's Disease Psychosis (PDP)

Parkinson's disease (PD) is a neurodegenerative disorder related to the neuronal accumulation of alpha-synuclein in histologically distinct complexes called Lewy bodies. The worldwide prevalence of PD is estimated at > 7 million, of which more than 50% will develop symptoms of Parkinson's disease psychosis (PDP). The prevalence of PDP increases to 75% of patients in those with PD and related dementia. In 2007 a consensus definition for PDP was elaborated that included the existence of hallucinations, delusions, illusions or false sense of presence for at least 1 month in a patient previously diagnosed with PD and in whom other etiologies have been ruled out (e.g. delirium) [58]. The development of PDP is associated with increased caregiver burden, increased likelihood of nursing home placement, and is associated with increased mortality [59].

For most of the twentieth century, PD was viewed primarily as a motor disease related to loss of dopamine neurons in the nigrostriatal pathway, but PD is now recognized as a multisystem disease associated with cognitive impairment related to loss of cholinergic neurons, depression due to loss of noradrenergic neurons, autonomic and other nonmotor symptoms [60]. In prior decades PDP was often referred to as levodopa psychosis under the belief that excessive dopaminergic stimulation from dopamine agonist treatment was the principal underlying cause. It is now understood that the pathophysiology of PDP is due to loss of serotonergic midbrain dorsal raphe neurons from the accumulated Lewy body burden in these cells. The loss of this serotonin signal results in upregulation and supersensitivity of postsynaptic $5HT_{2A}$ receptors, a finding confirmed by neuroimaging of PD patients with and without psychosis [61]. That increased stimulation of $5HT_{2A}$ receptors can induce psychotic symptoms has been known for decades based on elucidation of common mechanisms among hallucinogens such as psilocybin and lysergic acid diethylamide.

The therapeutic dilemma in treating PDP relates to the profound loss of dopamine neurons in the dorsal striatum, and the inability to tolerate antipsychotics that possess moderate D_2 affinity without significant worsening of motor symptoms. Recognition that clozapine was associated with extremely low risk for drug-induced parkinsonism led to a 1990 study exploring its tolerability in six PDP patients at doses ranging from 75 to 250 mg/day (mean 170.8 mg/day) [62]. This early study noted a 50% response rate, but 50% also experienced worsening motor symptoms at those doses. These findings informed the design of the two seminal PDP studies published in 1999, one from a French group and the second from a US consortium. Each study was a double-blind, placebo-controlled 4-week trial, and both enrolled a total of 60 subjects. Based on high rates of motoric worsening in the 1990 study, the starting clozapine dose in each trial was 6.25 mg/day, with titration every 3–4 days based on response and tolerability. In the French study mean endpoint clozapine dose was 36 mg/day, while it was 24.7 mg/day in the US-based **Psychosis and Clozapine in the treatment of Parkinsonism (PSYCLOPS)** trial [63,64]. At these low doses, clozapine was significantly more effective than placebo in both trials, and with large effect sizes; moreover, there was no exacerbation of parkinsonism in the PSYCLOPS study, while 22% of patients in the French trial noted mild or transient worsening of parkinsonism, although no patient discontinued the study for this reason. Results from the 12-week PSYCLOPS extension study ($n = 53$)

confirmed the efficacy of low-dose clozapine for PDP (mean 28.8 mg/day), again without worsening of underlying Parkinson's disease symptoms as noted by ratings of motor function or need for higher doses of dopamine agonist medications [65]. Recent naturalistic data are consistent with the clinical trials findings. A retrospective review of 36 PDP patients treated at one center (mean age 68 years) noted that 33% had complete response, and 33% a partial response to clozapine [66]. Highlighting the practical issues involved with clozapine administration, the overall retention rate on clozapine was only 41%, and the most common reasons for discontinuation were frequent blood testing (28%), refusal of medical staff to continue clozapine after nursing home placement (11%) and neutropenia (8%). Only 2.8% stopped clozapine due to worsening motor symptoms, and a similar proportion discontinued treatment due to orthostasis or delirium (2.8% for each). The possible benefit of clozapine for levodopa-induced dyskinesias (LID) was later studied in 50 PD patients without psychosis in a 10-week, double-blind, placebo-controlled, multicenter trial. The principal outcome was change in the LID "on" time (hours per day). At a mean clozapine dose of 39.4 mg/day, clozapine treatment was associated with reduction in the duration of "on" periods from 5.68 h/day to 3.98 h/day, while the placebo group slightly worsened from 4.54 h/day to 5.28 h/day [67].

Over the ensuing decade other atypical antipsychotics have been used in PDP patients with results primarily reported in case series. Most have proved ineffective and were associated with significant motoric worsening (olanzapine, risperidone, ziprasidone, aripiprazole) [68]. Only olanzapine and quetiapine were examined in double-blind studies as summarized in Table 1.6. In all trials olanzapine was ineffective, and in the largest studies olanzapine exacerbated parkinsonian symptoms. Quetiapine was generally ineffective, but did not induce motoric adverse effects. Despite widespread use for PDP, a recent meta-analysis concluded that: "Given the randomized controlled trial-derived evidence, quetiapine should not be used in this indication, unless further studies have clarified this issue" [69]. Concerns over quetiapine were further heightened by results of a large retrospective study exploring 180-day mortality rates in 7877 PD patients starting antipsychotic treatment and 7877 PD patients who did not take an antipsychotic matched for age, sex, race, year of treatment, presence and duration of dementia, duration of PD, delirium, medical comorbidity, and hospitalization. In this study, mortality was increased by a factor of 2.16 for quetiapine [70]. Unfortunately, the number of clozapine cases was too small to analyze separately.

Table 1.6 Summary of double-blind studies for Parkinson's disease psychosis [68].

Reference	Medication(N)	Effect on psychosis symptoms	Effect on motor symptoms
The French Clozapine Parkinson Study Group 1999 [64]	Clozapine (n = 60)	+++	0
Parkinson Study Group 1999 [63]	Clozapine (n = 60)	+++	0
Goetz et al., 2000 [78]	Olanzapine (n = 15)	0	−
Breier et al., 2002 [79]	Olanzapine (n = 160)	0	−
Ondo et al., 2002 [80]	Olanzapine (n = 30)	0	0
Ondo et al., 2005 [81]	Quetiapine (n = 31)	0	0
Rabey et al., 2007 [82]	Quetiapine (n = 58)	0	0
Shotbolt et al., 2009 [83]	Quetiapine (n = 24)	0	0
Fernandez et al., 2009 [84]	Quetiapine (n = 16)	+	0
Friedman et al., 2010 [85]	Pimavanserin (n = 298)	+	0
Cummings et al., 2014 [59]	Pimavanserin (n = 199)	++	0

Despite its efficacy data, a limiting factor in clozapine use for PDP relates to the mandatory hematological monitoring, as a weekly laboratory trip can prove daunting for a patient group comprised of older individuals with limited mobility. To obviate this issue, researchers have sought to harness clozapine's effectiveness in a molecule that does not require laboratory monitoring. At the low doses used for PDP one of clozapine's most prominent receptor actions is at $5HT_{2A}$, and this is likely the primary site of action based on the known pathophysiology of this disorder. This insight led to development of the potent selective $5HT_{2A}$ antagonist pimavanserin for PDP (Ki 0.087 nM), with US FDA approval granted in 2016 [59]. Pimavanserin lacks affinity for dopaminergic, cholinergic, alpha-adrenergic and histaminergic receptors, and in clinical trials had no impact on ratings of motor function. While pimavanserin is a promising development in PDP treatment, it is currently only available in the US, so clozapine remains the mainstay of PDP management worldwide, and for those who fail to respond to pimavanserin.

Box 1.4 Essential Facts about Use of Clozapine for Parkinson's Disease Psychosis

1. The initial starting dose is 6.25 mg PO QHS (*quaque hora somni* – every night at bedtime). The clozapine dose can be advanced in 6.25 mg increments as needed every 3–4 days, with most patients responding at doses < 50 mg/day. The mean doses reported in clinical studies range from 25 to 36 mg/day.

2. Routine hematological monitoring must be performed.

3. While generally well tolerated, sedation, orthostasis, worsening motor symptoms and constipation have been reported.

Summary Points

a. Clozapine is the only antipsychotic with compelling efficacy data in treatment-resistant schizophrenia, and in schizophrenia spectrum patients with psychogenic polydipsia, suicidality or aggression that does not respond to other antipsychotics.

b. Clozapine's effectiveness for suicidality and aggression is independent of the antipsychotic effect.

c. In real-world use clozapine reduces hospitalization rates, and is associated with lower mortality rates from unnatural causes (suicide, accidents) and from natural causes.

d. Clozapine's efficacy as an adjunctive agent for treatment-resistant mania is also independent of the antipsychotic effect.

e. Clozapine is a mainstay for the treatment of PDP, although pimavanserin is approved in the US for this indication. Quetiapine appears ineffective in most PDP trials and is associated with a 2.16-fold increased mortality risk over 180 days compared to PD patients on no antipsychotic.

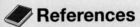

References

1. Meyer, J. M. and Leckband, S. G. (2013). A history of clozapine and concepts of atypicality. In E. F. Domino (Ed.), *History of Psychopharmacology*, vol. 2 (pp. 95–106). Arlington, MA: Domemtech/NPP Books.

2. Gross, H. and Langner, E. (1966). Das wirkungsprofil eines chemisch neuartigen breitbandneuroleptikums der dibenzodiazepingruppe. *Wiener Medizinische Wochenschrift*, 116, 814–816.

3. Amsler, H. A., Teerenhovi, L., Barth, E., et al. (1977). Agranulocytosis in patients treated with clozapine. A study of the Finnish epidemic. *Acta Psychiatrica Scandinavica*, 56, 241–248.

4. Claghorn, J., Honigfeld, G., Abuzzahab, F. S., Sr., et al. (1987). The risks and benefits of clozapine versus chlorpromazine. *Journal of Clinical Psychopharmacology*, 7, 377–384.

5. Fischer-Cornelssen, K. A. and Ferner, U. J. (1976). An example of European multicenter trials: Multispectral analysis of clozapine. *Psychopharmacology Bulletin*, 12, 34–39.

6. Kane, J., Honigfeld, G., Singer, J., et al. (1988). Clozapine for the treatment-resistant schizophrenic. A double-blind comparison with chlorpromazine. *Archives of General Psychiatry*, 45, 789–796.

7. Siskind, D., Siskind, V. and Kisely, S. (2017). Clozapine response rates among people with treatment-resistant schizophrenia: Data from a systematic review and meta-analysis. *Canadian Journal of Psychiatry*, 62, 772–777.

8. Canuso, C. M. and Goldman, M. B. (1999). Clozapine restores water balance in schizophrenic patients with polydipsia–hyponatremia syndrome. *Journal of Neuropsychiatry and Clinical Neuroscience*, 11, 86–90.

9. Conley, R. R., Tamminga, C. A., Bartko, J. J., et al. (1998). Olanzapine compared with chlorpromazine in treatment-resistant schizophrenia. *American Journal of Psychiatry*, 155, 914–920.

10. Conley, R. R., Kelly, D. L., Richardson, C. M., et al. (2003). The efficacy of high-dose olanzapine versus clozapine in treatment-resistant schizophrenia: A double-blind crossover study. *Journal of Clinical Psychopharmacology*, 23, 668–671.

11. Meltzer, H. Y., Bobo, W. V., Roy, A., et al. (2008). A randomized, double-blind comparison of clozapine and high-dose olanzapine in treatment-resistant patients with schizophrenia. *Journal of Clinical Psychiatry*, 69, 274–285.

12. Samara, M. T., Dold, M., Gianatsi, M., et al. (2016). Efficacy, acceptability, and tolerability of antipsychotics in treatment-resistant schizophrenia: A network meta-analysis. *JAMA Psychiatry*, 73, 199–210.

13. McCutcheon, R., Beck, K., D'Ambrosio, E., et al. (2018). Antipsychotic plasma levels in the assessment of poor treatment response in schizophrenia. *Acta Psychiatrica Scandinavica*, 137, 39–46.

14. Howes, O. D., McCutcheon, R., Agid, O., et al. (2017). Treatment-resistant schizophrenia: Treatment Response and Resistance in Psychosis (TRRIP) Working Group consensus guidelines on diagnosis and terminology. *American Journal of Psychiatry*, 174, 216–229.

15. Meyer, J. M. (2014). A rational approach to employing high plasma levels of antipsychotics for violence associated with schizophrenia: Case vignettes. *CNS Spectrums*, 19, 432–438.

16. Vanasse, A., Blais, L., Courteau, J., et al. (2016). Comparative effectiveness and safety of antipsychotic drugs in schizophrenia treatment: A real-world observational study. *Acta Psychiatrica Scandinavica*, 134, 374–384.

17. Tiihonen, J., Mittendorfer-Rutz, E., Majak, M., et al. (2017). Real-world effectiveness of antipsychotic treatments in a nationwide cohort of 29823 patients with schizophrenia. *JAMA Psychiatry*, 74, 686–693.

18. Stroup, T. S., Gerhard, T., Crystal, S., et al. (2016). Comparative effectiveness of clozapine and standard antipsychotic treatment in adults with schizophrenia. *American Journal of Psychiatry*, 173, 166–173.

19. Howes, O. D., Vergunst, F., Gee, S., et al. (2012). Adherence to treatment guidelines in clinical practice: Study of antipsychotic treatment prior to clozapine initiation. *British Journal of Psychiatry*, 201, 481–485.

20. Ucok, A., Cikrikcili, U., Karabulut, S., et al. (2015). Delayed initiation of clozapine may be related to poor response in treatment-resistant schizophrenia. *International Clinical Psychopharmacology*, 30, 290–295.

21. Yoshimura, B., Yada, Y., So, R., et al. (2017). The critical treatment window of clozapine in treatment-resistant schizophrenia: Secondary analysis of an observational study. *Psychiatry Research*, 250, 65–70.

22. Wimberley, T., MacCabe, J. H., Laursen, T. M., et al. (2017). Mortality and self-harm in association with clozapine in treatment-resistant schizophrenia. *American Journal of Psychiatry*, 174, 990–998.

23. Vermeulen, J. M., van Rooijen, G., van de Kerkhof, M. P. J., et al. (2019). Clozapine and long-term mortality risk in patients with schizophrenia: A systematic review and meta-analysis of studies lasting 1.1–12.5 years. *Schizophrenia Bulletin*, 45, 315–329.

24. Goldman, M. B. (2010). The assessment and treatment of water imbalance in patients with psychosis. *Clinical Schizophrenia & Related Psychoses*, 4, 115–123.

25. de Leon, J. (2003). Polydipsia – A study in a long-term psychiatric unit. *European Archives of Psychiatry and Clinical Neuroscience*, 253, 37–39.

26. Fuller, M. A., Jurjus, G., Kwon, K., et al. (1996). Clozapine reduces water-drinking behavior in schizophrenic patients with polydipsia. *Journal of Clinical Psychopharmacology*, 16, 329–332.

27. Simpson, G. M., Lee, J. H. and Shrivastava, R. K. (1978). Clozapine in tardive dyskinesia. *Psychopharmacology*, 56, 75–80.

28. Small, J. G., Milstein, V., Marhenke, J. D., et al. (1987). Treatment outcome with clozapine in tardive dyskinesia, neuroleptic sensitivity, and treatment-resistant psychosis. *Journal of Clinical Psychiatry*, 48, 263–267.

29. Sachdev, P., Kruk, J., Kneebone, M., et al. (1995). Clozapine-induced neuroleptic malignant syndrome: Review and report of new cases. *Journal of Clinical Psychopharmacology*, 15, 365–371.

30. Bhidayasiri, R., Fahn, S., Weiner, W. J., et al. (2013). Evidence-based guideline: treatment of tardive syndromes: Report of the Guideline Development Subcommittee of the American Academy of Neurology. *Neurology*, 81, 463–469.

31. Bergman, H., Rathbone, J., Agarwal, V., et al. (2018). Antipsychotic reduction and/or cessation and antipsychotics as specific treatments for tardive dyskinesia. *Cochrane Database of Systematic Reviews*, 2, Cd000459.

32. Tiihonen, J., Lonnqvist, J., Wahlbeck, K., et al. (2009). 11-year follow-up of mortality in patients with schizophrenia: A population-based cohort study (FIN11 study). *Lancet*, 374, 620–627.

33. Meyer, J. M., Cummings, M. A., Proctor, G., et al. (2016). Psychopharmacology of persistent violence and aggression. *Psychiatric Clinics of North America*, 39, 541–556.

34. Khan, A., Khan, S. R., Leventhal, R. M., et al. (2001). Symptom reduction and suicide risk among patients treated with placebo in antipsychotic clinical trials: An analysis of the food and drug administration database. *American Journal of Psychiatry*, 158, 1449–1454.

35. Osby, U., Correia, N., Brandt, L., et al. (2000). Mortality and causes of death in schizophrenia in Stockholm county, Sweden. *Schizophrenia Research*, 45, 21–28.

36. Palmer, B. A., Pankratz, V. S. and Bostwick, J. M. (2005). The lifetime risk of suicide in schizophrenia: A reexamination. *Archives of General Psychiatry*, 62, 247–253.

37. Meltzer, H. Y. and Okayli, G. (1995). Reduction of suicidality during clozapine treatment of neuroleptic-resistant schizophrenia: Impact on risk–benefit assessment. *American Journal of Psychiatry*, 152, 183–190.

38. Vangala, V. R., Brown, E. S. and Suppes, T. (1999). Clozapine associated with decreased suicidality in bipolar disorder: A case report. *Bipolar Disorders*, 1, 123–124.

39. Meltzer, H. Y. (2001). Treatment of suicidality in schizophrenia. *Annals of the New York Academy of Sciences*, 932, 44–58; discussion 58–60.

40. Meltzer, H. Y., Alphs, L., Green, A. I., et al. (2003). Clozapine treatment for suicidality in schizophrenia: International Suicide Prevention Trial (InterSePT). *Archives of General Psychiatry*, 60, 82–91.

41. Novartis Pharmaceuticals Corporation (2017). Clozaril package insert. East Hanover, NJ.

42. Rund, B. R. (2018). The association between schizophrenia and violence. *Schizophrenia Research*,

43. Fazel, S., Gulati, G., Linsell, L., et al. (2009). Schizophrenia and violence: Systematic review and meta-analysis. *PLoS Medicine*, 6, e1000120.

44. Fazel, S., Langstrom, N., Hjern, A., et al. (2009). Schizophrenia, substance abuse, and violent crime. *JAMA*, 301, 2016–2023.

45. Quanbeck, C. D., McDermott, B. E., Lam, J., et al. (2007). Categorization of aggressive acts committed by chronically assaultive state hospital patients. *Psychiatric Services*, 58, 521–528.

46. Frogley, C., Taylor, D., Dickens, G., et al. (2012). A systematic review of the evidence of clozapine's anti-aggressive effects. *International Journal of Neuropsychopharmacology*, 15, 1351–1371.

47. Krakowski, M. I., Czobor, P., Citrome, L., et al. (2006). Atypical antipsychotic agents in the treatment of violent patients with schizophrenia and schizoaffective disorder. *Archives of General Psychiatry*, 63, 622–629.

48. Krakowski, M. I. and Czobor, P. (2012). Executive function predicts response to antiaggression treatment in schizophrenia: A randomized controlled trial. *Journal of Clinical Psychiatry*, 73, 74–80.

49. Brown, D., Larkin, F., Sengupta, S., et al. (2014). Clozapine: An effective treatment for seriously violent and psychopathic men with antisocial personality disorder in a UK high-security hospital. *CNS Spectrums*, 19, 391–402.

50. Patchan, K., Vyas, G., Hackman, A. L., et al. (2018). Clozapine in reducing aggression and violence in forensic populations. *Psychiatric Quarterly*, 89, 157–168.

51. Muller, P. and Heipertz, R. (1977). [Treatment of manic psychosis with clozapine (author's transl)]. *Fortschritte der Neurologie, Psychiatrie und Ihrer Grenzgebiete*, 45, 420–424.

52. Kimmel, S. E., Calabrese, J. R., Woyshville, M. J., et al. (1994). Clozapine in treatment-refractory mood disorders. *Journal of Clinical Psychiatry*, 55, 91–93.

53. Suppes, T., Webb, A., Paul, B., et al. (1999). Clinical outcome in a randomized 1-year trial of clozapine versus treatment as usual for patients with treatment-resistant illness and a history of mania. *American Journal of Psychiatry*, 156, 1164–1169.

54. Green, A. I., Tohen, M., Patel, J. K., et al. (2000). Clozapine in the treatment of refractory psychotic mania. *American Journal of Psychiatry*, 157, 982–986.

55. Suppes, T., Ozcan, M. E. and Carmody, T. (2004). Response to clozapine of rapid cycling versus non-cycling patients with a history of mania. *Bipolar Disorders*, 6, 329–332.

56. Nielsen, J., Kane, J. M. and Correll, C. U. (2012). Real-world effectiveness of clozapine in patients with bipolar disorder: Results from a 2-year mirror-image study. *Bipolar Disorders*, 14, 863–869.

57. Wu, C. S., Wang, S. C. and Liu, S. K. (2015). Clozapine use reduced psychiatric hospitalization and emergency room visits in patients with bipolar disorder independent of improved treatment regularity in a three-year follow-up period. *Bipolar Disorders*, 17, 415–423.

58. Ravina, B., Marder, K., Fernandez, H. H., et al. (2007). Diagnostic criteria for psychosis in Parkinson's disease: Report of an NINDS, NIMH work group. *Movement Disorders*, 22, 1061–1068.

59. Cummings, J., Isaacson, S., Mills, R., et al. (2014). Pimavanserin for patients with Parkinson's disease psychosis: A randomised, placebo-controlled phase 3 trial. *Lancet*, 383, 533–540.

60. Giugni, J. C. and Okun, M. S. (2014). Treatment of advanced Parkinson's disease. *Current Opinion in Neurology*, 27, 450–460.

61. Ballanger, B., Strafella, A. P., van Eimeren, T., et al. (2010). Serotonin 2A receptors and visual hallucinations in Parkinson disease. *Archives of Neurology*, 67, 416–421.

62. Wolters, E. C., Hurwitz, T. A., Mak, E., et al. (1990). Clozapine in the treatment of parkinsonian patients with dopaminomimetic psychosis. *Neurology*, 40, 832–834.

63. Parkinson Study Group (1999). Low-dose clozapine for the treatment of drug-induced psychosis in Parkinson's disease. *New England Journal of Medicine*, 340, 757–763.

64. The French Clozapine Parkinson Study Group (1999). Clozapine in drug-induced psychosis in Parkinson's disease. The French Clozapine Parkinson Study Group. *Lancet*, 353, 2041–2042.

65. Factor, S. A., Friedman, J. H., Lannon, M. C., et al. (2001). Clozapine for the treatment of drug-induced psychosis in Parkinson's disease: Results of the 12 week open label extension in the PSYCLOPS trial. *Movement Disorders*, 16, 135–139.

66. Hack, N., Fayad, S. M., Monari, E. H., et al. (2014). An eight-year clinic experience with clozapine use in a Parkinson's disease clinic setting. *PLoS ONE*, 9, e91545.

67. Durif, F., Debilly, B., Galitzky, M., et al. (2004). Clozapine improves dyskinesias in Parkinson disease: a double-blind, placebo-controlled study. *Neurology*, 62, 381–388.

68. Borek, L. L. and Friedman, J. H. (2014). Treating psychosis in movement disorder patients: A review. *Expert Opinion on Pharmacotherapy*, 15, 1553–1564.

69. Frieling, H., Hillemacher, T., Ziegenbein, M., et al. (2007). Treating dopamimetic psychosis in Parkinson's disease: Structured review and meta-analysis. *European Neuropsychopharmacology*, 17, 165–171.

70. Weintraub, D., Chiang, C., Kim, H. M., et al. (2016). Association of antipsychotic use with mortality risk in patients with Parkinson Disease. *JAMA Neurology*, 73, 535–541.

71. Conley, R. R., Tamminga, C. A., Kelly, D. L., et al. (1999). Treatment-resistant schizophrenic patients respond to clozapine after olanzapine non-response. *Biological Psychiatry*, 46, 73–77.

72. Hayes, R. D., Downs, J., Chang, C. K., et al. (2015). The effect of clozapine on premature mortality: An assessment of clinical monitoring and other potential confounders. *Schizophrenia Bulletin*, 41, 644–655.

73. Niskanen, P., Achte, K. and Jaskari, M. (1974). Results of a comparative double blind study with clozapine and chlorpromazine in the treatment of schizophrenic patients. *Psychiatrica Fennica*, 4, 307–313.

74. Chow, E. W. C., Bury, A. S., Roy, R., et al. (1996). The effect of clozapine on aggression – A randomised controlled study. Presented at the 149th Annual Meeting of the American Psychiatric Association, May 1996.

75. Citrome, L., Volavka, J., Czobor, P., et al. (2001). Effects of clozapine, olanzapine, risperidone, and haloperidol on hostility among patients with schizophrenia. *Psychiatric Services*, 52, 1510–1514.

76. Volavka, J., Czobor, P., Sheitman, B., et al. (2002). Clozapine, olanzapine, risperidone, and haloperidol in the treatment of patients with chronic schizophrenia and schizoaffective disorder. *American Journal of Psychiatry*, 159, 255–262.

77. Volavka, J., Czobor, P., Nolan, K., et al. (2004). Overt aggression and psychotic symptoms in patients with schizophrenia treated with clozapine, olanzapine, risperidone, or haloperidol. *Journal of Clinical Psychopharmacology*, 24, 225–228.

78. Goetz, C. G., Blasucci, L. M., Leurgans, S., et al. (2000). Olanzapine and clozapine: comparative effects on motor function in hallucinating PD patients. *Neurology*, 55, 789–794.

79. Breier, A., Sutton, V. K., Feldman, P. D., et al. (2002). Olanzapine in the treatment of dopamimetic-induced psychosis in patients with Parkinson's disease. *Biological Psychiatry*, 52, 438–445.

80. Ondo, W. G., Levy, J. K., Vuong, K. D., et al. (2002). Olanzapine treatment for dopaminergic-induced hallucinations. *Movement Disorders*, 17, 1031–1035.

81. Ondo, W. G., Tintner, R., Voung, K. D., et al. (2005). Double-blind, placebo-controlled, unforced titration parallel trial of quetiapine for dopaminergic-induced hallucinations in Parkinson's disease. *Movement Disorders*, 20, 958–963.

82. Rabey, J. M., Prokhorov, T., Miniovitz, A., et al. (2007). Effect of quetiapine in psychotic Parkinson's disease patients: a double-blind labeled study of 3 months' duration. *Movement Disorders*, 22, 313–318.

83. Shotbolt, P., Samuel, M., Fox, C., et al. (2009). A randomized controlled trial of quetiapine for psychosis in Parkinson's disease. *Neuropsychiatric Disease and Treatment*, 5, 327–332.

84. Fernandez, H. H., Okun, M. S., Rodriguez, R. L., et al. (2009). Quetiapine improves visual hallucinations in Parkinson disease but not through normalization of sleep architecture: Results from a double-blind clinical-polysomnography study. *Internatioanl Journal of Neuroscience*, 119, 2196–2205.

85. Friedman, J. H., Ravina, B., Mills, R., et al. (2010). A multi-center placebo controlled trial to examine safety and efficacy of pimavanserin in the treatment of psychosis in Parkinson's disease. Program and abstracts of the 62nd American Academy of Neurology Annual Meeting, April 10–17, 2010, Toronto, Ontario, Canada.

2

Addressing Clozapine Positive Symptom Nonresponse in Schizophrenia Spectrum Patients

QUICK CHECK

INTRODUCTION

Clozapine provides the best option for treatment-resistant schizophrenia patients, but at least 40% will have suboptimal response. Although numerous adjunctive pharmacological strategies have been explored in clozapine nonresponders, none present a compelling picture of superior outcomes. Echoing this sentiment, a 2015 review on biological approaches notes that improvement is modest with medication strategies, although electroconvulsive therapy (ECT) is more promising despite the paucity of controlled studies [1]. These conclusions may engender a certain amount of therapeutic nihilism; however, before deciding that clozapine is ineffective and embarking on a litany of adjunctive options, there is a short list of strategies that may convert nonresponders into responders. Given the tepid response to adjunctive options, the best hope for most patients is optimizing clozapine exposure through assessment of plasma levels and addressing tolerability issues that impose barriers to titration.

2: CLOZAPINE POSITIVE SYMPTOM NONRESPONSE

- Medication nonadherence can occur with clozapine-treated patients and must be ruled out as a cause of inadequate response.

- Although a plasma clozapine level of 350 ng/ml (1070 nmol/l) is used as a threshold for response, many patients require levels substantially higher. If tolerated, levels as high as 1000 ng/ml (3057 nmol/l) should be pursued in search of efficacy.

- All tolerability issues that limit titration to higher doses (and plasma levels) must be addressed. The best hope for response will come from optimizing clozapine.

- Adjunctive antipsychotics with greater D_2 affinity can be tried in clozapine nonresponders, but effect sizes are small.

- Electroconvulsive therapy (ECT) is an effective adjunctive strategy for treatment-resistant schizophrenia, with greater effect sizes seen when combined with clozapine than with other antipsychotics.

- Nonantipsychotic adjunctive medications have limited efficacy data (e.g. minocycline, memantine, topiramate, high-dose famotidine), but can be tried if tolerated and there is insufficient efficacy from use of a D_2 antagonist and ECT.

 Is My Patient Adherent?

Medication nonadherence is common in schizophrenia, and a primary cause for antipsychotic failure (Figure 2.1). In an outpatient sample of 99 schizophrenia patients deemed treatment-resistant, 35% had plasma antipsychotic levels that were subtherapeutic [2]. Although the use of clozapine may be associated with better adherence than other antipsychotic treatments, the only method to unequivocally assess adherence is through measurement of plasma antipsychotic levels [3]. As noted in Chapter 3, up to 30% variation in trough plasma clozapine levels is not unusual even with adherent patients. When fluctuations exceed 50% nonadherence must be suspected, assuming no change in clozapine dose, or exposure to inhibitors or inducers. Oral dissolving tablet and liquid preparations should be considered in these circumstances, along with observed medication administration and routine measurement of plasma levels. (See Chapter 5 for more extensive discussion about use of clozapine plasma levels.) Like many antipsychotics, clozapine has a response threshold defined by plasma level, with the cut-off of 350 ng/ml (1070 nmol/l) chosen on the basis of numerous studies [4]. Although levels above this value do not guarantee response, patients with levels consistently below have lower response rates. The first goal for the poorly adherent patient is minimizing excessive fluctuations in plasma levels that suggest nonadherence, and achieving a trough plasma clozapine level consistently > 350 ng/ml (> 1070 nmol/l). Patients can be persistently nonadherent, so clinicians must be equally persistent in using all tools to maximize and verify adherence on an ongoing basis. Once nonadherence has been excluded as a cause for inadequate clozapine response, a systematic approach to further dose titration can be explored.

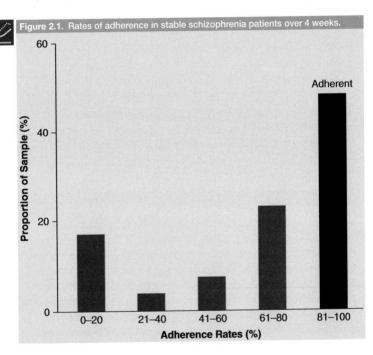

Figure 2.1. Rates of adherence in stable schizophrenia patients over 4 weeks.

(Adapted from: Remington, G., Teo, C., Mann, S., et al. (2013b). Examining levels of antipsychotic adherence to better understand nonadherence. *Journal of Clinical Psychopharmacology*, 33, 261–263 [31].)

B Should the Plasma Level Be Increased?

As discussed in Chapter 5, having a plasma clozapine level above the response threshold of 350 ng/ml or 1070 nmol/l increases the chance of response; however, some misinterpret this fact and incorrectly conclude that a patient who fails to respond at a level above threshold is a clozapine failure. For many patients the optimum plasma level for response is significantly higher than the threshold value [5]. The threshold level of 350 ng/ml or 1070 nmol/l was elaborated as a concept so that clinicians have an initial target in those not responding at a given dose for a reasonable period of time, typically 3 weeks based on recent clinical trials. In nonresponders without dose-limiting adverse effects, the literature clearly justifies exploring levels up to 1000 ng/ml or 3057 nmol/l if tolerated. Very few patients will respond at levels > 1000 ng/ml or > 3057 nmol/l (the so-called "point of futility"), although clinicians may encounter rare patients who tolerate and respond to such levels.

Box 2.1 Principles for Titrating Clozapine

1. The likelihood of response < 350 ng/ml or 1070 nmol/l is low (but not zero). If tolerated, this is a reasonable initial target.

2. Many laboratories report an "upper limit" for clozapine levels of 600 ng/ml (1834 nmol/l) or 700 ng/ml (2140 nmol/l), but there are clearly patients who benefit from and tolerate these high plasma levels [5]. Given the limited alternatives for resistant schizophrenia, patients must not be deprived of a clozapine trial with higher plasma levels, assuming tolerability.

3. Once the dose is increased, patients should be given 2–3 weeks to respond before further titration if adverse effects are not limiting. In a dose titration trial, time to response once the patient reached a dose where they responded was 17 days on average (range of 2–56 days). No late response was found among nonresponders despite a mean follow-up period of 75 weeks [32].

4. Nonresponders without dose-limiting adverse effects must not be left on the same dose and at the same plasma level for months on end hoping for "late response."

5. As levels reach the point of diminishing tolerability (> 700 ng/ml or > 2140 nmol/l), they should be rechecked after each dose increase of 50 mg/day. Very few patients will respond at levels > 1000 ng/ml or > 3057 nmol/l (the so called "point of futility"), but clinicians may encounter rare patients who seemingly tolerate and respond to such levels.

As discussed throughout this volume, effective treatment of dose-limiting adverse effects is critical to providing each patient an adequate clozapine trial. Due to concerns about QT issues and seizures, some may be reluctant to push plasma levels beyond what a local laboratory designates as the therapeutic range. As noted in Chapter 3, the older literature on QT prolongation with clozapine relied on data using the Bazett QT correction formula [6]. It is now clear that for patients with heart rates ≥ 80 BPM (a common occurrence with clozapine), the Bazett formula grossly overcorrects and provides a distorted picture of clozapine's impact on the QT interval [7]. Although the Fridericia and Framingham formulas are preferable to Bazett, most machine-generated QTc values still use the obsolete Bazett formula. For this reason, QTc values that look concerning (i.e. ≥ 400 ms) should be recalculated using a non-Bazett formula via web-based or smartphone app QT calculators [8]. The use of a modern QT correction method will help point out those cases of QT prolongation that are simply artifacts of outdated technology, thereby facilitating further clozapine dose increases. Chapter 10 provides an extensive discussion of seizure risk, and notes three important facts: slower titration may help mitigate risk; seizures occur uncommonly, even at high plasma levels; prophylactic anticonvulsants should not be used as these will be unnecessary in over 90% of patients. The development of intolerable adverse effects despite heroic countermeasures is a reason to limit clozapine titration; clinician fear of manageable problems such as seizures based on a misunderstanding of the risk is not [9].

 Antipsychotic Augmentation

Despite titration to maximum tolerable levels, a significant proportion of clozapine-treated schizophrenia patients may not respond adequately, prompting a search for any adjunctive strategy to manage persistent positive symptoms. Numerous antipsychotic and other biological strategies have been examined over the years using a variety of outcome measures to define response. In well-designed clinical trials, response is typically defined as symptom reduction exceeding a certain threshold (e.g. ≥ 30%) using a standard rating instrument such as the Positive and Negative Syndrome Scale (PANSS) or the Brief Psychiatric Rating Scale (BPRS). Anecdotes and small case series often lack an anchored measure of symptom reduction and are difficult to interpret for that reason.

Clozapine has low affinity for D_2, so the adjunctive use of a stronger D_2 antagonist makes pharmacological sense. Unfortunately, the road to clozapine for most patients is littered with failed trials of such agents, so the addition of risperidone to a prior haloperidol nonresponder lacks intuitive appeal. Nonetheless, this approach has been studied extensively and a 2012 meta-analysis of 14 studies ($n = 734$) by noted clozapine expert David Taylor, PharmD (Maudsley, London, UK) found a small effect size of 0.24 [10]. The antipsychotics used in these augmentation studies included amisulpride, aripiprazole, chlorpromazine, haloperidol, pimozide, risperidone, sertindole, and sulpiride. Since that review another double-blind, placebo-controlled adjunctive amisulpride trial (400 mg/day) was published ($n = 68$), but augmentation did not increase chance of response at the 12-week endpoint, and greater adverse effects were seen in the adjunctive amisulpride cohort [11].

There are few comparative studies with two antipsychotic augmentation arms, but one of the largest and longest studies examined outcomes between a D_2 antagonist (haloperidol) and a partial agonist antipsychotic (aripiprazole). In this 12-month, randomized, controlled, open-label trial, 106 Italian patients who were inadequate responders to clozapine at doses $\geq$ 400 mg/day for at least 6 months were enrolled. Starting from a median baseline BPRS score of 60, mean decrease in BPRS over the 12 months of treatment was under 13%, and was similar between the aripiprazole and haloperidol groups (7.0 vs. 7.9 point reduction, respectively; $p = 0.389$). All-cause withdrawal rates were also not significantly different between the two adjunctive arms: 37% vs. 28% in the aripiprazole and haloperidol groups, respectively ($p = 0.43$) (see Figure 2.2) [12].

A 2017 Cochrane review specifically examined trials with two different antipsychotic augmentation arms, incorporating the results of the Italian study with other smaller studies [13]. Using these inclusion criteria, five comparative studies with 309 participants were reviewable. The quality of the evidence was low, and no one antipsychotic appeared superior to any other for augmenting clozapine among a list that included amisulpride, aripiprazole, haloperidol, quetiapine, sulpiride, and ziprasidone. Based on these results and those from the Taylor 2012 review, the following conclusions should guide antipsychotic augmentation attempts.

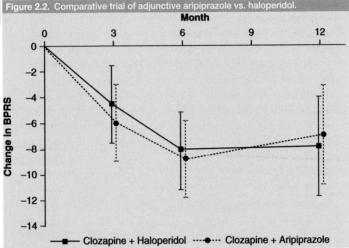

Figure 2.2. Comparative trial of adjunctive aripiprazole vs. haloperidol.

(Adapted from: Cipriani, A., Accordini, S., Nose, M., et al. (2013). Aripiprazole versus haloperidol in combination with clozapine for treatment-resistant schizophrenia: A 12-month, randomized, naturalistic trial. *Journal of Clinical Psychopharmacology*, 33, 533–537 [12].)

Box 2.2 Principles for Use of a Second Antipsychotic to Augment Clozapine

1. There is no compelling evidence that any one antipsychotic is superior for augmenting clozapine.

2. The effect size for antipsychotic augmentation is small (0.24), but the strategy is still worth pursuing.

3. Choice of antipsychotic should be based on avoidance of additive adverse effects with clozapine (e.g. orthostasis, sedation, constipation, metabolic), and a patient history of sensitivity to D_2 antagonism.

D **Electroconvulsive Therapy**

Electroconvulsive therapy (ECT) has proven efficacy for schizophrenia, but is not as commonly used for this purpose in Western countries as for treatment-resistant major depressive episodes. A 2005 Cochrane review commented that ECT was more effective than sham treatment for schizophrenia, but less so than antipsychotics; moreover, there was limited evidence at that time to suggest that ECT combined with antipsychotics resulted in greater improvement than antipsychotics alone [14]. Nonetheless, shortly after clozapine's approval a pioneer in ECT research, Max Fink, MD suggested adjunctive ECT for clozapine nonresponders, and case reports gradually emerged over the next decade [15]. While the addition of ECT to clozapine appeared safe and not associated with high rates of prolonged seizure as was feared, no controlled trials were published until the 2015 study by Petrides reignited interest in combining ECT with clozapine [16]. In this single-blind, 8-week trial, clozapine nonresponders were assigned to clozapine treatment as usual (TAU) ($n = 19$) or clozapine combined with bilateral ECT ($n = 20$) administered thrice-weekly for weeks 1–4, then twice-weekly for weeks 5–8. Response was rigorously defined: $\geq 40\%$ decrease in the psychotic symptom subscale of the BPRS, plus a Clinical Global Impression (CGI) severity rating < 3 (see Box 2.4), and a global impression of being much improved. None of the TAU group met response criteria, but 50% of the ECT + clozapine group were classified as responders (Figure 2.3). In the crossover phase, all 19 patients from the TAU group received 8 weeks of the ECT protocol and 47% met response criteria [16].

Box 2.3 Electroconvulsive Therapy (ECT) in Clozapine Nonresponders

1. ECT is effective as adjunctive treatment in schizophrenia, with retrospective data suggesting it is more effective when combined with clozapine that with other antipsychotics.

2. Prolonged seizure (< 5%) and delirium (< 5%) are uncommon when combined with clozapine. Post-treatment hypertension was noted in one study from India (17%). Mild cognitive impairment occurs in approximately 10% of patients and is not persistent. Severe impairment is not reported. Pre-ECT tachycardia must be managed.

3. The majority of papers reported use of bilateral electrode placement for schizophrenia (all antipsychotics). There is no consensus on whether bitemporal or bifrontal is more effective or induces less cognitive dysfunction.

4. In the one controlled trial of ECT + clozapine, the mean number of treatments over 8 weeks was 15. Retrospective case series report a mean of 14 treatments, with some responding in as few as five treatments.

5. Sustained response without additional ECT treatment is often noted, but some may need maintenance ECT.

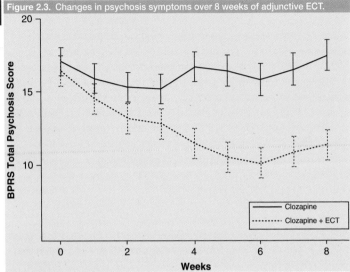

Figure 2.3. Changes in psychosis symptoms over 8 weeks of adjunctive ECT.

(Adapted from: Petrides, G., Malur, C., Braga, R. J., et al. (2015). Electroconvulsive therapy augmentation in clozapine-resistant schizophrenia: A prospective, randomized study. *American Journal of Psychiatry*, 172, 52–58 [16].)

Since 2015 there has been an explosion of interest regarding the addition of ECT to antipsychotic therapy for treatment-resistant schizophrenia patients, with nine papers published in 2017 alone [17]. The bulk of these are retrospective reviews, although one study randomized patients to one of three ECT electrode placements, but with no control group. The Petrides study provides the best efficacy data for ECT added to clozapine, but several conclusions can be gleaned from the newer papers as summarized in Box 2.3 [17]. The superiority of ECT + clozapine compared to ECT + other antipsychotics was found in one large retrospective inpatient study examining post-treatment hospital days over the following year, and a related review of all available studies [18,19]. Two case series comprised exclusively of clozapine-treated patients ($n = 66$) also noted no persistent cognitive adverse effects, or unusual patterns of prolonged seizure activity or delirium [20,21]. These conclusions are consistent with larger reviews summarizing all of the case literature for combined

ECT + clozapine treatment [22]. More controlled randomized trials will be helpful to resolve important questions about the choice of ECT electrode placement, unilateral vs. bilateral treatment, treatment parameters and schedules, the duration of sustained response, and any long-term cognitive impact compared to a control group [23]. Nonetheless, there is a compelling picture of efficacy and tolerability for adjunctive ECT in clozapine nonresponders, and this treatment modality should be pursued before the more questionable nonantipsychotic medication strategies mentioned below.

There are case reports and series for the use of repetitive transcranial magnetic stimulation (rTMS) for schizophrenia. While high-frequency rTMS over the dorsolateral prefrontal cortex and low-frequency rTMS over the temporoparietal cortex do appear safe in clozapine-treated patients, efficacy in clozapine-refractory patients remains uncertain [24].

 ## Nonantipsychotic Augmentation Strategies

Nonantipsychotic pharmacological augmentation strategies have been studied including anticonvulsants, glutamate signal modulators, and anti-inflammatory agents. For some molecules (e.g. lamotrigine, topiramate), the reduction in positive symptoms seen when added to other antipsychotics was not seen when combined with clozapine. As discussed in Chapter 5, clozapine is hypothesized to exert its unique benefit partly via interaction with the glycine co-agonist site on N-methyl-D-aspartate (NMDA) glutamate receptors [25]. Increasing glycinergic activity through agonists or glycine reuptake inhibitors improves efficacy of nonclozapine antipsychotics, but not clozapine. In three studies where glycine was administered in daily doses of 30–60 g to clozapine-treated patients, positive symptoms significantly worsened [26]. A comprehensive 2017 review of all randomized clinical trials for augmentation strategies used with antipsychotics found that no combinations with clozapine outperformed controls [27].

Aside from case reports, one is left with a group of trials that have methodological limitations, but may provide some glimpses of hope for those who fail antipsychotic augmentation or ECT. Table 2.1 lists options that pose no significant safety hazard, and can be considered. It must be noted that the meta-analyses endorsing divalproex/ valproate, topiramate and minocycline included a significant number of studies that were excluded from the 2017 review due to high risk of bias or other concerns. These are suggested mostly due to the accrued clinical experience that their use poses no immediate safety hazard. However, because of tolerability issues with divalproex (weight gain, neutropenia risk) and topiramate (sedation, cognitive dysfunction) these

Table 2.1 Nonantipsychotic pharmacological augmenting strategies to consider.

Medication	Comments
Divalproex/ valproate	Nine randomized, controlled studies with small effect on total psychopathology (*n* = 658). Generally well tolerated, but long-term neutropenia risk presents an issue at higher serum valproate levels. Modest kinetic interaction with clozapine – clozapine levels should be rechecked [33].
Topiramate	Some improvement in total psychopathology and positive symptoms across five randomized, controlled studies (*n* = 270) with mean dose 165 mg/day. Not well tolerated [33].
Minocycline	Eight double-blind, adjunctive, placebo-controlled studies, most 100 mg BID, (mean dose 172 mg/day). Mean duration 18.5 weeks. Improvements in total symptoms, negative symptoms and cognition seen, but marked differences between studies. Well-tolerated [34,35].
Memantine	Two randomized, double-blind, placebo-controlled 12-week studies of 20 mg/day (total *n* = 73). Improvement in positive symptoms, negative symptoms and cognition noted. One-year open-label extension found benefits in all symptom domains. Well tolerated in studies up to 12 months [36–38].
Famotidine	One double-blind, high-dose study at 100 mg BID, started without titration. Well tolerated over 4 weeks. 11/30 subjects in the trial were on clozapine. At endpoint, significant improvements in PANSS total score and general psychopathology subscores noted [39].
Sodium benzoate	One double-blind, 6-week, three-arm study of 1g/day, 2g/day or placebo added to clozapine (*n* = 60). Well tolerated. Both doses of sodium benzoate were superior to placebo for negative symptoms, and 2 g/day was better than placebo for PANSS total score, and positive subscore [40].

agents should not be continued longer than 8 weeks as augmenting medications if clinically significant impact on positive symptoms is not seen. Minocycline is an antibiotic hypothesized to work via an anti-inflammatory mechanism and is well tolerated as an adjunctive agent, although perhaps not very effective. Memantine, a low-affinity uncompetitive NMDA antagonist, and sodium benzoate, a D-amino acid oxidase inhibitor, are thought to exert their effects via glutamate modulation, somewhat contrary to the theory proposed above. At NMDA receptors, the amino acid D-serine acts as a co-agonist at the glycine site. By blocking the enzyme responsible for its metabolism (D-amino acid oxidase), sodium benzoate will increase the D-serine signal at the glycinergic site on the NMDA receptor. Because there is only one study of adjunctive sodium benzoate with clozapine, more data will help clarify whether this is effective. Famotidine's efficacy is based on hypotheses regarding brain histamine signaling. Although well tolerated, the local pharmacy may be perplexed by the dose, although patients with Zollinger–Ellison syndrome (ulcers due to gastrinoma) take doses up to 800 mg/day with no ill effects [28].

Before embarking on any of these nonantipsychotic strategies, an effort should be made to rate baseline symptoms, especially as the trial might extend over many months and new providers may not have a sense of the pretreatment baseline. The one-item Clinical Global Impression (CGI) severity scale is very easy to use, and correlates extremely well with gold-standard schizophrenia rating scales during antipsychotic trials of acutely ill schizophrenia patients [29]. On pages 743–744 of the *Diagnostic & Statistical Manual of Mental Disorders*, 5th Edition (DSM-5) there is a proposed dimensional scoring instrument for psychosis that captures positive symptoms, negative symptoms and cognition [30]. The DSM-5 assessment should not be used for research purposes as the psychometric properties are not known, but the anchored definitions may be helpful in a clinical setting.

Box 2.4 The Clinical Global Impression (CGI) Severity Scale

1. Normal
2. Borderline mentally ill, not at all ill
3. Mildly ill
4. Moderately ill
5. Markedly ill
6. Severely ill
7. Among the most extremely ill patients

Except for the two anticonvulsants divalproex and topiramate, it is not unreasonable to consider a trial of up to 26 weeks for these nonantipsychotic medications, assuming no tolerability concerns emerge. It is important that no other substantial medication changes be made during that time to better assess whether the new molecule has any value. Although many of these medications are inexpensive, there is no point in subjecting a patient to years of an ineffective agent, especially given the number of medications that might be needed to manage the mental illness and clozapine-related adverse effects.

Summary Points

a. Before concluding that a patient is a clozapine failure, one must rule out adherence issues, and push plasma levels to the point of significant response, intolerability or futility.

b. Tolerability issues that limit titration to higher doses must be addressed. Fear of adverse effects (e.g. seizures) is not a valid reason to avoid pursuing higher plasma clozapine levels.

c. Adjunctive antipsychotics with greater D_2 affinity can be tried in clozapine nonresponders, albeit with small effect sizes.

d. Adjunctive electroconvulsive therapy (ECT) is an effective strategy for treatment-resistant schizophrenia patients on clozapine, and is well tolerated.

e. Nonantipsychotic adjunctive medications that have limited efficacy data can be tried if adjunctive antipsychotics or ECT do not yield sufficient benefit.

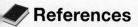
References

1. Miyamoto, S., Jarskog, L. F. and Fleischhacker, W. W. (2015). Schizophrenia: When clozapine fails. *Current Opinion in Psychiatry*, 28, 243–248.

2. McCutcheon, R., Beck, K., D'Ambrosio, E., et al. (2018). Antipsychotic plasma levels in the assessment of poor treatment response in schizophrenia. *Acta Psychiatrica Scandinavica*, 137, 39–46.

3. Weiss, K. A., Smith, T. E., Hull, J. W., et al. (2002). Predictors of risk of nonadherence in outpatients with schizophrenia and other psychotic disorders. *Schizophrenia Bulletin*, 28, 341–349.

4. Suzuki, T., Uchida, H., Watanabe, K., et al. (2011). Factors associated with response to clozapine in schizophrenia: A review. *Psychopharmacology Bulletin*, 44, 32–60.

5. Remington, G., Agid, O., Foussias, G., et al. (2013). Clozapine and therapeutic drug monitoring: Is there sufficient evidence for an upper threshold? *Psychopharmacology (Berlin)*, 225, 505–518.

6. Nielsen, J. (2012). QTc prolongation and clozapine: Fact or artefact? *Australian & New Zealand Journal of Psychiatry*, 46, 793–794.

7. Vandenberk, B., Vandael, E., Robyns, T., et al. (2016). Which QT correction formulae to use for QT monitoring? *Journal of the American Heart Association*, 5, e003264.

8. Kim, D. D., White, R. F., Barr, A. M., et al. (2018). Clozapine, elevated heart rate and QTc prolongation. *Journal of Psychiatry and Neuroscience*, 43, 71–72.

9. Gee, S., Vergunst, F., Howes, O., et al. (2014). Practitioner attitudes to clozapine initiation. *Acta Psychiatrica Scandinavica*, 130, 16–24.

10. Taylor, D. M., Smith, L., Gee, S. H., et al. (2012). Augmentation of clozapine with a second antipsychotic – A meta-analysis. *Acta Psychiatrica Scandinavica*, 125, 15–24.

11. Barnes, T. R., Leeson, V. C., Paton, C., et al. (2017). Amisulpride augmentation in clozapine-unresponsive schizophrenia (AMICUS): A double-blind, placebo-controlled, randomised trial of clinical effectiveness and cost-effectiveness. *Health Technology Assessment*, 21, 1–56.

12. Cipriani, A., Accordini, S., Nose, M., et al. (2013). Aripiprazole versus haloperidol in combination with clozapine for treatment-resistant schizophrenia: A 12-month, randomized, naturalistic trial. *Journal of Clinical Psychopharmacology*, 33, 533–537.

13. Barber, S., Olotu, U., Corsi, M., et al. (2017). Clozapine combined with different antipsychotic drugs for treatment-resistant schizophrenia. *Cochrane Database of Systematic Reviews*, 3, Cd006324.

14. Tharyan, P. and Adams, C. E. (2005). Electroconvulsive therapy for schizophrenia. *Cochrane Database of Systematic Reviews*, 2, Cd000076.

15. Fink, M. (1990). Clozapine and electroconvulsive therapy. *Archives of General Psychiatry*, 47, 290–291.

16. Petrides, G., Malur, C., Braga, R. J., et al. (2015). Electroconvulsive therapy augmentation in clozapine-resistant schizophrenia: A prospective, randomized study. *American Journal of Psychiatry*, 172, 52–58.

17. Sanghani, S. N., Petrides, G. and Kellner, C. H. (2018). Electroconvulsive therapy (ECT) in schizophrenia: A review of recent literature. *Current Opinion in Psychiatry*, 31, 213–222.

18. Ahmed, S., Khan, A. M., Mekala, H. M., et al. (2017). Combined use of electroconvulsive therapy and antipsychotics (both clozapine and non-clozapine) in treatment resistant schizophrenia: A comparative meta-analysis. *Heliyon*, 3, e00429.

19. Lin, H. T., Liu, S. K., Hsieh, M. H., et al. (2018). Impacts of electroconvulsive therapy on 1-year outcomes in patients with schizophrenia: A controlled, population-based mirror-image study. *Schizophrenia Bulletin*, 44, 798–806.

20. Grover, S., Chakrabarti, S., Hazari, N., et al. (2017). Effectiveness of electroconvulsive therapy in patients with treatment resistant schizophrenia: A retrospective study. *Psychiatry Research*, 249, 349–353.

21. Kim, H. S., Kim, S. H., Lee, N. Y., et al. (2017). Effectiveness of electroconvulsive therapy augmentation on clozapine-resistant schizophrenia. *Psychiatry Investigations*, 14, 58–62.

22. Lally, J., Tully, J., Robertson, D., et al. (2016). Augmentation of clozapine with electroconvulsive therapy in treatment resistant schizophrenia: A systematic review and meta-analysis. *Schizophrenia Research*, 171, 215–224.

23. Kaster, T. S., Daskalakis, Z. J. and Blumberger, D. M. (2017). Clinical effectiveness and cognitive impact of electroconvulsive therapy for schizophrenia: A large retrospective study. *Journal of Clinical Psychiatry*, 78, e383-e389.

24. Arumugham, S. S., Thirthalli, J. and Andrade, C. (2016). Efficacy and safety of combining clozapine with electrical or magnetic brain stimulation in treatment-refractory schizophrenia. *Expert Reviews in Clinical Pharmacology*, 9, 1245–1252.

25. Schwieler, L., Linderholm, K. R., Nilsson-Todd, L. K., et al. (2008). Clozapine interacts with the glycine site of the NMDA receptor: Electrophysiological studies of dopamine neurons in the rat ventral tegmental area. *Life Science*, 83, 170–175.

26. Veerman, S. R., Schulte, P. F., Begemann, M. J., et al. (2014). Clozapine augmented with glutamate modulators in refractory schizophrenia: A review and metaanalysis. *Pharmacopsychiatry*, 47, 185–194.

27. Correll, C. U., Rubio, J. M., Inczedy-Farkas, G., et al. (2017). Efficacy of 42 pharmacologic cotreatment strategies added to antipsychotic monotherapy in schizophrenia: Systematic overview and quality appraisal of the meta-analytic evidence. *JAMA Psychiatry*, 74, 675–684.

28. Howden, C. W. and Tytgat, G. N. (1996). The tolerability and safety profile of famotidine. *Clinical Therapeutics*, 18, 36–54; discussion 35.

29. Leucht, S., Kane, J. M., Etschel, E., et al. (2006). Linking the PANSS, BPRS, and CGI: Clinical implications. *Neuropsychopharmacology*, 31, 2318–2325.

30. American Psychiatric Association (2013). *Diagnostic & Statistical Manual of Mental Disorders*, 5th edition. Washington, DC: American Psychiatric Press, Inc.

31. Remington, G., Teo, C., Mann, S., et al. (2013). Examining levels of antipsychotic adherence to better understand nonadherence. *Journal of Clinical Psychopharmacology*, 33, 261–263.

32. Conley, R. R., Carpenter, W. T., Jr. and Tamminga, C. A. (1997). Time to clozapine response in a standardized trial. *American Journal of Psychiatry*, 154, 1243–1247.

33. Zheng, W., Xiang, Y. T., Yang, X. H., et al. (2017). Clozapine augmentation with antiepileptic drugs for treatment-resistant schizophrenia: A meta-analysis of randomized controlled trials. *Journal of Clinical Psychiatry*, 78, e498-e505.

34. Kelly, D. L., Sullivan, K. M., McEvoy, J. P., et al. (2015). Adjunctive minocycline in clozapine-treated schizophrenia patients with persistent symptoms. *Journal of Clinical Psychopharmacology*, 35, 374–381.

35. Xiang, Y. Q., Zheng, W., Wang, S. B., et al. (2017). Adjunctive minocycline for schizophrenia: A meta-analysis of randomized controlled trials. *European Neuropsychopharmacology*, 27, 8–18.

36. de Lucena, D., Fernandes, B. S., Berk, M., et al. (2009). Improvement of negative and positive symptoms in treatment-refractory schizophrenia: A double-blind, randomized, placebo-controlled trial with memantine as add-on therapy to clozapine. *Journal of Clinical Psychiatry*, 70, 1416–1423.

37. Veerman, S. R., Schulte, P. F., Smith, J. D., et al. (2016). Memantine augmentation in clozapine-refractory schizophrenia: A randomized, double-blind, placebo-controlled crossover study. *Psychological Medicine*, 46, 1909–1921.

38. Veerman, S. R., Schulte, P. F., Deijen, J. B., et al. (2017). Adjunctive memantine in clozapine-treated refractory schizophrenia: An open-label 1-year extension study. *Psychological Medicine*, 47, 363–375.

39. Meskanen, K., Ekelund, H., Laitinen, J., et al. (2013). A randomized clinical trial of histamine 2 receptor antagonism in treatment-resistant schizophrenia. *Journal of Clinical Psychopharmacology*, 33, 472–478.

40. Lin, C. H., Lin, C. H., Chang, Y. C., et al. (2018). Sodium benzoate, a D-amino acid oxidase inhibitor, added to clozapine for the treatment of schizophrenia: A randomized, double-blind, placebo-controlled trial. *Biological Psychiatry*, 84, 422–432.

3 Initiating Clozapine

INTRODUCTION

The decision to start clozapine therapy derives from the accepted, evidence-based uses for this medication including treatment-resistant schizophrenia spectrum disorders, schizophrenia patients with a history of suicidality, schizophrenia spectrum patients with persistent aggression, treatment-resistant mania, and psychosis associated with Parkinson's disease (see Chapter 1). As was discussed in Chapter 1, the greatest conundrum in determining whether a schizophrenia patient is truly resistant to other treatment is high rates of nonadherence, with subtherapeutic plasma antipsychotic levels seen in 35–44% of outpatients deemed to have treatment-resistant illness [1]. Once a patient is a candidate based on clinical criteria, patients and caregivers must be educated about the unique benefits of clozapine, its common adverse effects, and the demands of monitoring. With many

PRINCIPLES

- The work-up is limited to common labs, EKG, and usually a physical examination

- Evaluation of QT intervals requires the appropriate heart rate correction formula

- Registration of clozapine with the appropriate system for each country is required

- Titration of clozapine is geared towards the indication (e.g. schizophrenia, Parkinson's disease psychosis, etc.), acuity, age, the treatment setting (inpatient vs. outpatient), concurrent medications, and the presence of variables that influence clozapine disposition (e.g. smoking, use of cytochrome P450 inhibitors or inducers, functional cytochrome P450 polymorphisms)

outpatients this is a conversation that is often performed over an extended period as patients try and fail other options and come to trust the clinician's suggestion that the benefits of clozapine outweigh the burdens of treatment. An important principle to guide these discussions is that significant delays in starting clozapine may reduce the likelihood of response in treatment-resistant schizophrenia. A review of response rates among 90 patients who remained on clozapine for at least 3 months found that the response rate was 82% for those who started clozapine within 2.8 years of meeting clinical criteria for treatment resistance, but fell to 31% when clozapine was started > 2.8 years after reaching this benchmark [2].

At times clozapine is started in an inpatient setting; if so, enlisting the support of outpatient caregivers is crucial to treatment success, as they too will share the burdens of monitoring and treatment. The alacrity with which a caregiver can alert clinicians about adverse effects, and the caregiver's ability to convincingly reassure a patient that clozapine's benefits outweigh its burdens, may forestall unnecessary treatment termination. For certain outpatients, difficulties encountered in traveling may be the biggest barrier to treatment, but highly motivated caregivers may work with clinic personnel to troubleshoot these obstacles and devise strategies to facilitate transporting a patient to necessary laboratory and clinic appointments. Even with compulsory inpatient treatment, a discussion is critical to inform the patient about the reason clozapine is being utilized (e.g. persistent aggression despite high plasma levels of standard antipsychotics), the goals of treatment, and the frequency of monitoring. As with outpatient caregivers, educated hospital personnel will also be more motivated to work with resistant patients in obtaining laboratory measures with the understanding that clozapine is the best option to bring symptomatic relief or reduce violent behavior [3].

Baseline Work-Up

The approved indications for clozapine treatment and definitions of treatment resistance vary between countries, so clinicians must be alert to local regulations regarding "off-label" use of clozapine and any additional paperwork required [4]. A baseline work-up must be performed for all patients starting clozapine even if the patient has prior experience with clozapine. The purpose of this evaluation is to establish that hematological thresholds are met and to document baseline physical health status. For patients who have recently been discontinued from clozapine (e.g. < 90 days) and are candidates to resume treatment, hematological measures are sufficient, but as the time from last treatment lengthens (e.g. ≥ 12 months) prudence dictates a more thorough evaluation. In some parts of the world, elements of this baseline work-up are mandated by the local health trust, regulatory authority, clinic or hospital policy, but in many instances clinicians are left to choose what seems best from a myriad of conflicting recommendations. The sections below outline the minimum necessary items to be obtained prior to commencing clozapine therapy (see Tables 3.1–3.3).

Table 3.1 Baseline vital signs.

Measure	Rationale	Response to abnormal results
Temperature	Up to 20% incidence of benign fever during early weeks of clozapine therapy.	Appropriate work-up for fever etiology if temperature is ≥ 38°C. Hold clozapine initiation until resolved.
Resting heart rate	Tachycardia is a common adverse effect from clozapine.	Work-up to determine whether etiology is due to hypovolemia, or orthostasis due to effects of current medications. Hold clozapine initiation until resolved.
Blood pressure	Orthostasis is a common adverse effect from clozapine. Consider adding orthostatic BP measurements to routine seated BP in those with complaints of dizziness on standing.	If orthostatic changes are present upon standing, work-up to determine whether etiology is due to hypovolemia or medication related orthostasis. Hold clozapine initiation until resolved.

continued overleaf

Table 3.1 continued

Measure	Rationale	Response to abnormal results
Weight and body mass index (BMI)	Weight gain is a common adverse effect from clozapine.	Obesity by itself is not a contraindication to clozapine use, but may prompt use of more aggressive measures (e.g. lifestyle, metformin) to mitigate weight gain at the start of clozapine treatment.
Physical examination	Both the physical examination and the history obtained prior to the exam provide important data. For example, questions regarding symptoms of heart failure or constipation elicit information that could possibly be missed from vital signs, ECG or laboratory measures. Smoking status and history of seizures must be noted.	The nature of the response depends on the abnormalities found during the history or exam. Of particular concern is a history of, or physical findings consistent with, persistent constipation, poorly controlled seizure disorder or congestive heart failure, all of which must be addressed prior to clozapine initiation.

Table 3.2 Baseline laboratory measures.

Measure	Rationale	Response to abnormal results
Complete blood count (CBC) with differential	Baseline absolute neutrophil count (ANC) is required to commence clozapine. Some countries still require a total white blood cell count (WBC), but only ANC is tracked in the US. Baseline eosinophil is useful as eosinophilia may occur during treatment with clozapine.	Those with baseline ANC below treatment thresholds must be investigated for potential causes, including medications (e.g. antipsychotics, divalproex) and benign ethnic neutropenia (BEN).
Chemistry panel	Rule out previously undiagnosed physical ailments such as renal or hepatic dysfunction, or electrolyte disturbances.	Appropriate work-up depending on the abnormality found. Baseline creatinine is necessary should the patient later be suspected of developing clozapine-induced interstitial nephritis.
A1C	Rule out untreated diabetes mellitus (DM) and to establish a baseline, especially for those with known DM.	A1C values ≥ 6.5% are diagnostic of diabetes. In those with known DM, values > 7.0% represent less than ideal control and need to be addressed.
Lipid panel	Rule out untreated dyslipidemia and establish baseline, especially for those with known dyslipidemia.	Significant abnormalities must be addressed, particularly markedly elevated fasting triglycerides, given clozapine's known effects on insulin resistance.

Table 3.3 Additional baseline measures for consideration.

Measure	Rationale	Response to abnormal results
ECG	Rule out untreated conduction or other cardiac issues. Often required.	Cardiology consultation for abnormal findings. As noted below the appropriate QT correction formula should be applied if the resting heart rate (HR) is > 72 beats per minute (BPM). *(See discussion on QT.)*
Abdominal X-ray	Rule out undocumented constipation among patients with a history of constipation, or who are poor historians. May be required in some locales.	Address current issues impacting gastrointestinal motility prior to treatment if X-ray suggests significant constipation.

Box 3.1 Which QT Correction Formula to Use for QT Monitoring?

Tachycardia is often associated with QT prolongation due to the persistent use of the Bazett rate correction formula on most ECG machines. This formula was derived in 1920 from 39 healthy male controls and significantly overcorrects the QTc for faster heart rates [21]. For this reason, American Heart Association guidelines for ECG interpretation recommend against using Bazett's formula with high heart rates, as the "adjusted QT values may be substantially in error" [22]. A recent analysis of 6600 adults mean age 60 years old also found that Bazett performed worst of all formulas even among patients with HR < 90 BPM [23].

Bazett Formula: $QTcB = QT/\sqrt{RR}$ (Note: RR is expressed in seconds.)

Fridericia Formula: $QTcFri = QT/\sqrt[3]{RR}$ (Note: RR is expressed in seconds.)

Framingham Formula: $QTcFra = QT + 0.154(1 - RR)$ (Note: RR is expressed in seconds.)

Examples on how to use each formula (HR 80 BPM, RR = 0.75 sec, QT uncorrected = 400 ms or 0.4 sec):

a. Bazett: 0.400 sec$/(0.75)^{1/2} = 0.462$ sec $= 462$ ms

b. Fridericia: 0.400 sec$/(0.75)^{1/3} = 0.440$ sec $= 440$ ms

c. Framingham: 0.400 sec $+ 0.154(1 - 0.75) = 0.439$ sec $= 439$ ms

Table 3.4 Results of various QT rate correction formulas (example: uncorrected QT = 400 ms).

Heart rate (BPM)	RR interval (sec)	QTcB (Bazett) (ms)	QTcF (Fridericia) (ms)	QTcFra (Framingham) (ms)
60	1.00	400	400	400
72	0.83	438	425	426
80	0.75	462	440	439
90	0.67	490	458	451
100	0.60	516	474	462
110	0.56	542	490	470
120	0.50	566	504	477

Box 3.2 Comments on the Baseline Work-Up

a. *Why no waist circumference?* Although waist circumference is a criterion for the metabolic syndrome, in clinical practice there is significant variability in measurements between examiners to an extent that does not exist with BMI. Changes in BMI thus serve as a more accurate measure of changes in weight. In many analyses BMI values that are in the specific obesity range for that ethnic group (e.g. ≥ 30 kg/m^2 for Europid individuals) are excellent surrogate markers for the waist circumference criterion of metabolic syndrome. One can adequately monitor for the presence of the metabolic syndrome using the standard laboratory values and blood pressure combined with BMI.

b. *Is an ECG necessary?* The high prevalence of tachycardia combined with the common use of the Bazett QT correction formula present a skewed picture of clozapine's risk for cardiac adverse effects. A recent analysis of cardiovascular outcomes among 3262 Danish outpatients commencing clozapine found that cardiovascular adverse effects were rare and no greater than for other antipsychotic agents [24]. Despite these recent data, an ECG is typically required in most health-care settings as part of the baseline work-up. For older patients there may be considerable value in the baseline ECG to document existing abnormalities that might later be inaccurately ascribed to clozapine.

c. *Are a baseline troponin I/T, C-reactive protein and an echocardiogram necessary?* As will be discussed in Chapter 12, myocarditis is an uncommon (reported rates 0.1–3.0%) but potentially fatal complication of clozapine treatment seen during the first 6 weeks of treatment. While troponin I/T, C-reactive protein (CRP) and echocardiogram are considered standard care in those suspected of myocarditis, one group of Australian researchers has suggested obtaining these labs and an echocardiogram at baseline [18]. Without further research into the value of the baseline echocardiogram, given cost and feasibility issues this recommendation has not seen widespread adoption. Troponin and CRP levels may be useful during the first 6 weeks of treatment to screen for myocarditis (see Chapter 12).

Registration

Most countries have a coordinated system for registering patients prior to receiving clozapine treatment. There are several purposes: (a) to track neutrophil counts so that ongoing patients have clozapine withheld when counts are below dispensing thresholds; (b) to ensure that patients are not rechallenged without the clinician's explicit knowledge of prior episodes of severe neutropenia; (c) to help clinicians find periods of prior clozapine exposure, particularly when clozapine may have been terminated for unclear reasons; and (d) to limit clozapine prescribing to those with presumed expertise. Clinicians must also be registered to prescribe clozapine in nearly every country, and in some countries (e.g. US) may be required to pass a brief online examination to ensure they understand the hematologic monitoring scheme and are aware of the existence of benign ethnic neutropenia (BEN).

In some countries a separate registry may be overseen by each manufacturer, a process that causes two types of problems: (a) all registries must be checked prior to commencing clozapine; and (b) patients must be reregistered if they move to an area that uses a different supplier, or require a formulation from a different manufacturer. In the US, this problem was resolved in 2013 by creation of a central site that consolidated data from each of six manufacturers within the US (see Table 3.5) [4].

Table 3.5 Clozapine registry resources for Canada, the US, UK, and Australia.

Country	Clozapine registration
Canada[1]	a. Auro-Pharma: AA-Clozapine Risk Management Program www.aaclozapine.ca b. Mylan Pharmaceuticals GenCAN www.gencan.ca c. Novartis: Clozaril Support and Assistance Network (CSAN) https://psp-force-com.pspgw.ca
United States[2]	Clozapine Risk Evaluation & Mitigation Strategy (Clozapine REMS) www.clozapinerems.com
United Kingdom[1]	a. Britannia Pharmaceuticals Denzapine Monitoring System www.denzapine.co.uk b. Mylan Pharmaceuticals Clozaril Patient Monitoring Service CPMS) www.clozaril.co.uk c. Zaponex Treatment Access System (ZTAS) www.ztas.co.uk
Australia[1,3]	a. Novartis Clozaril Patient Monitoring System www.ecpms.com.au b. Pfizer Australia Clopine Central www.clopine.com.au/ClopineCentral/

1. Manufacturer specific registry; 2. Central registry for all manufacturers; 3. Prior to acquisition by Pfizer, Hospira created a joint database with Novartis, the Clozapine Exclusion Database (www.clozapine.com.au). Pfizer now has its own site.

C | Titration

The concept of a standard clozapine titration is a myth. A rapid titration might be tolerable and safe for a highly symptomatic or aggressive younger inpatient where vital signs are monitored routinely, and adverse effects noted immediately [5], but not for an older outpatient with a history of orthostasis. Smoking status must be factored into any titration schedule, as nonsmokers will achieve plasma clozapine levels 50% greater than will smokers for any given dose [6]. The patient's heritage also dictates dose targets during the first 3 weeks of treatment to adjust for anticipated differences in clozapine metabolism. A 2022 consensus paper recommended that Asian or indigenous American patients be exposed to initial doses that are 1/4 to 1/2 of those used in European or US patients without those backgrounds [7]. Even with excellent clinician rapport and caregiver support patients may refuse to continue with clozapine for treatable issues such as sialorrhea, sedation and orthostasis, issues that can result from overly ambitious titration schedules. As clozapine remains the treatment of choice for resistant schizophrenia, and for suicidal or aggressive schizophrenia spectrum patients, clozapine refusal for these adverse effects is a clinical outcome to be avoided. With these considerations in mind, Box 3.3 lists some principles that govern any clozapine initiation.

Box 3.3 Basic Principles for Initiating Clozapine

1. "Standard" clozapine titration schedules recommended by the institution, clinic or presented in the literature must be individualized with smoking status and heritage being paramount concerns. Prolonged titration should be avoided, but schedules must be adjusted based on tolerability and the clinical scenario (e.g. inpatient).

2. Aggressive management of early adverse effects such as constipation (see Chapter 7), sialorrhea (see Chapter 9), sedation and orthostasis (see Chapter 8) is important to maximize the likelihood of a successful trial.

3. Timely tapering of concurrent medications whose adverse effects overlap with that of clozapine is necessary to minimize adverse effects.

Given these caveats, below are suggested titrations broken down into *more* or *less* aggressive schedules based on smoking status and patient heritage as suggested by recent literature [7] (see Tables 3.6 and 3.7). While smoking is generally precluded on inpatient units, this is not universally true, so each table has a dosing modifier for those who continue to smoke, bearing in mind that consumption of as few as seven cigarettes per day may be sufficient to fully induce cytochrome P450 1A2 [8]. Clozapine's peripheral half-life ranges from 9 to 17 hours [9], leading many to

Table 3.6 Adult Inpatient Titration With Options Based on Patient Heritage (single bedtime dosing)

Day	Dose (smoker)[a]	Dose (nonsmoker)[a]	Dose (smoker)[b]	Dose (nonsmoker)[b]
1	25 mg	12.5 mg	12.5 mg	6.25 mg
2	50 mg	25 mg	12.5 mg	6.25 mg
3	100 mg	50 mg	25 mg	12.5 mg
5	150 mg	75 mg	37.5 mg	18.75 mg
7	200 mg	100 mg	50 mg	25 mg
9	250 mg	125 mg	62.5 mg	31.25 mg
11	300 mg	150 mg	75 mg	37.5 mg
14	350 mg	200 mg	100 mg	50 mg

[a] Appropriate for extensive metabolizers of European or US heritage (other than eastern Asian or indigenous American heritage)

[b] Appropriate for extensive metabolizers of eastern Asian or indigenous American heritage

Continued titration based on steady state plasma level obtained approximately 5-7 days after the increase on Day 14 and the clinical response (see **Target Plasma Levels** below)

Table 3.7 Adult Outpatient Titration With Options Based on Patient Heritage (single bedtime dosing)

Day	Dose (smoker)[a]	Dose (nonsmoker)[a]	Dose (smoker)[b]	Dose (nonsmoker)[b]
1	25 mg	12.5 mg	12.5 mg	6.25 mg
2	50 mg	25 mg	12.5 mg	6.25 mg
3	75 mg	37.5 mg	25 mg	12.5 mg
5	100 mg	50 mg	37.5 mg	18.75 mg
7	150 mg	75 mg	50 mg	25 mg
9	200 mg	100 mg	62.5 mg	31.25 mg
11	250 mg	125 mg	75 mg	37.5 mg
14	300 mg	150 mg	100 mg	50 mg

[a] Appropriate for extensive metabolizers of European or US heritage (other than eastern Asian or indigenous American heritage)

[b] Appropriate for extensive metabolizers of eastern Asian or indigenous American heritage

Continued titration based on steady state plasma level obtained approximately 5-7 days after the increase on Day 14 and the clinical response (see **Target Plasma Levels** below)

advocate for BID dosing; however, several facts need to be considered: (a) the half-life of the active metabolite norclozapine is nearly 20 hours [10]; (b) in North America clozapine is prescribed once daily in 75% of schizophrenia patients without loss of efficacy [11]; (c) clozapine and norclozapine are high-affinity antagonists at histamine H_1 (Ki values: 2.0 and 3.4 nM, respectively), and clozapine is also an antagonist at multiple muscarinic receptors, resulting in significant sedation. For these reasons, the suggested schedules recommend bedtime dosing. (For a detailed discussion of clozapine initiation in children or adolescents, see Chapter 15).

● **Minimizing Cytochrome P450 Inhibitors or Inducers Prior to Starting Clozapine**

As discussed in Chapter 5, clozapine's metabolism is primarily through cytochrome P450 (CYP) 1A2, especially at lower plasma levels, with contributions from CYP 2C19, 3A4, 2C9, and 2D6 that are 24%, 22%, 12% and 6%, respectively [12]. In particular, the combination of clozapine with the strong 1A2 inhibitors fluvoxamine or ciprofloxacin has been associated with reported fatalities, and these agents should not be routinely combined with clozapine. Strong inhibitors of the other isoenzymes listed may double clozapine plasma levels, so a 50% downward adjustment to the titration doses must be made if these agents cannot be discontinued prior to starting clozapine. Carbamazepine and omeprazole decrease clozapine exposure as much as 50% through induction of CYP 3A4 and P-glycoprotein (carbamazepine) or CYP 1A2 (omeprazole). Alternatives to these agents must be sought and commenced prior to starting clozapine, with a preference for using divalproex given its superiority to other anticonvulsants for those rare patients who develop clozapine-related myoclonic or generalized seizures.

Rapid Titration: Two studies of extremely rapid titration exist in the literature, with patients achieving mean daily doses of 100 mg in the first 4 hours, 260 mg by day 5, and 400 mg by day 7 [5,13]. It is worth noting that 90% of the patients in one study were smokers, as were 54% in the second study. While one study ($n = 38$) had no patients with seizures, severe hypotension or other significant adverse effects, in the second study, 36% of the rapid titration group ($n = 25$) developed hypotension compared to 19% of a standard titration group ($n = 26$) (number needed to harm (NNH) = 6), although only 12% of the rapid titration group developed excessive sedation compared to 19% of the standard titration group [13].

Comments: Faster titrations may be acceptable for younger patients, those who reside close to a clinic, and those who have reliable caregiver support.

Plasma Levels: Obtaining plasma levels early in treatment allows for an assessment of progress towards minimum response thresholds, as well as problems with adherence or unusually rapid metabolism. Particularly when levels are markedly below what might be expected for the given dose, bearing in mind smoking status and interacting medications, repeating levels can help determine whether adherence or genetic factors are the cause, or there are laboratory issues with the assay [6]. (See Chapter 5 for an extensive discussion of factors influencing clozapine metabolism and the use of plasma levels.) For schizophrenia spectrum disorders, there is an extensive literature on the minimum response threshold. The 12-hour trough plasma level (obtained prior to administration of morning clozapine if on divided doses) is used to assess clozapine exposure. The response threshold of 350 ng/ml or 1070 nmol/l is cited most commonly in the literature [14], although some may respond at lower levels, and many may require levels more than twofold higher.

Parkinson's Disease Psychosis (see Chapter 1 for more discussion): Pimavanserin, a potent and selective $5HT_{2A}$ inverse agonist, has been approved for the treatment of Parkinson's disease psychosis (PDP) [15], but it may not be available in all countries, and may prove inadequate for some patients. Clozapine has proven effective for PDP, with mean daily doses in the range of 25–36 mg/day in the two pivotal double-blind, placebo-controlled trials [16,17]. Daily doses as low as 6.25 mg may be effective for PDP, and this is the recommended starting dose given at bedtime. Doses can be advanced by 6.25 mg increments every 3–4 days based on tolerability and symptomatic response. Rarely are doses ≥ 50 mg/day required.

● **Patient Discussions Prior To Initiation**

Many hospitals or clinics have mandated informed consent or information forms to document discussions with the patient about aspects of clozapine treatment.

Table 3.8 Suggested checklist of patient and caregiver information prior to starting treatment.

Item	Date
1. The indication for clozapine has been explained.	
2. The reasons for clozapine monitoring have been explained.	
3. Clozapine's common side effects have been explained and actions to take should they occur.	
4. Signs and symptoms of infection have been explained and what to do should they occur.	
5. The importance of regular blood tests has been discussed and what may happen if they miss their blood test.	
6. Discuss the importance of continuing clozapine.	
7. Document that dietary and lifestyle advice has been given to the patient.	
8. What to do if they miss a dose, especially if more than 48 hours has elapsed.	
9. Explain how smoking can affect clozapine levels and the importance of letting the prescriber know if they intend to stop or cut down smoking, or start smoking.	
10. Whom to contact in an emergency both during and after office hours.	

Whether a checklist or special consent form is required or not, it is important to demonstrate that the patient has been informed about the important considerations in their treatment. A review of various practices worldwide notes common elements that ought to be documented by the prescribing clinician, typically via checklist (see Table 3.8). Items 1–8 are appropriate for inpatients and outpatients, while items 9 and 10 will apply to outpatients.

● Monitoring During Initiation

The only mandatory laboratory monitoring during the first few months of clozapine treatment is the routine CBC used to determine the absolute neutrophil count. However, a number of clinical outcomes ought to be tracked during the first 3 months of clozapine therapy, both to manage signs of intolerability that might cause a patient to refuse clozapine, and to monitor for myocarditis, which presents predominantly during weeks 1–7 of treatment, with most cases occurring within 28 days of initiation [18].

● Choice of Formulation

Clozapine is available in tablet and orally disintegrating tablet (ODT) forms, and in some countries also exists as an oral suspension (50 mg/ml), and as an intramuscular (IM) formulation. All orally administered forms, including the suspension, are bioequivalent on a milligram basis, as are different tablets made by various manufacturers [19]. The oral bioavailability is 60–70%. A significant decrease in plasma clozapine level when switching between oral formulations, especially when transitioning from suspension or ODT forms to tablets, ought to raise suspicion of nonadherence, unless obvious supervening issues are noted (e.g. resumption of smoking, addition of a CYP inducer such as omeprazole). ODT and suspension forms are typically reserved for those with adherence issues, but there may be other reasons that these formulations are utilized. The IM formulation is primarily for inpatient use, and employed almost exclusively to initiate treatment because administering higher daily maintenance doses would require multiple injections. The strength of the IM formulation is 25 mg/ml and ampoules usually contain 5 ml (125 mg). The IM preparation is painful and must be administered by deep intramuscular injection in the gluteus, with a maximum injection volume of 4 ml. As the bioavailability of the IM form is 100%, doses used are 50% of the comparable oral dose.

Clinical inpatient monitoring following initiation: Most hospitals have established protocols for clozapine initiation that include daily observation for sedation, sialorrhea, and constipation, and routine monitoring of orthostatic vital signs and temperature. Orthostatic blood pressures are obtained first after having the patient lay flat for 5 minutes, then 1 minute and 3 minutes after standing. Orthostatic hypotension is defined as a fall in systolic blood pressure of ≥ 20 mmHg or in diastolic blood pressure of ≥ 10 mmHg upon standing, often with compensatory tachycardia. The frequency at which orthostatic vital signs are checked is higher during the first 3–4 weeks of titration, and may be obtained as often as multiple times per day depending on institutional mandates, patient age, history of orthostasis, or presence of medications that increase likelihood for orthostasis. The frequency tapers off after the first few weeks to a monthly assessment, especially as the patient achieves stable plasma levels and establishes tolerability. The frequency of temperature assessments parallels that of blood pressure, with once- to thrice-daily readings in the early weeks of treatment. Unlike blood pressure, routine temperature readings are often stopped after 8 weeks of treatment because the patient has passed the highest risk period for myocarditis and interstitial nephritis.

Clinical outpatient monitoring following initiation: There is enormous variation in the degree of recommended monitoring. Many clinics having established protocols that mandate frequent daily contacts with a nurse or other clinically trained personnel during the first week of initiation, with vital signs and other assessments performed. These are tapered to twice-daily assessments in week 2, and then weekly for the first 4 months of treatment. However, in many countries patients are started on treatment by private providers, in clinics that do not have staff or nursing personnel to perform daily contacts, or in parts of the world where the distance to a clinic is 15–25 km, precluding the type of frequent attention that is possible in a highly staffed urban setting. In these instances, the caregiver must have a firm grasp on the signs or symptoms of interest, and must be provided with a contact number that can reach a clinician 24 hours per day. Dizziness, sedation, fever or malaise, constipation > 48 hours, other bodily complaints (e.g. chest pain), and sialorrhea all represent instances where close contact with the clinician can immediately address the situation. Automated blood pressure cuffs can be considered for caregivers to track orthostatic vital signs during the early weeks of treatment (with proper instruction and demonstration of competence); daily temperature readings can also be performed by caregivers. The goal is to not deprive patients in need of clozapine of this important medication due to logistical or other circumstances that might not be considered ideal in well-funded urban clinics. There are no data to indicate that commencing clozapine treatment in patients who reside with motivated and competent caregivers increases the risk for adverse outcomes in instances where daily clinical contact is not possible. When clinical contact is made during the first 2 months of treatment, a complete set of vital signs ought to be obtained that includes one assessment of orthostatic blood pressure, especially if tachycardia is present or if there is any complaint of dizziness.

● Tapering Concomitant Medications

Minimizing the pharmacodynamic interactions that can contribute to constipation, sedation or orthostasis risk is crucial to improving the success of a clozapine trial. Box 3.5 lists some strategies focusing on pharmacodynamic interactions by benzodiazepines and anticholinergic agents.

Box 3.5 Handling Benzodiazepines and Anticholinergic Medications When Commencing Clozapine

Benzodiazepines: These agents should not be commenced just prior to or concurrent with clozapine initiation, as the combined sedating effects may result in delirium, with reported cases of respiratory arrest. In patients who have been on stable benzodiazepine doses without evidence of sedation, every effort must be made to taper down the benzodiazepine (and ideally off) prior to commencing clozapine, especially if the patient is on high daily doses. If the patient on long-standing benzodiazepine therapy cannot be completely weaned off benzodiazepines prior to starting clozapine, titration schedules may need to be modified to minimize oversedation, the patient observed carefully for evidence of sedation, and the benzodiazepine taper continued at a rate that the patient can tolerate.

Anticholinergics: Clozapine is strongly antimuscarinic, with 50–100 mg of oral clozapine equaling the anticholinergic potency of 1 mg of benztropine [25]. Clozapine therapy is associated with constipation and a risk for ileus, and the ileus risk is doubled with the concurrent use of strongly anticholinergic agents (see Table 3.9) [26].

Table 3.9 List of common strongly anticholinergic medications.

Psychotropics	Chlorpromazine, olanzapine, quetiapine (> 600 mg/day), amitriptyline, nortriptyline, clomipramine, imipramine, desipramine
Antiparkinsonian medications	Benztropine, diphenhydramine, trihexyphenidyl
Nonpsychiatric medications	Oxybutynin, tolterodine, darifenacin, solifenacin, trospium, glycopyrrolate

Among all antipsychotics, chlorpromazine presents the greatest risk for ileus when combined with clozapine, as it is strongly antimuscarinic. If possible, convert chlorpromazine to an equivalent dose of a medium- or high-potency antipsychotic prior to starting clozapine. If not possible, use aggressive measures to minimize risks of severe constipation (see Chapter 7), and cross-taper with clozapine in a chlorpromazine:clozapine ratio of approximately 100 mg:100 mg for nonsmokers, and a chlorpromazine:clozapine ratio of 100 mg:200 mg for smokers. For quetiapine, the taper can proceed with a quetiapine:clozapine ratio of approximately 200 mg:100 mg for nonsmokers, and 100 mg:100 mg for smokers. For olanzapine, an approximate taper is a olanzapine:clozapine ratio of approximately 10 mg:100 mg for nonsmokers, and 10 mg:200 mg for smokers. It is worth recalling that some treatment-resistant patients derive modest benefit from D_2 antagonism despite therapeutic clozapine levels. If the removal of chlorpromazine or olanzapine results in decompensation despite optimization of clozapine levels [20], add a source of D_2 antagonism in a form that does not increase risk for constipation, orthostasis or sedation. For patients on antipsychotics lacking receptor affinities that increase risk for constipation, orthostasis or sedation (e.g. aripiprazole), the current antipsychotic dose can be maintained until clozapine is at a minimum therapeutic plasma level. At that juncture, the antipsychotic can be tapered off, again bearing in mind that the patient my have realized some benefit from the prior agent, albeit limited in nature. If the patient becomes symptomatically worse as the prior antipsychotic is tapered, resume the prior dose that maintained stability, titrate clozapine further, and then try again to taper the prior antipsychotic.

Any tricyclic antidepressants should be tapered off in lieu of other agents, preferably those that will not have pharmacokinetic interactions with clozapine (see Chapter 5). Antiparkinsonian medications can be cross-tapered with clozapine in the manner shown in Box 3.6.

Box 3.6 Approximate Anticholinergic Equivalents

Nonsmokers: 50 mg clozapine = 1 mg benztropine = 2.5 mg trihexyphenidyl = 25 mg diphenhydramine

Smokers: 100 mg clozapine = 1 mg benztropine = 2.5 mg trihexyphenidyl = 25 mg diphenhydramine

It is important to recall that a number of medications used for overactive bladder are potent antimuscarinic agents. If possible, taper these medications off prior to or during the early initiation period of clozapine treatment to minimize the risk of constipation and ileus. The presence of other constipating agents such as oral iron supplements and opioids (see below) must be minimized or eliminated completely prior to starting clozapine.

Other Constipating Medications: iron (ferrous sulfate or gluconate), hydrocodone, oxycodone, codeine, hydromorphone, morphine, fentanyl, methadone, oxymorphone, tramadol.

Orthostasis Inducing Medications: certain psychotropics (low-potency antipsychotics, iloperidone), medications for benign prostatic hypertrophy (prazosin, terazosin), and antihypertensives may all contribute to increased risk of orthostasis during clozapine initiation through a variety of mechanisms. In particular, antipsychotics that are strong alpha$_1$-adrenergic antagonists need to be tapered as clozapine is started, with consideration given to tapering other alpha$_1$-adrenergic antagonists (prazosin, terazosin) or substituting an agent such as tamsulosin with lower hypotension risk (if being used for urinary symptoms). For antihypertensive medications, close consultation with the primary care provider is important to reach a joint decision on which medications to taper if orthostasis becomes a clinical problem.

Summary Points

a. Clozapine titration must be individualized based on clinical setting (inpatient or outpatient), patient variables (age, heritage), the presence of kinetic interactions with medications or smoking behavior.

b. ECG machines using a linear QT rate correction formula such as Framingham are preferable.

c. Tapering off medications that cause pharmacodynamic interactions (e.g. anticholinergics, benzodiazepines, alpha$_1$-adrenergic antagonists, constipating medications) or unsafe kinetic interactions (fluvoxamine, ciprofloxacin) prior to commencing clozapine decreases risk of adverse outcomes that might result in clozapine discontinuation.

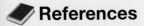

References

1. McCutcheon, R., Beck, K., D'Ambrosio, E., et al. (2018). Antipsychotic plasma levels in the assessment of poor treatment response in schizophrenia. *Acta Psychiatrica Scandinavica*, 137, 39–46.

2. Yoshimura, B., Yada, Y., So, R., et al. (2017). The critical treatment window of clozapine in treatment-resistant schizophrenia: Secondary analysis of an observational study. *Psychiatry Research*, 250, 65–70.

3. Krakowski, M. I., Czobor, P., Citrome, L., et al. (2006). Atypical antipsychotic agents in the treatment of violent patients with schizophrenia and schizoaffective disorder. *Archives of General Psychiatry*, 63, 622–629.

4. Nielsen, J., Young, C., Ifteni, P., et al. (2016). Worldwide differences in regulations of clozapine use. *CNS Drugs*, 30, 149–161.

5. Ifteni, P., Nielsen, J., Burtea, V., et al. (2014). Effectiveness and safety of rapid clozapine titration in schizophrenia. *Acta Psychiatrica Scandinavica*, 130, 25–29.

6. Rostami-Hodjegan, A., Amin, A. M., Spencer, E. P., et al. (2004). Influence of dose, cigarette smoking, age, sex, and metabolic activity on plasma clozapine concentrations: A predictive model and nomograms to aid clozapine dose adjustment and to assess compliance in individual patients. *Journal of Clinical Psychopharmacology*, 24, 70–78.

7. de Leon, J., Schoretsanitis, G., Smith, R. L., et al. (2022). An international adult guideline for making clozapine titration safer by using six ancestry-based personalized dosing titrations, CRP, and clozapine levels. Pharmacopsychiatry, 55, 73-86.

8. Haslemo, T., Eikeseth, P. H., Tanum, L., et al. (2006). The effect of variable cigarette consumption on the interaction with clozapine and olanzapine. *European Journal of Clinical Pharmacology*, 62, 1049–1053.

9. Jann, M. W., Grimsley, S. R., Gray, E. C., et al. (1993). Pharmacokinetics and pharmacodynamics of clozapine. *Clinical Pharmacokinetics*, 24, 161–176.

10. Guitton, C., Kinowski, J. M., Abbar, M., et al. (1999). Clozapine and metabolite concentrations during treatment of patients with chronic schizophrenia. *Journal of Clinical Pharmacology*, 39, 721–728.

11. Takeuchi, H., Powell, V., Geisler, S., et al. (2016). Clozapine administration in clinical practice: Once-daily versus divided dosing. *Acta Psychiatrica Scandinavica*, 134, 234–240.

12. Olesen, O. V. and Linnet, K. (2001). Contributions of five human cytochrome P450 isoforms to the *N*-demethylation of clozapine in vitro at low and high concentrations. *Journal of Clinical Pharmacology*, 41, 823–832.

13. Poyraz, C. A., Ozdemir, A., Saglam, N. G., et al. (2016). Rapid clozapine titration in patients with treatment refractory schizophrenia. *Psychiatry Quarterly*, 87, 315–322.

14. Suzuki, T., Uchida, H., Watanabe, K., et al. (2011). Factors associated with response to clozapine in schizophrenia: A review. *Psychopharmacology Bulletin*, 44, 32–60.

15. Cummings, J., Isaacson, S., Mills, R., et al. (2014). Pimavanserin for patients with Parkinson's disease psychosis: A randomised, placebo-controlled phase 3 trial. *Lancet*, 383, 533–540.

16. Parkinson Study Group. (1999). Low-dose clozapine for the treatment of drug-induced psychosis in Parkinson's disease. *New England Journal of Medicine*, 340, 757–763.

17. The French Clozapine Parkinson Study Group. (1999). Clozapine in drug-induced psychosis in Parkinson's disease. The French Clozapine Parkinson Study Group. *Lancet*, 353, 2041–2042.

18. Ronaldson, K. J., Fitzgerald, P. B. and McNeil, J. J. (2015). Clozapine-induced myocarditis, a widely overlooked adverse reaction. *Acta Psychiatrica Scandinavica*, 132, 231–240.

19. Golden, G. and Honigfeld, G. (2008). Bioequivalence of clozapine orally disintegrating 100-mg tablets compared with clozapine solid oral 100-mg tablets after multiple doses in patients with schizophrenia. *Clinical Drug Investigation*, 28, 231–239.

20. Taylor, D. M., Smith, L., Gee, S. H., et al. (2012). Augmentation of clozapine with a second antipsychotic – A meta-analysis. *Acta Psychiatrica Scandinavica*, 125, 15–24.

21. Luo, S., Michler, K., Johnston, P., et al. (2004). A comparison of commonly used QT correction formulae: The effect of heart rate on the QTc of normal ECGs. *Journal of Electrocardiology*, 37(Suppl), 81–90.

22. Kim, D. D., White, R. F., Barr, A. M., et al. (2018). Clozapine, elevated heart rate and QTc prolongation. *Journal of Psychiatry and Neuroscience*, 43, 71–72.

23. Vandenberk, B., Vandael, E., Robyns, T., et al. (2016). Which QT correction formulae to use for QT monitoring? *Journal of the American Heart Association*, 5, e003264.

24. Rohde, C., Polcwiartek, C., Kragholm, K., et al. (2018). Adverse cardiac events in out-patients initiating clozapine treatment: a nationwide register-based study. *Acta Psychiatrica Scandinavica*, 137, 47–53.

25. de Leon, J. (2005). Benztropine equivalents for antimuscarinic medication. *American Journal of Psychiatry*, 162, 627.

26. Nielsen, J. and Meyer, J. M. (2012). Risk factors for ileus in patients with schizophrenia. *Schizophrenia Bulletin*, 38, 592–598.

4

Discontinuing Clozapine and Management of Cholinergic Rebound

QUICK CHECK

INTRODUCTION

The need to discontinue clozapine is a lamentable but medically necessary event in certain circumstances, and at times must be accomplished abruptly. In instances when the patient can be tapered off gradually (e.g. dilated cardiomyopathy), the risk of cholinergic rebound symptoms is lessened and the clinician can focus on making an informed choice about antipsychotic treatment. Although no agent equals clozapine's efficacy for treatment-resistant schizophrenia, 35% of a group of schizophrenia outpatients with poor antipsychotic response ($n = 99$) who were considered candidates for clozapine had subtherapeutic plasma levels of their current antipsychotic [1]. Thus, a certain fraction of patients who end up on clozapine were failures due to inadequate dosing of prior antipsychotics, poor adherence or kinetic issues. As will be discussed below, this is an important consideration for patients deemed treatment-resistant but who did not experience adverse effects of prior antipsychotic treatment, particularly those related to D_2 antagonism. This understanding may open the door to revisiting prior antipsychotics, but with careful monitoring of adherence and drug exposure via use of plasma levels [2].

A withdrawal syndrome following abrupt discontinuation of chlorpromazine (including some on concurrent anticholinergic antiparkinsonian medications) was

- During abrupt discontinuation, management of cholinergic rebound is critical to prevent central nervous system and peripheral adverse effects.

- The decision on which antipsychotic to start in lieu of clozapine is based on detailed knowledge of prior response and tolerability.

- Previous antipsychotic trials previously deemed treatment failures must be reassessed for evidence of inadequate dosing or nonadherence, especially when there was no documentation of adverse effects related to D_2 antagonism.

- ECT is an underutilized but effective treatment for schizophrenia and must be considered when pharmacotherapy is inadequate.

- Parkinson's disease psychosis (PDP) patients have limited options. In areas where it is available, pimavanserin is a potent, selective $5HT_{2A}$ antagonist approved for PDP that lacks any activity at dopamine receptors. Despite weak efficacy data, lack of approved indication, and a twofold increase in mortality rates, the weak D_2 antagonist quetiapine is commonly used.

first described in a 1959 study ($n = 28$). The cluster of symptoms comprised "acute, uncomfortable reactions characterized by tension, fear, restlessness, insomnia, increased perspiration, and vomiting" [3]. For the 17 patients who developed clinically significant withdrawal reactions, three developed symptoms on the second day, nine on the third day, three on the fourth day, and two on the fifth day. The author also noted: "The symptoms had not entirely subsided until two weeks after the sudden withdrawal" [3]. This classic description of cholinergic rebound was not recognized for many years as the product of cholinergic supersensitivity due to the complex pharmacology of chlorpromazine, combined with the prevalent use of anticholinergic antiparkinsonian agents with higher-potency antipsychotics. Twenty years later it finally became clear that the central nervous system (CNS) and systemic symptoms described in 1959 were related to removal of potent muscarinic antagonism, and not the dopaminergic property of the antipsychotic [4]. Lieberman introduced the term "cholinergic rebound" in 1981 to reinforce the concept that this is a phenomenon related to tolerance of and abrupt withdrawal of a muscarinic antagonist, with the severity related to the prior anticholinergic load [5].

Clozapine possesses over sevenfold higher affinity for the muscarinic M_1 receptor than does chlorpromazine, and by 1974 early reports of a clozapine withdrawal syndrome were alluded to; however, not until wider commercial release in 1989 was the problem recognized, with five case reports emerging by 1994. In 1996 a dedicated study of clozapine withdrawal symptoms was performed in 28 clozapine-treated inpatients enrolled in a kinetic study, all of whom received 200 mg/day for 1 month. No adjunctive psychotropics were allowed aside from benzodiazepines or chloral hydrate for sleep. Over the week after abrupt discontinuation 12 patients experienced mild withdrawal symptoms (agitation, headache, nausea), four had moderate symptoms (nausea, vomiting, diarrhea) and one patient experienced a rapid-onset psychotic episode with manic features requiring hospitalization [6]. The use of anticholinergics was effective for the mild and moderate symptoms, which were ascribed to cholinergic rebound, although most were not symptom-free until 5–7 days after onset of the withdrawal syndrome. The manic episode was also deemed related to cholinergic rebound, although it did not respond to anticholinergic medications as did somatic symptoms. (NB: Case reports and one clinical trial of the acetylcholinesterase inhibitor donepezil support the cholinergic hypothesis for mania. In a double-blind, placebo-controlled study of adjunctive donepezil for treatment-resistant mania, the donepezil cohort had twofold higher Young Mania Rating Scale scores than the placebo group after 6 weeks: 20.17 ± 3.66 vs. 11.20 ± 4.60 ($p = 0.01$) [7]. As has been discussed throughout this handbook, effective management of common adverse effects such as tachycardia, sialorrhea and constipation, and a timely approach to fever presenting in the first 2 months of treatment, can minimize the need to discontinue clozapine treatment, the complex decisions that ensue regarding antipsychotic options, and need to address cholinergic rebound symptoms.

Box 4.1 Cholinergic Rebound Symptoms*

Mild: sleep disturbance, vivid dreams, nightmares

Moderate: anxiety, nausea, diarrhea, sweating, urinary urgency

Severe: confusion, delirium, catatonia

* Comment: By its actions at striatal cholinergic interneurons, cholinergic rebound may also induce parkinsonism, akathisia or dystonia if the patient is being exposed to another source of D_2 antagonism. In this context the effect of cholinergic rebound can be thought of as "anti-benztropine" [15].

A Management of Cholinergic Rebound

When a clinician has the luxury of time, the best method for managing cholinergic rebound is to prevent its occurrence by slowly tapering clozapine. For patients on full therapeutic doses (typically ≥ 300 mg/day) the taper can proceed up to 100 mg each week until a dose of 100 mg/day is reached. At that point, the clozapine dose can be consolidated to bedtime (if not already), and the taper proceed by 25 mg increments every 4–7 days until discontinued. Mild cholinergic rebound symptoms in the form of sleep disturbance can be managed with modest diphenhydramine doses (25–50 mg) at bedtime.

In cases where clozapine must be stopped abruptly and will not be resumed at full dose within 48 hours, anticholinergic medication must be used to prevent cholinergic rebound. The literature over the past two decades is replete with cases of severe rebound with delirium when appropriate anticholinergic therapy was not administered [8]. Not only is clozapine a potent antimuscarinic medication, it is used in high milligram doses, thus exposing patients to a systemic anticholinergic burden not seen with other antipsychotics or even high doses of antiparkinsonian medications [9]. Based on studies of serum anticholinergicity, a clozapine dose in the range of 50–100 mg/day is approximately equivalent to benztropine 1 mg/day [10]. The use of an anticholinergic atypical antipsychotic to cover cholinergic rebound and underlying psychotic disorder seems appealing, and olanzapine is touted as the leading candidate based in part on slightly greater efficacy in a small fraction (7–9%) of treatment-resistant schizophrenia patients [11,12]. While olanzapine has high *in vitro* muscarinic M_1 affinity (Ki 2.5 nM), it provides nowhere near the anticholinergic activity of clozapine (M_1 Ki 6.2 nM) due to the larger clozapine doses used in nearly every application except Parkinson's disease psychosis (PDP). Assays of patients taking olanzapine (mean dose 15 mg/day) show serum anticholinergic activity less than 20% of that seen with patients on clozapine (mean dose 444 mg/day) [13]. Thus, an abrupt switch from clozapine to olanzapine can result in rebound symptoms including delirium, and this has been reported in the literature [14]. Chlorpromazine is a weaker M_1 antagonist than clozapine, may not adequately manage rebound symptoms, and may be an unappealing choice for patients with a history of sensitivity to D_2 antagonism. The use of a separate anticholinergic medication to manage rebound symptoms allows this agent to be tapered off over time, and also allows the clinician flexibility in the antipsychotic chosen to manage the psychiatric disorder. Benztropine or other strongly anticholinergic medications used for cholinergic rebound must be started in the first 24 hours after clozapine is discontinued, using the dosing equivalence in Box 4.2.

Nonsmokers: 50 mg clozapine = 1 mg benztropine = 2.5 mg trihexyphenidyl = 25 mg diphenhydramine

Smokers: 100 mg clozapine = 1 mg benztropine = 2.5 mg trihexyphenidyl = 25 mg diphenhydramine

Comments:

1. Benztropine is the preferred agent for managing cholinergic rebound, but diphenhydramine can also be used. Trihexyphenidyl has greater abuse potential and may not be available in certain forensic settings. Other atypical antipsychotics (e.g. olanzapine) do not provide sufficient anticholinergic activity to mitigate rebound for patients on therapeutic doses of clozapine [14]. Chlorpromazine is one option for those without marked sensitivity to D_2 antagonism; however, use of a separate anticholinergic medication provides maximum flexibility in antipsychotic choice.

2. Local guidelines may limit the maximum daily benztropine dose to 6 or 8 mg/day. Although these doses may not equal the anticholinergic load from clozapine, they should be sufficient to forestall moderate and severe cholinergic rebound symptoms. Due to the short half-life, benztropine (and other anticholinergics) must be administered at least twice per day.

3. Benztropine (or other anticholinergic medication) should not be tapered for at least 2 weeks after clozapine discontinuation unless the clozapine dose was ≤ 50 mg/day, and the taper should not start until all withdrawal symptoms have abated for at least 1 week. A slow taper of no more than 1 mg/day (benztropine equivalent) per week will minimize the risk of rebound symptoms. Once a benztropine equivalent dose of 1 mg/day is reached, the taper should proceed by 0.5 mg/day each week. If mild withdrawal symptoms occur (e.g. sleep disturbance, vivid dreams), the prior anticholinergic dose must be resumed, and the taper commenced the subsequent week at a slower rate (e.g. 0.5 mg/day each week).

Exact equivalent doses to that provided by clozapine may not be possible due to the daily maximum limits for anticholinergic medications. (In the US these are: benztropine 6 mg/day, trihexyphenidyl 15 mg/day, diphenhydramine 300 mg/day.) Nonetheless, the use of an anticholinergic agent will greatly decrease the severity of, or completely abate the development of cholinergic rebound. Cholinergic rebound symptoms from higher clozapine doses may not resolve for 2–3 weeks. For this reason, the anticholinergic medication must not be discontinued abruptly, but instead tapered very slowly over several weeks starting no sooner than 2 weeks after clozapine was abruptly discontinued unless the clozapine dose was very low (e.g. ≤ 50 mg/day). In patients who are receiving another source of D_2 antagonism (e.g. haloperidol, risperidone), abruptly stopping the anticholinergic agent may itself induce rebound effects including the tendency to promote parkinsonism, acute dystonia and akathisia [15]. If a patient develops sleep disturbance (i.e. vivid dreams, nightmares) or systemic symptoms (e.g. gastrointestinal disturbance) during the taper, the most recent higher dose should be resumed, and the taper slowed.

B Provision of Appropriate Antipsychotic Therapy

Patients often require clozapine treatment due to treatment-resistant schizophrenia, schizophrenia with suicidality or schizophrenia with aggression, and by definition were considered failures on other antipsychotics. However, prior treatment failure may have been due to a number of factors including inadequate doses prescribed by the clinician, substance use, treatment nonadherence, or kinetic reasons (e.g. unrecognized exposure to cytochrome P450 inducers, or presence of cytochrome P450 ultrarapid metabolizer status). When patients were deemed treatment-resistant despite never manifesting common D_2 antagonism adverse effects, significant questions must be raised about the adequacy of prior antipsychotic trials. The approach to those patients will be very different than for individuals with a history of extreme sensitivity to dopamine D_2 antagonism in the form of neuroleptic malignant syndrome, parkinsonism, akathisia or dystonia from other antipsychotics. For the latter group, there is no debate about the adequacy of prior antipsychotic exposure, and the treatment options are considerably narrower.

Although clozapine was initially approved in 1989 based on efficacy in treatment-resistant schizophrenia, one of its common uses was for patients intolerant of D_2 antagonism from first-generation antipsychotics. Patients with exquisite sensitivity to D_2 blockade still exist, but represent a smaller pool of clozapine-treated patients since the advent of atypical antipsychotics. If a patient with history of marked intolerance of D_2 antagonism must be discontinued from clozapine, one can consider weak antagonists such as quetiapine, agents with low rates of acute movement disorders such as iloperidone, and electroconvulsive therapy (ECT). In some cases, novel strategies must be considered, including off-label adjunctive use of newer medications without D_2 activity such as pimavanserin, a selective and potent $5HT_{2A}$ antagonist (Ki 0.087 nM). Pimavanserin is indicated for PDP, but in a double-blind schizophrenia study enhanced the efficacy of risperidone 2 mg/day to the extent that symptom reduction for this combination strategy was equivalent to that for risperidone monotherapy at the dose of 6 mg/day [16]. The presence of potent $5HT_{2A}$ antagonism also helps mitigate the development of akathisia or parkinsonism, and this property is the basis for trials of mirtazapine, a moderate $5HT_{2A}$ antagonist, added to antipsychotics for akathisia management [17].

1. Included in this group are patients with a documented history of acute parkinsonism, dystonia or akathisia after modest exposure to D_2 antagonists.

2. Quetiapine is a weak D_2 antagonist (Ki 380 nM) and the most likely agent to be tolerated. Moreover, there are two large studies of doses up to 1200 mg/day if such dosing is permitted by local guidelines [26,27]. Iloperidone had low rates of acute parkinsonism, dystonia or akathisia in clinical trials up to the maximum dose of 12 mg BID, and can also be considered [28]. Titration should proceed more cautiously than with quetiapine as iloperidone is a more potent D_2 antagonist (Ki 6.3 nM), although other properties of the molecule may help mitigate risk for D_2-related adverse effects. Rates of orthostasis with iloperidone noted in the package insert may be somewhat lessened in this context as patients have developed tolerance to alpha$_1$-adrenergic antagonism from exposure to clozapine. Nonetheless, rapid titration should be avoided.

3. Given the paucity of therapeutic options, one could consider the off-label use of pimavanserin in combination with quetiapine or iloperidone. Pimavanserin is a potent serotonin $5HT_{2A}$ inverse agonist (Ki 0.087 nM) approved for treatment of Parkinson's disease psychosis, and is devoid of affinity for any dopamine receptors [20]. Moreover, pimavanserin has been shown to enhance the efficacy of risperidone but not haloperidol, implying that its most plausible use as an augmenting agent might be in the context of a relatively weaker D_2 antagonist [16].

4. ECT remains an evidence-based but often underutilized option for schizophrenia, and at times is employed successfully in clozapine nonresponders [29].

In patients where D_2 sensitivity is not an issue, one must rely on the prior pattern of response and tolerability to guide treatment. Bearing in mind that 35–44% of schizophrenia outpatients deemed treatment-resistant had subtherapeutic plasma antipsychotic levels when measured, strong consideration should be given to using plasma levels to guide future antipsychotic therapy, and to exploring higher plasma levels if tolerability is not an issue [1]. While decidedly inferior to clozapine for resistant schizophrenia, olanzapine may have slightly greater efficacy than other antipsychotics, and clinical trials have demonstrated adequate tolerability up to plasma levels of 200 ng/ml (640 mmol/l), with the major adverse effect being constipation [18]. In general, antipsychotic doses should be advanced when tolerability is not limiting until one of two hard endpoints is reached: significant symptomatic improvement or intolerability. There is a small subset of patients who will never develop D_2-related adverse effects, so plasma levels must be tracked to avoid proceeding past the point of futility where the likelihood of response is remote [19].

Box 4.4 Antipsychotic Options for Schizophrenia Spectrum Patients Without a History of Marked Sensitivity to D_2 Antagonism

1. Included in this group are patients without a documented history of acute parkinsonism, dystonia or akathisia, or who only experienced these events with higher doses of D_2 antagonists.

2. At least 35% of outpatients deemed treatment-resistant have subtherapeutic plasma antipsychotic levels. For patients who have never experienced parkinsonism, dystonia or akathisia, scour the clinical record for evidence of treatment nonadherence (or occasionally cytochrome P450 ultrarapid metabolizer status). Plasma antipsychotic levels on oral antipsychotic therapy prior to the clozapine trial will be very helpful.

3. Whether the prior failure was due to inadequate dosing, kinetic reasons or nonadherence, tracking the subsequent antipsychotic trial with plasma levels will help resolve these issues. The following two options are appealing due to the extensive body of data on concentration/oral dose relationships and response thresholds.

   a. The response threshold for haloperidol is 3–5 ng/ml (8.0–13.3 nmol/l), with few patients tolerating levels > 20 ng/ml (80 nmol/l), although levels up to 30 ng/ml (80 nmol/l) can be pursued if tolerated [19].

   Haloperidol Concentration/Oral Dose Relationships in CYP 2D6 Extensive Metabolizers [30]

   2 mg/day –> 1.57 ± 1.42 ng/ml (4.18 ± 3.78 nmol/l)
   10 mg/day –> 7.79 ± 4.79 ng/ml (20.72 ± 12.74 nmol/l)

   b. Olanzapine may capture 7–9% more responders among treatment-resistant schizophrenia patients compared to nonclozapine antipsychotics [11,12]. The response threshold for olanzapine is 23 ng/ml (74 nmol/l), and tolerability threshold is close to 200 ng/ml (640 nmol/l), with constipation being the primary adverse effect at high plasma levels [18,19].

   Olanzapine Concentration/Oral Dose Relationships in CYP 1A2 Extensive Metabolizers [30]

   10 mg –> 20 ng/ml (64 nmol/l) (nonsmokers)
   14 mg –> 20 ng/ml (64 nmol/l) (smokers)

4. ECT remains an evidence-based but often underutilized option for schizophrenia, and at times is employed successfully in clozapine nonresponders [29].

Parkinson's Disease Psychosis

More than 50% of patients with Parkinson's disease develop psychosis as a consequence of pathologic processes related to the disease itself, and not primarily due to D_2 agonist therapy as previously hypothesized. Psychosis is the most common cause of nursing home placement in nondemented PD patients, and has enormous impact on patients and caregivers [20]. The pathophysiology of psychosis in PDP is due to the accumulation of subcortical Lewy body burden that causes death of serotonin-producing dorsal raphe neurons. This loss of the serotonin signal results in upregulation of postsynaptic $5HT_{2A}$ receptors and receptor supersensitivity. The concept that excessive $5HT_{2A}$ receptor stimulation may cause psychosis with prominent visual hallucinations had been known from studies of lysergic acid diethylamide (LSD) and other hallucinogenic compounds whose activity is blocked by $5HT_{2A}$ antagonists. PD patients are notoriously intolerant of D_2 antagonism, and respond in a robust manner to only one antipsychotic, low-dose clozapine. In the two widely cited 4-week, double-blind, placebo-controlled trials, the mean doses were 25–36 mg/day with a large effect size [21,22]. No significant motoric effects were seen during low-dose clozapine treatment. There are numerous failed trials for other atypical antipsychotics, including quetiapine, and recent data indicate that quetiapine and atypical antipsychotics (except clozapine) are associated with twofold increased mortality rates when used in PD patients [23].

Based on the finding that clozapine in low doses acts primarily at $5HT_{2A}$ receptors, a novel compound pimavanserin was designed as a potent $5HT_{2A}$ antagonist (Ki 0.087 nM) (technically an inverse agonist), with no appreciable affinity for adrenergic, dopaminergic, muscarinic, histaminergic, adrenergic or GABA-ergic receptors. Because it is devoid of affinity for dopamine receptors, pimavanserin avoids the motoric worsening seen with most antipsychotics, and was approved by the US FDA in 2016 for treatment of PDP [20]. For PDP patients who must be removed from clozapine, consultation with a neurologist specializing in movement disorders should be considered, as these specialists have the greatest experience with this clinical scenario. Based on the history, one can consider modest adjustments to dopamine agonist exposure to see if this improves psychosis symptoms; however, the PDP patient who needs clozapine has usually exhausted this option early in the course of their psychosis, often due to intolerable motoric exacerbation when dopamine agonist therapy was lessened. When clozapine needs to be discontinued, pimavanserin represents the best of the remaining choices, although it may not be available outside of the US. The approved dose is 34 mg once daily, and separation from placebo appeared at week 2 of the pivotal 6-week trial, so patients should be advised that efficacy may not be seen for several weeks [20]. As pimavanserin lacks histaminic or muscarinic antagonism, clozapine should ideally be tapered off by 12.5 mg/day each week, or diphenhydramine used to mitigate rebound insomnia, because this symptom may worsen PDP symptoms. When pimavanserin is not accessible, many clinicians have resorted to quetiapine, mostly due to the paucity of other viable options. Quetiapine's advantage over other antipsychotics is that it is a very weak D_2 antagonist, and should not worsen motor symptoms; however, it did not prove effective in three of four clinical trials, although some patients do report benefit [24]. Moreover, naturalistic data from over 15,000 PD patients found that quetiapine increased mortality twofold compared to matched PD patients not receiving antipsychotic treatment (OR 2.16, 95% CI 1.88–2.48) [23]. As with schizophrenia, ECT remains an option for PD patients, and may produce improvements in psychosis, mood and motor symptoms [25].

Summary Points

a. Management of cholinergic rebound must start within 24 hours after clozapine discontinuation, using appropriate equivalent doses of benztropine. Olanzapine is not sufficiently anticholinergic to prevent cholinergic rebound.

b. After abrupt clozapine discontinuation, the anticholinergic agent should not be tapered for 2–3 weeks unless the clozapine dose was ≤ 50 mg/day, and then at no more than the equivalent of 1 mg/day of benztropine each week.

c. For schizophrenia spectrum patients the antipsychotic choice to replace clozapine depends on whether there is a documented history of significant sensitivity to D_2 antagonism. Patients who are exquisitely sensitive to D_2 blockade have many fewer options.

d. ECT is an effective treatment for schizophrenia, including some treatment-resistant cases.

e. The viable options for Parkinson's disease psychosis patients who must stop clozapine include pimavanserin, possibly quetiapine and ECT.

References

1. McCutcheon, R., Beck, K., D'Ambrosio, E., et al. (2018). Antipsychotic plasma levels in the assessment of poor treatment response in schizophrenia. *Acta Psychiatrica Scandinavica*, 137, 39–46.

2. Horvitz-Lennon, M., Mattke, S., Predmore, Z., et al. (2017). The role of antipsychotic plasma levels in the treatment of schizophrenia. *American Journal of Psychiatry*, 174, 421–426.

3. Brooks, G. W. (1959). Withdrawal from neuroleptic drugs. *American Journal of Psychiatry*, 115, 931–932.

4. Luchins, D. J., Freed, W. J. and Wyatt, R. J. (1980). The role of cholinergic supersensitivity in the medical symptoms associated with withdrawal of antipsychotic drugs. *American Journal of Psychiatry*, 137, 1395–1398.

5. Lieberman, J. (1981). Cholinergic rebound in neuroleptic withdrawal syndromes. *Psychosomatics*, 22, 253–254.

6. Shiovitz, T. M., Welke, T. L., Tigel, P. D., et al. (1996). Cholinergic rebound and rapid onset psychosis following abrupt clozapine withdrawal. *Schizophrenia Bulletin*, 22, 591–595.

7. Eden Evins, A., Demopulos, C., Nierenberg, A., et al. (2006). A double-blind, placebo-controlled trial of adjunctive donepezil in treatment-resistant mania. *Bipolar Disorders*, 8, 75–80.

8. Stanilla, J. K., de Leon, J. and Simpson, G. M. (1997). Clozapine withdrawal resulting in delirium with psychosis: A report of three cases. *Journal of Clinical Psychiatry*, 58, 252–255.

9. de Leon, J., Odom-White, A., Josiassen, R. C., et al. (2003). Serum antimuscarinic activity during clozapine treatment. *Journal of Clinical Psychopharmacology*, 23, 336–341.

10. de Leon, J. (2005). Benztropine equivalents for antimuscarinic medication. *American Journal of Psychiatry*, 162, 627.

11. Conley, R. R., Tamminga, C. A., Bartko, J. J., et al. (1998). Olanzapine compared with chlorpromazine in treatment-resistant schizophrenia. *American Journal of Psychiatry*, 155, 914–920.

12. Lindenmayer, J. P., Czobor, P., Volavka, J., et al. (2002). Olanzapine in refractory schizophrenia after failure of typical or atypical antipsychotic treatment: An open-label switch study. *Journal of Clinical Psychiatry*, 63, 931–935.

13. Chengappa, K. N., Pollock, B. G., Parepally, H., et al. (2000). Anticholinergic differences among patients receiving standard clinical doses of olanzapine or clozapine. *Journal of Clinical Psychopharmacology*, 20, 311–316.

14. Delassus-Guenault, N., Jegouzo, A., Odou, P., et al. (1999). Clozapine–olanzapine: A potentially dangerous switch. A report of two cases. *Journal of Clinical Pharmacy and Therapeutics*, 24, 191–195.

15. Simpson, G. M. and Meyer, J. M. (1996). Dystonia while changing from clozapine to risperidone. *Journal of Clinical Psychopharmacology*, 16, 260–261.

16. Meltzer, H. Y., Elkis, H., Vanover, K., et al. (2012). Pimavanserin, a selective serotonin (5-HT)2A-inverse agonist, enhances the efficacy and safety of risperidone, 2 mg/day, but does not enhance efficacy of haloperidol, 2 mg/day: Comparison with reference dose risperidone, 6 mg/day. *Schizophrenia Research*, 141, 144–152.

17. Hieber, R., Dellenbaugh, T. and Nelson, L. A. (2008). Role of mirtazapine in the treatment of antipsychotic-induced akathisia. *Annals of Pharmacotherapy*, 42, 841–846.

18. Kelly, D. L., Richardson, C. M., Yu, Y., et al. (2006). Plasma concentrations of high-dose olanzapine in a double-blind crossover study. *Human Psychopharmacology*, 21, 393–398.

19. Meyer, J. M. (2014). A rational approach to employing high plasma levels of antipsychotics for violence associated with schizophrenia: Case vignettes. *CNS Spectrums*, 19, 432–438.

20. Cummings, J., Isaacson, S., Mills, R., et al. (2014). Pimavanserin for patients with Parkinson's disease psychosis: A randomised, placebo-controlled phase 3 trial. *Lancet*, 383, 533–540.

21. Parkinson Study Group. (1999). Low-dose clozapine for the treatment of drug-induced psychosis in Parkinson's disease. *New England Journal of Medicine*, 340, 757–763.

22. The French Clozapine Parkinson Study Group. (1999). Clozapine in drug-induced psychosis in Parkinson's disease. The French Clozapine Parkinson Study Group. *Lancet*, 353, 2041–2042.

23. Weintraub, D., Chiang, C., Kim, H. M., et al. (2016). Association of antipsychotic use with mortality risk in patients with Parkinson Disease. *JAMA Neurology*, 73, 535–541.

24. Borek, L. L. and Friedman, J. H. (2014). Treating psychosis in movement disorder patients: A review. *Expert Opinion on Pharmacotherapy*, 15, 1553–1564.

25. Usui, C., Hatta, K., Doi, N., et al. (2011). Improvements in both psychosis and motor signs in Parkinson's disease, and changes in regional cerebral blood flow after electroconvulsive therapy. *Progress in Neuropsychopharmacology and Biological Psychiatry*, 35, 1704–1708.

26. Lindenmayer, J. P., Citrome, L., Khan, A., et al. (2011). A randomized, double-blind, parallel-group, fixed-dose, clinical trial of quetiapine at 600 versus 1200 mg/d for patients with treatment-resistant schizophrenia or schizoaffective disorder. *Journal of Clinical Psychopharmacology*, 31, 160–168.

27. Honer, W. G., MacEwan, G. W., Gendron, A., et al. (2012). A randomized, double-blind, placebo-controlled study of the safety and tolerability of high-dose quetiapine in patients with persistent symptoms of schizophrenia or schizoaffective disorder. *Journal of Clinical Psychiatry*, 73, 13–20.

28. Tonin, F. S., Wiens, A., Fernandez-Llimos, F., et al. (2016). Iloperidone in the treatment of schizophrenia: An evidence-based review of its place in therapy. *Core Evidence*, 11, 49–61.

29. Miyamoto, S., Jarskog, L. F. and Fleischhacker, W. W. (2015). Schizophrenia: When clozapine fails. *Current Opinion in Psychiatry*, 28, 243–248.

30. Meyer, J. M. (2017). Converting oral to long acting injectable antipsychotics: A guide for the perplexed. *CNS Spectrums*, 22, 14–28.

4

5

Binding Profile, Metabolism, Kinetics, Drug Interactions and Use of Plasma Levels

 QUICK CHECK

 INTRODUCTION

    Clinicians must be knowledgeable about the mechanisms, metabolic pathways, and kinetics of all prescribed medications, but this is especially true for agents with narrower therapeutic indices such as clozapine. Armed with this information, one can maximize the potential for a successful clozapine trial in a patient who may lack other viable therapeutic options. While the properties underlying clozapine's unique efficacy profile are not fully elucidated, there are extensive data on peripheral and central nervous system (CNS) kinetics, drug–drug and environmental interactions, and plasma levels to inform routine clinical care. (Throughout this volume clozapine plasma levels

PRINCIPLES

- Clozapine's high affinity for muscarinic, histaminic and alpha$_1$-adrenergic receptors is associated with risk for constipation, sedation and orthostasis. Norclozapine's muscarinic agonism is responsible for sialorrhea.

- Clinicians must be aware of environmental (e.g. smoking), drug interaction and genetic influences on clozapine metabolism. The mean population plasma clozapine:norclozapine ratio of 1.32 will be altered when subjected to significant kinetic effects.

- Plasma clozapine levels must be tracked to determine adherence and adequacy of the treatment trial. Response correlates best with the 12-hour trough clozapine level and not the combined concentration of clozapine + norclozapine. Likelihood of response in schizophrenia spectrum patients is low with trough clozapine levels below 350 ng/ml or 1070 nmol/l.

- Serious bacterial or viral infections can be associated with downregulation of cytochrome P450 1A2 activity. The net result is a marked jump in plasma clozapine levels, metabolic ratio and clozapine-related adverse effects.

5

will be presented in ng/ml and nmol/l units. Some laboratories may report levels in μg/l, which is exactly equivalent to ng/ml.)

 Clozapine Metabolism and Kinetics

Clozapine is predominantly administered in the form of tablets, suspension or orally dissolving tablets (ODT), all of which are considered bioequivalent when studied by comparative assays [1,2]. Nonetheless, clinicians are advised to routinely check plasma clozapine levels 1 week after changing preparations to make sure levels have remained stable, and to account for the possibility of improved patient adherence when going from tablets to ODT or oral suspension. The bioavailability for all oral forms is 60%, without apparent impact from food. An intramuscular (IM) formulation (25 mg/ml) is available in a limited number of countries and it is 100% bioavailable, so IM doses are approximately half of the intended oral doses.

As seen in Figure 5.1, clozapine is converted to an active metabolite, norclozapine (also called *N*-desmethylclozapine), and the inactive clozapine-*N*-oxide, along with other minor metabolites without known clinical significance.

Figure 5.1. Structure of clozapine and its primary metabolites.

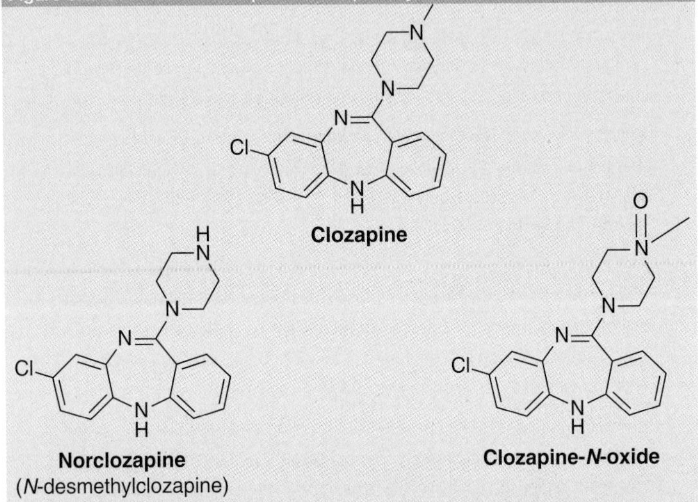

Clozapine

Norclozapine
(*N*-desmethylclozapine)

Clozapine-*N*-oxide

Clozapine exhibits linear pharmacokinetics within the usual therapeutic range and is a substrate for multiple cytochrome P450 (CYP) isoenzymes, and also for the efflux transporter P-glycoprotein (PGP). Among the CYP isoenzymes that contribute to its metabolism, CYP 1A2 is the most important, especially at lower plasma concentrations (Table 5.1). In addition to being susceptible to inhibition by other medications, CYP 1A2 is also inducible, and has a number of functional polymorphisms. Among the most useful facts to remember, the ratio of clozapine to norclozapine plasma levels (also called the *metabolic ratio* or MR) is 1.32 in patients who are extensive metabolizers at all relevant CYP isoenzymes, and who are not being exposed to inhibitors or inducers. This MR reference value is derived from an analysis of nearly 5000 samples obtained from over 2000 patients [3]. Values significantly greater than 1.32 (e.g. > 2.00) reflect a nontrough value, slow metabolism or the presence of inhibitors [4]. Similarly, metabolic ratios ≤ 1.00 reflect the presence of inducers (e.g. smoking, omeprazole, carbamazepine) (see section C, Plasma Levels). As will be discussed in section C, Plasma Levels, it may be difficult to predict the net effect of multiple concurrent medications or environmental agents (e.g. smoking) that influence CYP activity, making plasma level monitoring critical to documenting clozapine exposure. Importantly, assuming there is no change in the use of concomitant medications or smoking behavior (e.g. cessation or resumption), the MR will remain unchanged during periods of poor adherence unless the patient takes the clozapine

Table 5.1 Fast facts about clozapine metabolism and kinetics [29].

Formulations	• Tablets • Oral dissolving tablet (ODT) • Oral suspension (50 mg/ml) • Intramuscular (25 mg/ml) (in some countries)
Bioavailability (oral)	• Bioavailability: 60% • No impact of food on bioavailability
Kinetics	• Half-life: 12 (4–66) hours • T_{Max} 2.5 hours • Dose adjustments may be necessary in patients with significant renal impairment (CrCl < 30 ml/min) or severe hepatic impairment (Child–Pugh Class C)*
Metabolism	• The mean contributions of CYPs 1A2, 2C19, 3A4, 2C9, and 2D6 are 30%, 24%, 22%, 12%, and 6%, respectively. In some studies CYP 1A2 is responsible for 40–55% of clozapine biotransformation • CYP 1A2 is the most important form at low concentrations, which is in agreement with clinical findings • The population ratio of clozapine to norclozapine trough plasma concentrations is 1.32 but papers show a range from 1.19 to 3.37, with a weighted mean of 1.73 in one meta-analysis. [3]
CYP inhibitor effects	• Fluvoxamine increases serum levels 5–10-fold** • Strong 2D6 or 3A4 inhibitors may increase clozapine levels as much as 100%**
CYP/PGP inducer effects	• Loss of smoking-related 1A2 induction results in ≥ 50% increase in serum levels • Carbamazepine, phenytoin, and omeprazole decrease levels on average by 50%**

*   Child–Pugh criteria: low serum albumin, high total bilirubin, elevated INR (derived from plasma prothrombin time), and the presence of ascites or hepatic encephalopathy. Class C patients have severe advanced liver disease with 1-year survival under 50% and are rarely encountered in routine psychiatric practice. Alanine aminotransferase (ALT) and aspartate aminotransferase (AST) are not part of the criteria and are not a basis for adjustment of medication dosages [30].

** See Table 5.2 for guidance on dosing adjustments with inhibitors and inducers.

just prior to obtaining a plasma level. Nonadherence with oral clozapine will result in low and erratic trough levels, as will be mentioned in section C, but does not alter the MR.

Given the narrow therapeutic index for clozapine, including case reports of fatality with concomitant use of clozapine and strong CYP 1A2 inhibitors, most package inserts provide detailed information about adjustment of clozapine in the context of the addition or removal of drugs with known kinetic interactions [5]. Often lacking from these advisories are standard definitions for what distinguishes a strong, moderate or weak inhibitor or inducer, and these are included in Box 5.1.

The updated US clozapine prescribing guidelines contain a useful table addressing the clinical scenario, and the nature and magnitude of the kinetic interaction (Table 5.2). Based on the standard definitions, Table 5.3 provides a list of CYP inhibitors and inducers among commonly encountered medications. Although divalproex is a known inhibitor of the phase II enzyme UGT1A4, its presence may modestly increase or decrease clozapine levels depending on smoking status, and possibly serum valproate levels [6,7]. In large kinetic modeling studies, valproic acid was estimated to increase levels in nonsmokers (effect size +16%), but reduce levels in smokers (effect size −22%) [6]. When starting clozapine, clinicians must consult the latest information about interactions with concomitant medications, and check plasma clozapine levels early in treatment (e.g. at a dose of 100 mg/day). Similarly, when medications with potential kinetic interactions are added to or removed from the regimen of a patient on clozapine, a repeat clozapine level needs to be obtained once the new medication is at steady state.

● CYP 1A2: Impact of Smoking, Caffeine and Genetic Polymorphisms

CYP 1A2 accounts for about 13% of the total CYP content in human liver, but is the primary isoenzyme regulating clozapine metabolism, accounting for 30–55% of CYP-mediated metabolism. Throughout the population there are more than 15-fold differences in CYP 1A2 messenger RNA levels and more than 40-fold differences in its expression [8]. Polymorphisms not only impact baseline activity, but also the response to inducers such as those present in cigarette smoke. When unexpectedly high plasma clozapine levels and metabolic ratios (i.e. > 2.00) are encountered without exposure to known inhibitors, and these are replicated with a repeat plasma level, it is likely due to

Table 5.2 US guidelines on dose adjustment in patients taking concomitant medications.

Comedications	Scenarios	
	Initiating clozapine while taking a comedication *OR* *Adding a comedication while taking clozapine*	*Discontinuing a comedication while continuing clozapine*
Strong CYP 1A2 inhibitors	Use one-third of the clozapine dose.	Increase clozapine dose based on clinical response.
Moderate or weak CYP 1A2 inhibitors	Monitor for adverse reactions. Consider reducing the clozapine dose if necessary.	Monitor for lack of effectiveness. Consider increasing clozapine dose if necessary.
Strong CYP 2D6 or 3A4 inhibitors*	Monitor for adverse reactions. Consider reducing the clozapine dose if necessary.	Monitor for lack of effectiveness. Consider increasing clozapine dose if necessary.
Strong CYP 3A4 inducers	Concomitant use is not recommended. However, if the inducer is necessary, it may be necessary to increase the clozapine dose. Monitor for decreased effectiveness.	Reduce clozapine dose based on clinical response.
Moderate or weak CYP 1A2 or 3A4 inducers	Monitor for decreased effectiveness. Consider increasing the clozapine dose if necessary.	Monitor for adverse reactions. Consider reducing the clozapine dose if necessary.

* Dose adjustments may be necessary in patients who are CYP2D6 poor metabolizers.

Table 5.3 Selected list of common CYP inhibitors and inducers.

	Strong	Moderate/weak
CYP 1A2 inhibitors	Fluvoxamine, ciprofloxacin, enoxacin	Oral contraceptives, caffeine
CYP 2D6 inhibitors	Paroxetine, bupropion, fluoxetine, quinidine	Duloxetine
CYP 3A4 inhibitors	Ketoconazole, itraconazole, posaconazole, clarithromycin, nefazodone, ritonavir, saquinavir, nelfinavir, indinavir, boceprevir, telaprevir, telithromycin, conivaptan	Amprenavir, aprepitant, atazanavir, diltiazem, erythromycin, fluconazole, fosamprenavir, grapefruit juice, imatinib, verapamil
CYP 1A2 inducers	Smoking, omeprazole	
CYP 3A4 inducers	Phenytoin, carbamazepine, phenobarbital, rifampin	Oxcarbazepine, St. John's wort

the presence of one or more nonfunctional CYP 1A2 alleles [4]. Genetic testing for CYP polymorphisms may miss new variants not included in commercial panels. (see Table 5.4). The MR is much more helpful in deciding on a course of action.

Table 5.4 List of functional CYP 1A2 single nucleotide polymorphisms (SNP).
(Source: www.snpedia.com/index.php/SNPedia; accessed September 30, 2018.)

Allele	rs SNP designation	Nucleotide change (older nomenclature)	Functional effect
*1		Wild type	Extensive metabolizer (normal)
*1C	rs2069514	−3860G>A	Decreased activity
*1F	rs762551	−163C>A	Increased inducibility
*1 K	rs12720461	−729C>T	Decreased activity and inducibility
*1 K	rs2069526	−739T>G	Decreased activity
*3	rs56276455	2385G>A	Decreased activity
*4	rs72547516	2499A>T	Decreased activity
*6	rs28399424	5090C>T	No activity
*7	no identifier	3533G>A	No activity
*11	rs72547513	558C>A	Decreased activity

Smoking induces CYP 1A2 activity by the action of aryl hydrocarbons at the aromatic hydrocarbon receptor (AhR). Nicotine itself plays no role in this process. The AhR is a cytosolic transcription factor that remains inactive and bound to a protein complex in the absence of a ligand. Upon binding of an appropriate ligand (e.g. aryl hydrocarbons from smoke), an interacting protein is released from the complex and translocated to the nucleus where it binds to the CYP 1A2 promoter region and increases expression of messenger RNA [8]. CYP 1A2 appears to be fully induced after regular use of only 7–12 cigarettes per day [9], and this induction results in a mean 1.66-fold increase in CYP 1A2 activity [8]. The higher clozapine dose required for smokers to achieve comparable plasma levels as nonsmokers is fully explained by this phenomenon. Upon *complete* cessation of smoking, the induction effects are lost and CYP 1A2 levels return gradually to baseline. When studied in a sample of 12 individuals who smoked at least 20 cigarettes per day, the half-life of the CYP 1A2 activity decrease following smoking cessation was 38.6 hours (range 27.4–54.4 hours) [10].

Caffeine is a substrate for CYP 1A2 and historically has been used as a probe to measure CYP 1A2 activity. While not an inhibitor, caffeine in large doses may compete with clozapine for CYP 1A2, thereby increasing plasma clozapine levels. In a sample

Box 5.2 Smoking and Clozapine

1. Smoking as few as 7–12 cigarettes/day is sufficient to fully induce CYP 1A2, with a net increase of 1.66-fold in enzyme activity. Aryl hydrocarbons induce CYP 1A2 expression. **Nicotine plays no role.**

2. Upon smoking cessation the CYP 1A2 activity declines with a half-life of 38.6 hours (range 27.4–54.4 h). CYP 1A2 activity will therefore return to baseline after 5 half-lives, or 8 days on average.

3. Plasma clozapine levels must be rechecked after any change in smoking status, ideally after 7 days and 14 days, and doses adjusted.

4. When outpatient smokers treated with clozapine are placed in situations without access to cigarettes for more than 48 hours, doses ought to be lowered by 10% every 48 hours to a maximum reduction of 50%. Plasma levels on days 7 and 14 can be used to guide further dose adjustments.

5. The loss of induction from smoking will increase plasma clozapine levels at least 50%. In patients whose clozapine level as a smoker was in the high therapeutic range (600–1000 ng/ml or 1800–3000 nmol/l) this can result in severe toxicity as clozapine levels rise and CYP 1A2 becomes saturated, resulting in nonlinear kinetics.

of *nonsmoking* volunteers who ingested 400–1000 mg/day of caffeine, there was a 19% increase in mean total clozapine exposure ($p = 0.05$) and a 14% decrease in mean oral clozapine clearance ($p = 0.05$) compared to values without caffeine [11]. While the effect of caffeine may not be clinically significant in most individuals, there are case reports of patients increasing their clozapine levels twofold or more during periods of excessive caffeine intake. As will be discussed in section C, Plasma Levels, if there is doubt about the kinetic effect of an increase in caffeine intake, a repeat trough plasma clozapine level is useful.

● **BID vs. QD Dosing and Relationship to Hypotheses About Clozapine's Efficacy**

Due to the short peripheral half-life, low levels of D_2 occupancy even at peak plasma levels, and concerns about the tolerability of large single doses, clozapine was brought to market with recommendations for multiple daily dosing, typically BID. As practice has evolved over the ensuing decades, the standard in many parts of the world is to commence clozapine with a single daily QHS dose. A 2016 review of nearly 1000 clozapine-treated individuals managed at academic centers in Toronto and New York noted that once daily dosing was employed in 75% of patients without an apparent loss of efficacy, even though doses exceeding 200 mg/day were administered in over 84% of the samples from each site [12]. Moreover, among nonsmokers in state hospital settings within California, single QHS doses up to 500 mg are well tolerated. Putative advantages of QHS dosing including possibly lower rates of daytime sedation, and improved adherence among outpatients. Nonetheless, there is an absence of controlled comparative data, so clinicians can tailor dosing schedules to patient needs, bearing in mind that many patients do well with QHS dosing, but that others may respond better with BID dosing.

B Binding Profile of Clozapine and Its Primary Active Metabolite Norclozapine

The clinical effects of clozapine are related to the activities of clozapine and its primary metabolite norclozapine. The activity of norclozapine is distinct enough from clozapine that it was studied by itself as a potential antipsychotic [13]. That the trials of norclozapine were not successful may relate to methodological issues, but it may also relate to the concept that the combined actions of clozapine and norclozapine may be necessary to achieve the antipsychotic benefit. Although *in vitro* assays indicate that clozapine-*N*-oxide has high affinity for both M_1 and $5HT_{2A}$ receptors, it represents < 10% of the active moiety (clozapine + metabolites) [14]. Moreover, data from primate studies indicate clozapine-*N*-oxide has high affinity for the PGP efflux transporter, which limits CNS penetration [15]. Unfortunately, the mechanisms that underlie clozapine's unique efficacy are not explained by the affinity of clozapine or norclozapine for monoamine receptors. Nonetheless, the monoamine receptor affinities (Table 5.5) and intrinsic activity at muscarinic receptors (Table 5.6) correlate with several features of clozapine treatment.

Table 5.5 Binding profile at cloned human receptors (Ki nM) [13] and PDSP Ki database.

	D_2	$5HT_{2A}$	$5HT_{2C}$	$5HT_{1A}$	M_1	M_3	α_{1A}	α_{1B}	H_1	Brain/plasma ratio in PGP KO vs. WT
Clozapine	20	5.0	39.8	123.7	6.17	6.31	7.9	7.0	0.32	1.6 [31]
Norclozapine	63	5.0	15.9	13.9	67.6	158	5.0	85.2	6.3	?

(Source: pdsp.med.unc.edu/pdsp.php; accessed September 30, 2018.)

KO, knockout; WT, wild-type.

Table 5.6 Muscarinic intrinsic activity relative to the full agonist carbachol [13].

	M_1	M_2	M_3	M_4	M_5
Clozapine	24 ± 3%	65 ± 8%	NR	57 ± 5%	NR
Norclozapine	72 ± 5%	106 ± 9%	27 ± 4%	87 ± 8%	48 ± 6%
Carbachol	101 ± 2%	101 ± 5%	102 ± 3%	96 ± 3%	105 ± 3%

Box 5.3 Properties Related to Known Receptor Affinities

D_2 antagonism: both clozapine and norclozapine have low affinity for this receptor, and this is associated with extremely low risk for parkinsonism and akathisia.

M_1 and M_3 antagonism: clozapine has high affinity for both of these muscarinic receptors, and weak intrinsic activity at M_1, and therefore acts as an antagonist. This significant antagonist activity is associated with high rates of constipation and other peripheral anticholinergic adverse effects.

M_1–M_5 agonism: norclozapine has significant intrinsic agonist activity at multiple muscarinic receptors except for M_3. While these agonist properties are not sufficient to mitigate most peripheral anticholinergic effects of clozapine, they are hypothesized to be responsible for inducing sialorrhea.

H_1 antagonism: clozapine and to a lesser extent norclozapine have significant affinity, contributing to sedation and impaired satiety.

α_1 antagonism: clozapine and norclozapine have significant affinity resulting in risk for orthostasis.

$5HT_{2A}$ inverse agonism: clozapine and norclozapine have significant affinity, and are *inverse agonists*. G-protein-coupled receptors have low levels of basal activity even in the absence of a ligand. While a potent antagonist will block ligand actions, it does not alter the level of basal activity. An inverse agonist will reduce the level of basal activity below baseline. The clinical implications of potent $5HT_{2A}$ inverse agonism include: (a) increased presynaptic dopamine release in nigrostriatal neurons, thereby decreasing risk for parkinsonism, akathisia, acute dystonia; and (b) decreased dopamine neurotransmission in the limbic portions of the striatum, possibly contributing to the antipsychotic effect.

The discovery that clozapine possesses potent $5HT_{2A}$ binding led to the development of other atypical antipsychotics, although none have approached clozapine's efficacy in resistant schizophrenia. Inverse agonists at $5HT_{2A}$ receptors mitigate the development of antipsychotic-induced parkinsonism and akathisia through binding to presynaptic dopaminergic neurons in the nigrostriatal pathway.

Blocking the inhibitor signal from serotonin facilitates increased synaptic release of dopamine. This action is the basis for the use of mirtazapine to treat akathisia: mirtazapine has moderate affinity for $5HT_{2A}$ receptors (Ki 69 nM), but this is sufficient at doses of 30–60 mg/day to relieve the akathisia associated with D_2 antagonism.

That potent $5HT_{2A}$ inverse agonism has antipsychotic effects was proven in successful trials of pimavanserin for Parkinson's disease psychosis (PDP). Pimavanserin has subnanomolar $5HT_{2A}$ affinity (Ki 0.87 nM) with no appreciable binding at dopaminergic, adrenergic, muscarinic, histaminergic, GABAergic or glutamatergic receptors [16]. Although potent $5HT_{2A}$ inverse agonism by itself is effective for PDP, it may not be sufficient to treat the more complex illness of schizophrenia. Nonetheless, there is one clinical trial showing that the combination of pimavanserin plus risperidone 2 mg/day achieved efficacy comparable to risperidone 6 mg/day without pimavanserin [17]. Both clozapine and norclozapine are weaker D_2 antagonists than risperidone, with D_2 occupancy only transiently exceeding 50%, so it is biologically plausible that the significant $5HT_{2A}$ inverse agonism of these molecules contributes appreciably to the antipsychotic effect. Moreover, the time course of $5HT_{2A}$ receptor occupancy demonstrates a longer half-life than that seen for D_2 binding (Figures 5.2 and 5.3). This property that may help explain the efficacy seen with once-daily dosing [18].

While not crucial to routine practice, clinicians ought to be aware of another theory for clozapine's efficacy – its putative impact on glutamate neurotransmission. The glutamate hypofunction hypothesis of schizophrenia derives from the known psychotomimetic and cognitive disrupting effects of N-methyl-D-aspartate (NMDA) glutamate receptor antagonists such as phencyclidine (PCP). Based on this finding, it is hypothesized that NMDA receptor hypofunction might be inherent to schizophrenia pathophysiology [19]. The NMDA receptor has binding sites for both glutamate and a co-agonist glycine, and clinical trials have been conducted with agents that act as NMDA agonists through various mechanisms, including inhibition of CNS glycine transporters (GlyT1). While the addition of the GlyT1 inhibitor sarcosine to nonclozapine antipsychotics improves schizophrenia symptoms, it was not beneficial when added to clozapine, implying that clozapine possessed an optimal level of glycinergic activity [20]. Supporting this concept are *in vitro* data demonstrating that clozapine has selective activity at GlyT1 in a manner not seen with other antipsychotics or norclozapine, and *in vivo* animal data supporting a glycinergic mechanism [21,22]. In the few trials when glycine itself was given to

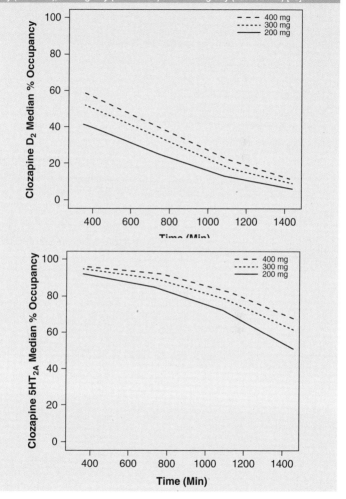

Figures 5.2 and 5.3. Predicted D_2 and $5HT_{2A}$ occupancy with clozapine 200 mg/day (solid line), 300 mg/day (dotted line) and 400 mg/day (dashed line) [18].

(Adapted from: Li, C. H., Stratford, R. E., Jr., Velez de Mendizabal, N., et al. (2014). Prediction of brain clozapine and norclozapine concentrations in humans from a scaled pharmacokinetic model for rat brain and plasma pharmacokinetics. *Journal of Translational Medicine*, 12, 203 [18].)

clozapine patients in doses of 30–60 g/day, it worsened the positive symptoms of schizophrenia [23].

 Plasma Levels

Given the varied binding properties and actions of clozapine and norclozapine there was a healthy debate in the literature whether clinicians should track the summed levels of both molecules or each one individually. The accumulated data over the past 30 years points to the following conclusions.

1. Plasma clozapine levels, and not the concentration of clozapine + norclozapine, best correlate with efficacy.

2. With proper sample storage both serum and plasma clozapine levels are acceptable and highly correlated, with serum levels on average only 3% higher than hematocrit corrected plasma levels [24]. [NB: Throughout this volume "plasma level" will be used as the default term for the sake of simplicity.]

3. The primary use of norclozapine levels is to track CYP 1A2 activity. Assuming that trough plasma levels are obtained consistently at approximately the same time since the evening dose (± 2 hours), the ratio of clozapine to norclozapine levels (the *metabolic ratio* or *MR*) ought not to change significantly between determinations. **Significant changes in MR therefore reflect the addition or removal of an inhibitor or inducer.** The one exception to this rule (discussed below) is a marked increase in clozapine plasma levels and MR accompanying severe bacterial or viral infections [25]. When the timing of trough levels is consistent, dose adjustments or nonadherence should also not alter MR, with the exception of overdose situations where CYP 1A2 may become saturated, and clozapine levels increase disproportionately compared to norclozapine levels. Box 5.4 details some rough guidelines for interpreting changes in MR.

There is increasing enthusiasm over the use of plasma level monitoring to track patient exposure to antipsychotic agents, explore problems of nonadherence or kinetic interactions, and determine a future course of treatment when inadequate response or significant adverse effects arise. The principles that govern obtaining useful plasma levels are very similar to those employed for monitoring of lithium and many other oral medications, and are given in Box 5.5.

Box 5.4 Guidelines for Interpreting the Metabolic Ratio (MR)

1. MR = 1.32: The expected mean value for nonsmokers who are CYP 1A2 extensive metabolizers.

2. MR << 1.32: Trough values of 1.00 or less reflect exposure to an inducer (e.g. smoking, carbamazepine, omeprazole), or CYP 1A2 ultrarapid metabolizer status.

3. MR >> 1.32: Trough values greater than 2.00 reflect exposure to inhibitors of the main CYP enzymes involved in clozapine metabolism: 1A2, 2C19, 2D6 or 3A4, or poor metabolizer status, especially at CYP 1A2 or CYP 2D6. As clozapine is principally metabolized via CYP 1A2, strong CYP 2D6 or 3A4 inhibitors will typically increase clozapine levels by 40–100%, generating MR values in the range of 1.80–2.60. Conversely, strong 1A2 inhibitors (e.g. fluvoxamine, ciprofloxacin) may increase clozapine levels up to 10-fold, with resulting MR values of 3.00 or greater. CYP poor metabolizers will typically have MR values comparable to those seen with use of strong 2D6 or 3A4 inhibitors.

4. MR ≥ 3.0 during medical illness. A marked increase in MR from baseline in the context of serious bacterial or viral infections may occur, with MR values on average around 3.0 (range 1.4–8.6). This change in clozapine metabolism reflects an inhibitory effect of inflammatory cytokines on CYP 1A2 activity [25]. (See Box 5.6.)

● **Response to Levels Markedly Above or Below Expected Values, and Suspected Nonadherence**

For patients starting on clozapine, an initial level is best obtained early in therapy to gain a sense of drug metabolism and possible nonadherence. Many clinicians choose a round number such as 100 mg QHS or 200 mg QHS as the point at which they obtain plasma levels during titration, waiting at least 5–7 days on that dose so clozapine will be at steady state. Issues with drug metabolism will be reflected in MR values that differ markedly from that expected based on the patient's current exposure to inhibitors or inducers (especially smoking). A good rule of thumb when the results do not jive with the clinical scenario is to repeat the level, preferably on the same dose. If it is not possible to recheck on the same dose due to slow laboratory turnaround (in some instances 7–14 days or more), try choosing another multiple of 100 mg to make the math easier, as clozapine exhibits linear pharmacokinetics within the usual therapeutic range. The presence of two data points will greatly clarify the appropriate course of action. In particular, poor adherence will be reflected by

Box 5.5 Principles for Obtaining Clozapine levels

1. **Timing:** The gold standard is a 12-hour (± 2 h) trough value obtained at steady state (i.e. after 5–7 days), but consistency is also important. If a patient who receives their daily clozapine at 8 pm cannot make it to a laboratory until 10 am, this should be the agreed upon time for future levels to be drawn. Samples obtained within a time span of approximately 4 hours (10–14 h postdose) do not show significant median differences [32]. However, as the timing of blood draws deviates significantly (e.g. > 4 h) the levels will be more difficult to interpret, as will the MR, as more (or less) time has elapsed for the formation of norclozapine. While a 16-hour trough is less than ideal, it is preferable to having no documentation of plasma levels.

2. **Divided doses:** For patients who receive their clozapine in two (or occasionally three) daily doses, the morning dose must be held until the level is drawn. Communication of this with outpatients and caregivers is crucial. If the patient and caregiver are unsure whether the morning dose was administered prior to the laboratory visit, then simply repeat the level. When clozapine is administered shortly before a level is obtained the MR will be much higher than baseline values because little time has passed for clozapine's metabolism. The morning dose ought to be taken as soon as possible after the level is drawn.

3. **Interpreting the result:** Using a nomogram or online calculator, the clinician can generate a rough estimate of what the expected plasma level will be for the administered dose, bearing in mind important patient variables (age, gender, smoking status, weight), and the presence of known inhibitors or inducers [3].

4. **Variability of results:** Using 723 samples from 61 patients, the mean coefficient of variation for sequential plasma concentrations of clozapine and of norclozapine were both approximately 30% [33]. Given this level of variability of ± 30% between determinations, clinicians are advised that more than one plasma level may be necessary to make an appropriate clinical decision. Importantly, clinicians must be alert to the possibility of laboratory error, as some laboratories may be more expert than others in performing clozapine and norclozapine assays [34].

marked fluctuations (> 50%) in plasma clozapine levels for a given dose between determinations.

   a. **Plasma levels significantly below what is expected:** When there are no prior plasma levels for the patient and the value is more than 50% below that predicted using a nomogram or calculator that adjusts for dose and demographic variables (especially smoking), nonadherence is the likely culprit. As noted above, a repeat level will be instructive. Marked plasma level fluctuations (> 50%) on the same dose will indicate nonadherence, while consistent levels (especially with multiple data points) with limited fluctuation may indicate absorption issues. For patients with an established baseline, fluctuations up to 30% are to be expected. When fluctuations exceed 50% nonadherence must be suspected, again assuming no change in dose, or exposure to inhibitors or inducers.

b. **Plasma levels significantly higher than expected:** The first rule of thumb is patient safety as determined by clinical evaluation. When no prior levels are available, many clinicians become alarmed when very high levels are returned from the laboratory (e.g. > 1000 ng/ml or > 3000 nmol/l) and reflexively reduce doses without first determining whether the level fits the clinical picture. Most patients with very high plasma concentrations typically exhibit adverse effects consistent with the level including sedation, orthostasis, tachycardia or sialorrhea. As will be discussed below, very high clozapine levels are also seen in in the context of severe bacterial or viral infections due to the impact of cytokines on CYP 1A2 activity. Before any actions are taken, a few steps need to be performed. (a) The patient must be evaluated in person, including consideration of an ECG if deemed appropriate (using the appropriate rate correction formula if tachycardic) (see Chapter 3), assessment of the possibility of serious infection, and the presence or absence of adverse effects noted. (b) For those on divided daily doses, an attempt ought to be made to determine if the level was a true trough, or if a morning dose was inadvertently given prior to the blood draw. (c) An estimated plasma level needs to be calculated based on dose, presence of inhibitors/inducers, and demographics to assess how far the obtained value is from the expected result. When there are adverse effects, the dose ought to be reduced to bring levels below 1000 ng/ml or 3000 nmol/l, and perhaps lower depending on the severity of the adverse effect. Abrupt discontinuation should be avoided, as it will cause marked cholinergic rebound and possible delirium. Dose reduction is preferable. When there is a complete absence of adverse effects, evidence of a serious infection or ECG findings, a suspicion of laboratory error needs to be raised and this hypothesis noted in the record as the reason for not changing the dose and for ordering a repeat level for the next morning. Occasional patients will also be encountered who both tolerate and respond to very high plasma levels (1000–1200 ng/ml or 3057–3669 nmol/l), and who decompensate at lower plasma levels.

When baseline plasma levels are available, and no significant change has occurred with respect to kinetically interfering medications or habits (e.g. smoking cessation), a level markedly higher than expected raises three possibilities. (a) The morning dose was inadvertently given prior to the blood draw. This will result in an increase in the MR compared to prior baseline values because limited time has elapsed for clozapine to be converted to norclozapine. (b) There is a serious infection that has markedly increased plasma clozapine levels (see below). (c) The high plasma level is due to laboratory error. As noted above, the patient must be evaluated and systemic complaints or adverse effects noted, particularly if they have changed in severity. When there is a complete absence of systemic symptoms of infection, adverse effects or ECG findings, or the patient appears to be at baseline, the suspicion of laboratory error ought to be raised and noted as the reason for not changing the dose and for ordering a repeat level the next morning.

● Serious Bacterial or Viral Infections: Impact on Clozapine Levels and Metabolic Ratio

Even prior to the COVID-19 pandemic there were numerous case reports documenting unexpected increases in plasma clozapine levels associated with serious bacterial, and occasionally viral, infections. The changes in clozapine metabolism are substantial, and not related to the use of antibiotics or other medications with kinetic effects. A 2018 review of the 40 existing cases noted that the median baseline level (in the 25 cases where reported) was 550 ng/ml (1681 nmol/l), but jumped to a mean level of 1811 ng/ml (5536 nmol/l) during the period of infection [25]. Not all patients exhibited signs of excessive clozapine exposure, but adverse effects were common with sedation occurring in 48%, delirium 20%, speech disturbance 15%, and gait disturbance 12.5%. Myoclonus ($n = 7$) or generalized seizures ($n = 1$) were also reported. Nearly every patient was hospitalized due to the seriousness of the underlying medical problem, with 57.5% having a respiratory infection, 32.5% urinary, 7.5% gastrointestinal and 5% orthopedic, with three cases (0.75%) having concurrent respiratory and urinary tract infections [25]. Of note, 30% of cases did not have fever at the time of presentation.

Norclozapine levels obtained during the infection were available for half of the cases, and the mean MR was markedly elevated at 3.0 (range 1.4–8.6). This

1. Any inflammatory process of sufficient severity to induce marked cytokine release (including COVID-19 infection with systemic symptoms that do not merit hospitalization, and after COVID-19 vaccination) will downregulate CYP 1A2 activity, and this will increase plasma clozapine levels and also the MR.

2. Educate patients, caregivers and nonpsychiatric clinicians involved with the patient's care to be vigilant for the development of signs consistent with high clozapine levels during periods of acute or chronic serious infections or after COVID-19 vaccination. All parties should be particularly sensitive to new-onset sedation, and not to assume that tiredness is solely due to the medical condition.

3. Obtain a trough clozapine level immediately upon any medical hospitalization, especially when the admission is for infection. Although the plasma level result may not be available for a week or more, it can be useful in adjusting clozapine doses.

4. Only 50% of published cases involving plasma level increases during infection had clinical symptoms [25], so the clozapine dose need not be reflexively decreased in all hospitalized patients. However, those who exhibit any new or worsening adverse effects should have the clozapine dose reduced by approximately 50%, bearing in mind that further dose reduction may be needed if adverse effects persist several days after the dose reduction. Abrupt discontinuation should be avoided due to the risks associated with cholinergic rebound and rebound psychosis. A repeat trough plasma level should be drawn at steady state 5 days after any dosage change to help guide future decision-making.

5. Although acute signs of sepsis or infection may resolve quickly during treatment for the underlying condition, the levels of inflammatory cytokines can remain elevated for longer periods, thereby prolonging the time course of subnormal CYP 1A2 capacity. Patients can remain on lower than normal clozapine doses for an extended time (e.g. weeks) while CYP 1A2 activity slowly returns to normal, with the caveat that plasma levels are equivalent to pre-infection values.

6. Weekly monitoring of plasma clozapine levels can document the resolution of infection-mediated impact on clozapine metabolism. During this time, the MR will gradually return to its baseline value. Clozapine doses should be increased if breakthrough psychiatric symptoms develop, or levels have dropped below pre-infection values.

combination of elevated MR coincident with a tripling of the plasma clozapine level points to a process impacting CYP 1A2-mediated clozapine metabolism. The leading hypothesis is that inflammatory cytokines mobilized due to the infection and related stress can downregulate CYP 1A2 expression as much as 90%, resulting in a marked decrease in CYP 1A2 capacity in the same manner as would be seen with administration of a strong CYP 1A2 inhibitor [25]. The true prevalence of this problem in clozapine-treated patients with serious infections is unknown, but likely is underreported as plasma clozapine levels are often not drawn during periods of infection. Thus, in the absence of documented changes in plasma clozapine levels and MR, the most common complaint (sedation) may be ascribed to tiredness from the medical illness itself. Given the potential seriousness of clozapine toxicity in the context of a severe medical illness, clinicians should keep in mind the following principles outlined in Box 5.6. The goal is to adjust clozapine doses in patients who require such intervention, but avoid complete discontinuation of clozapine, especially abrupt cessation that can result in cholinergic rebound and rebound psychosis.

● Use of Levels to Monitor Efficacy

Depending on the country in which one resides, clozapine levels may be reported in ng/ml or nmol/l. Units as µg/l are occasionally used and are identical to values in ng/ml. For the mathematically inclined, conversion formulas between these two units are provided below which rely on the molecular weight of clozapine (326.83 g/mol). Table 5.7 provides comparable values for a range of commonly encountered plasma levels.

a. Converting to nmol/l to ng/ml: level (nmol/l) × 0.32683

b. Converting ng/ml to nmol/l: level (ng/ml) × 3.057

Table 5.7 Clozapine plasma levels in ng/ml and nmol/l.

Level in ng/ml	Level in nmol/l
200	611
300	917
400	1223
500	1528
600	1834
700	2140
800	2446
900	2571
1000	3057

Table 5.8 Clozapine plasma level ranges for resistant schizophrenia.

	Response threshold	Diminishing tolerability	Point of futility
Level in ng/ml	350	700–1000	> 1000
Level in nmol/l	1070	2140–3057	> 3057

Table 5.8 is informed by numerous reviews that document a mean threshold for response in resistant schizophrenia around 350 ng/ml or 1070 nmol/l, and a therapeutic range up to 1000 ng/ml or roughly 3000 nmol/l [27]. Patients treated for Parkinson's disease psychosis typically require such minute doses (6.25–50 mg/day) that plasma levels are not useful.

While many laboratories report an "upper limit" of 600 ng/ml (1834 nmol/l) or 700 ng/ml (2140 nmol/l), there are clearly patients who benefit from and tolerate these high plasma levels [27]. Given the lack of viable alternatives for resistant schizophrenia and other common uses, patients must not be deprived of a trial of clozapine with higher plasma levels, assuming tolerability up to that point.

Once the trough plasma level has crossed the therapeutic threshold, patients need to be given 2–3 weeks to look for any signals of response before deciding on further titration, assuming adverse effects are not limiting. In a dose titration trial, the mean time to response (± SD) once a patient reached the dose (and level) at which they finally responded was 17 (± 14) days, with a range of 2–56 days. Importantly, no late response was found among nonresponders despite a mean follow-up period of 75 weeks [28]. While some clinicians cite old literature touting very late response (6 months or longer), these nonsystematic data do not stand up to the rigorous methods used in later trials. Nonresponders without dose-limiting adverse effects must not be left at the same plasma level for months on end hoping for "late response." Titration ought to proceed even when levels exceed what a particular laboratory has arbitrarily decided is the upper threshold, as the literature clearly justifies exploring levels up to 1000 ng/ml or 3057 nmol/l if tolerated. As levels reach the point of diminishing tolerability, they need to be rechecked after each dose increase of 50 mg/day. Very few patients will respond at levels > 1000 ng/ml or > 3057 nmol/l (the so called "point of futility"), but clinicians may encounter rare patients who seemingly tolerate and respond to such levels. Documentation of response after careful titration, and the absence of significant adverse effects, is important so that other clinicians understand the context for maintaining a patient with seemingly heroic plasma concentrations.

Box 5.7 Principles for Titrating Clozapine

1. The likelihood of response < 350 ng/ml or 1070 nmol/l is low (but not zero). If tolerated, this is a reasonable initial target.

2. Many laboratories report an "upper limit" for clozapine levels of 600 ng/ml (1834 nmol/l) or 700 ng/ml (2140 nmol/l), but there are clearly patients who benefit from and tolerate these high plasma levels [27]. Given the limited alternatives for resistant schizophrenia, patients must not be deprived of a clozapine trial with higher plasma levels, assuming tolerability.

3. Once the dose is increased, patients should be given 2–3 weeks to respond before further titration if adverse effects are not limiting. In a dose titration trial, time to response once the patient reached a dose where they responded was 17 days on average (range of 2–56 days). No late response was found among nonresponders despite a mean follow-up period of 75 weeks [28].

4. Nonresponders without dose-limiting adverse effects must not be left on the same dose and at the same plasma level for months on end hoping for "late response."

5. As levels reach the point of diminishing tolerability (> 700 ng/ml or > 2140 nmol/l), they should be rechecked after each dose increase of 50 mg/day. Very few patients will respond at levels > 1000 ng/ml or > 3057 nmol/l (the so-called "point of futility"), but clinicians may encounter rare patients who seemingly tolerate and respond to such levels.

6. Concentration oral dose relationships (assuming MR = 1.32) [3]:
   40 year old male, weight 80 kg:
   Concentration (ng/ml) = 1.08 x oral dose (mg/d) (nonsmoker)
   Concentration (ng/ml) = 0.67 x oral dose (mg/d) (smoker)
   40 year old female, weight 70 kg:
   Concentration (ng/ml) = 1.32 x oral dose (mg/d) (nonsmoker)
   Concentration (ng/ml) = 0.80 x oral dose (mg/d) (smoker)

Summary Points

a. The mechanisms underlying clozapine's unique efficacy are not clear, but many of the adverse effects can be predicted by receptor binding and activity at certain sites: α_1 antagonism (orthostasis), H_1 antagonism (sedation and weight gain), M_1 and M_3 antagonism (constipation), and M_1–M_5 agonism (sialorrhea).

b. Single daily bedtime dosing is the norm in many parts of the world without apparent loss of efficacy. Single QHS doses up to 500 mg are routinely employed.

c. Familiarity with interpreting the metabolic ratio (ratio of clozapine:norclozapine plasma levels) is very helpful in making clinical decisions.

d. Serious bacterial or viral infections can result in downregulation of cytochrome P450 1A2 activity by inflammatory cytokines, with a resultant increase in clozapine levels up to threefold, and an increase in the MR to 3.0. Even milder infections with COVID-19 may increase plasma clozapine levels to the point that the patient experiences new or worse adverse effects. The cytokine release from COVID-19 vaccination has also been reported to impair clozapine metabolism in some patients. Plasma levels and clinical symptoms of clozapine toxicity should be monitored for during any hospitalization for infection. Patients, caregivers and other clinicians involved with the patient must be alerted to the potential jump in plasma clozapine levels during serious infections, and the most common symptoms seen at higher plasma levels. For patients hospitalized with COVID-19, a trough level should be drawn on admission. Clozapine dose decreases of 50% or more may be needed depending on the emergence of adverse effects related to higher plasma clozapine levels. Levels should be obtained periodically to guide treatment even if the result may not return for 7 days or more.

e. Plasma clozapine levels correlate better with efficacy than the sum of clozapine + norclozapine levels. Tracking plasma (or serum) levels is crucial to a successful clozapine trial.

f. Nicotine itself plays no role in CYP 1A2 induction, it is the aryl hydrocarbons generated from burning the tobacco leaf. After smoking cessation or switching from cigarettes to an e-cigarette, a patient will lose their CYP 1A2 induction over the next week, and clozapine levels may rise 50% or more.

5

References

1. Golden, G. and Honigfeld, G. (2008). Bioequivalence of clozapine orally disintegrating 100-mg tablets compared with clozapine solid oral 100-mg tablets after multiple doses in patients with schizophrenia. *Clinical Drug Investigation*, 28, 231–239.

2. Couchman, L., Morgan, P. E., Spencer, E. P., et al. (2010). Plasma clozapine and norclozapine in patients prescribed different brands of clozapine (Clozaril, Denzapine, and Zaponex). *Therapeutic Drug Monitoring*, 32, 624–627.

3. Rostami-Hodjegan, A., Amin, A. M., Spencer, E. P., et al. (2004). Influence of dose, cigarette smoking, age, sex, and metabolic activity on plasma clozapine concentrations: A predictive model and nomograms to aid clozapine dose adjustment and to assess compliance in individual patients. *Journal of Clinical Psychopharmacology*, 24, 70–78.

4. Couchman, L., Morgan, P. E., Spencer, E. P., et al. (2010). Plasma clozapine, norclozapine, and the clozapine:norclozapine ratio in relation to prescribed dose and other factors: Data from a therapeutic drug monitoring service, 1993–2007. *Therapeutic Drug Monitoring*, 32, 438–447.

5. Meyer, J. M., Proctor, G., Cummings, M., et al. (2016). Ciprofloxacin and clozapine – A potentially fatal but underappreciated interaction. *Case Reports in Psychiatry*, 2016, 5606098.

6. Diaz, F. J., Santoro, V., Spina, E., et al. (2008). Estimating the size of the effects of co-medications on plasma clozapine concentrations using a model that controls for clozapine doses and confounding variables. *Pharmacopsychiatry*, 41, 81–91.

7. Diaz, F. J., Eap, C. B., Ansermot, N., et al. (2014). Can valproic acid be an inducer of clozapine metabolism? *Pharmacopsychiatry*, 47, 89–96.

8. Zhou, S. F., Wang, B., Yang, L. P., et al. (2010). Structure, function, regulation and polymorphism and the clinical significance of human cytochrome P450 1A2. *Drug Metabolism Reviews*, 42, 268–354.

9. Haslemo, T., Eikeseth, P. H., Tanum, L., et al. (2006). The effect of variable cigarette consumption on the interaction with clozapine and olanzapine. *European Journal of Clinical Pharmacology*, 62, 1049–1053.

10. Faber, M. S. and Fuhr, U. (2004). Time response of cytochrome P450 1A2 activity on cessation of heavy smoking. *Clinical Pharmacology & Therapeutics*, 76, 178–184.

11. Hagg, S., Spigset, O., Mjorndal, T., et al. (2000). Effect of caffeine on clozapine pharmacokinetics in healthy volunteers. *British Journal of Clinical Pharmacology*, 49, 59–63.

12. Takeuchi, H., Powell, V., Geisler, S., et al. (2016). Clozapine administration in clinical practice: Once-daily versus divided dosing. *Acta Psychiatrica Scandinavica*, 134, 234–240.

13. Weiner, D. M., Meltzer, H. Y., Veinbergs, I., et al. (2004). The role of M1 muscarinic receptor agonism of *N*-desmethylclozapine in the unique clinical effects of clozapine. *Psychopharmacology*, 177, 207–216.

14. Frazier, J. A., Cohen, L. G., Jacobsen, L., et al. (2003). Clozapine pharmacokinetics in children and adolescents with childhood-onset schizophrenia. *Journal of Clinical Psychopharmacology*, 23, 87–91.

15. Raper, J., Morrison, R. D., Daniels, J. S., et al. (2017). Metabolism and distribution of clozapine-*N*-oxide: Implications for nonhuman primate chemogenetics. *ACS Chemical Neuroscience*, 8, 1570–1576.

16. Cummings, J., Isaacson, S., Mills, R., et al. (2014). Pimavanserin for patients with Parkinson's disease psychosis: A randomised, placebo-controlled phase 3 trial. *Lancet*, 383, 533–540.

17. Meltzer, H. Y., Elkis, H., Vanover, K., et al. (2012). Pimavanserin, a selective serotonin (5-HT)2A-inverse agonist, enhances the efficacy and safety of risperidone, 2mg/day, but does not enhance efficacy of haloperidol, 2mg/day: Comparison with reference dose risperidone, 6mg/day. *Schizophrenia Research*, 141, 144–152.

18. Li, C. H., Stratford, R. E., Jr., Velez de Mendizabal, N., et al. (2014). Prediction of brain clozapine and norclozapine concentrations in humans from a scaled pharmacokinetic model for rat brain and plasma pharmacokinetics. *Journal of Translational Medicine*, 12, 203.

19. Coyle, J. T., Tsai, G. and Goff, D. C. (2002). Ionotropic glutamate receptors as therapeutic targets in schizophrenia. *Current Drug Targets – CNS & Neurological Disorders*, 1, 183–189.

20. Lane, H. Y., Huang, C. L., Wu, P. L., et al. (2006). Glycine transporter I inhibitor, *N*-methylglycine (sarcosine), added to clozapine for the treatment of schizophrenia. *Biological Psychiatry*, 60, 645–649.

21. Williams, J. B., Mallorga, P. J., Jeffrey Conn, P., et al. (2004). Effects of typical and atypical antipsychotics on human glycine transporters. *Schizophrenia Research*, 71, 103–112.

22. Schwieler, L., Linderholm, K. R., Nilsson-Todd, L. K., et al. (2008). Clozapine interacts with the glycine site of the NMDA receptor: Electrophysiological studies of dopamine neurons in the rat ventral tegmental area. *Life Sciences*, 83, 170–175.

23. Veerman, S. R., Schulte, P. F., Begemann, M. J., et al. (2014). Clozapine augmented with glutamate modulators in refractory schizophrenia: A review and metaanalysis. *Pharmacopsychiatry*, 47, 185–194.

24. Hermida, J., Paz, E. and Tutor, J. C. (2008). Clozapine and norclozapine concentrations in serum and plasma samples from schizophrenic patients. *Therapeutic Drug Monitoring*, 30, 41–45.

25. Clark, S. R., Warren, N. S., Kim, G., et al. (2018). Elevated clozapine levels associated with infection: A systematic review. *Schizophrenia Research*, 192, 50–56.

26. Tio, N., Schulte, P. F. J. and Martens, H. J. M. (2021). Clozapine intoxication in COVID-19. *Am J Psychiatry*, 178, 123–127.

27. Meyer, J. M. and Stahl, S. M. (2021). The Clinical Use of Antipsychotic Plasma Levels - Stahl's Handbooks. New York, NY, Cambridge University Press; 382 pp.

28. Conley, R. R., Carpenter, W. T., Jr. and Tamminga, C. A. (1997). Time to clozapine response in a standardized trial. *American Journal of Psychiatry*, 154, 1243–1247.

29. Meyer, J. M. (2018). Pharmacotherapy of psychosis and mania. In L. L. Brunton, R. Hilal-Dandan and B. C. Knollmann (Eds.), *Goodman & Gilman's The Pharmacological Basis of Therapeutics*, 13th Edition, pp. 279–302. Chicago, IL: McGraw-Hill.

30. Verbeeck, R. K. (2008). Pharmacokinetics and dosage adjustment in patients with hepatic dysfunction. *European Journal of Clinical Pharmacology*, 64, 1147–1161.

31. Doran, A., Obach, R. S., Smith, B. J., et al. (2005). The impact of P-glycoprotein on the disposition of drugs targeted for indications of the central nervous system: Evaluation using the MDR1A/1B knockout mouse model. *Drug Metabolism and Disposition*, 33, 165–174.

32. Jakobsen, M. I., Larsen, J. R., Svensson, C. K., et al. (2017). The significance of sampling time in therapeutic drug monitoring of clozapine. *Acta Psychiatrica Scandinavica*, 135, 159–169.

33. Lee, J., Bies, R., Takeuchi, H., et al. (2016). Quantifying intraindividual variations in plasma clozapine levels: A population pharmacokinetic approach. *Journal of Clinical Psychiatry*, 77, 681–687.

34. Oo, T. Z., Wilson, J. F., Naidoo, D., et al. (2006). Therapeutic monitoring of clozapine in Australia: The need for consensus. *Therapeutic Drug Monitoring*, 28, 696–699.

5

6 Understanding Hematologic Monitoring and Benign Ethnic Neutropenia

INTRODUCTION

Many nonchemotherapy medications are associated with neutropenia risk [1], but it was the cluster of 16 severe clozapine-related neutropenia cases reported from Finland in mid-summer 1975 with a 50% fatality rate that prompted clozapine's withdrawal [2]. Clozapine was subsequently reintroduced to the world market in the late 1980s based on demonstrable efficacy in treatment-resistant schizophrenia, albeit with mandatory hematologic monitoring and patient tracking.

PRINCIPLES

- Absolute neutrophil count (ANC) monitoring requirements have changed in the past half-decade, and now differ between the US and other countries.

- The possibility of benign ethnic neutropenia (BEN) must be ruled out in individuals with low baseline ANC. Individuals with BEN have lower ANC thresholds for starting and remaining on clozapine. Patients with BEN are at lower risk for the development of severe neutropenia.

- Other causes of neutropenia, especially medications such as valproate, must be explored in those who do not have BEN but who have subnormal ANC values.

- Lithium and filgrastim must be considered for individuals with or without BEN who have ANC below the threshold for commencing clozapine, or who experience treatment interruptions due to low ANC values.

- The period of greatest risk for neutropenia occurs during the first 6 months, but most countries mandate monthly ANC monitoring starting at week 52 for as long as the patient remains on clozapine.

- The median time to resolution of severe neutropenia from clozapine is 12 days.

Despite common elements around the world, clinicians must be mindful of variations in country-specific monitoring details including frequency of blood draws, whether a complete blood count (CBC) with differential or only the absolute neutrophil count (ANC) is tracked, how benign ethnic neutropenia (BEN) is managed, and the response to laboratory abnormalities [3]. Table 6.1 illustrates some basic differences in US and UK programs, including the change in US terminology from *agranulocytosis* for ANC values < 500/mm³ to *severe neutropenia.*

The purpose of this chapter is to provide clinicians with the core principles that underlie all clozapine monitoring schemes, including the period of highest neutropenia risk, hypothesized mechanisms and risk factors for neutropenia, the diagnosis of BEN, time course and management of severe neutropenia, and the use of lithium and filgrastim to stimulate neutrophil production. Throughout this chapter and others in this handbook *severe neutropenia* will replace the older terminology of *agranulocytosis* to denote ANC counts < 500/mm³.

	UK	US
Table 6.1 Some differences in US and UK clozapine hematologic monitoring.		
WBC parameters	Total WBC and ANC	ANC
Threshold for starting clozapine	1. WBC ≥ 3500/mm³ and ANC ≥ 2000/mm³ 2. BEN WBC ≥ 3000/mm³ and ANC ≥ 1500/mm³	1. ANC ≥ 1500/mm³ 2. BEN ANC ≥ 1000/mm³
Basic monitoring frequency	1. Weekly through week 18 2. Biweekly through week 52 3. Monthly after week 52 4. Up to 4 weeks after discontinuation	1. Weekly through week 26 2. Biweekly through week 52 3. Monthly after week 52 4. Up to 4 weeks after discontinuation
Terminology for neutropenia	Based on WBC and ANC, counts are classified using Green, Amber and Red indicators	Neutropenia is classified as mild, moderate, or severe based on ANC. "Severe neutropenia" replaces the previous terms severe leukopenia, severe granulocytopenia, or agranulocytosis
Rechallenge possible after severe neutropenia (agranulocytosis)	No	Yes
Benign ethnic neutropenia	1. Written confirmation of the BEN diagnosis is required from a consultant hematologist and completion of "Confirmation of Benign Ethnic Neutropenia Monitoring Criteria Approval Form" 2. BEN-specific WBC and ANC thresholds for commencing, holding and stopping clozapine	1. Consider hematology consultation before initiating or during treatment as necessary 2. BEN-specific ANC thresholds for commencing, holding and stopping clozapine 3. Package insert notes that BEN patients are not at increased risk for developing neutropenia
Eosinophil and platelet counts	1. Eosinophilia defined as > 1000/mm³ pretreatment and > 3000/mm³ while on treatment. Initiation or continuation of treatment not recommended if detected 2. Biweekly monitoring for high eosinophil (> 3000/mm³) or low platelet counts (< 50 K)	1. Eosinophilia defined as > 700/mm³. Clinicians alerted to evaluate promptly for signs/symptoms of systemic reactions, rash or other allergic symptoms, myocarditis, or other organ specific disease associated with eosinophilia 2. Mention of drug reaction with eosinophilia and systemic symptoms syndrome (DRESS), also known as drug-induced hypersensitivity syndrome (DIHS) 3. No specified reference ranges for platelet counts or response to aberrant values

Neutropenia Time Course and Risk Factors

Within the US all antipsychotics carry package insert warnings about risk for leukopenia and neutropenia, but these occurrences are considered too infrequent to necessitate routine laboratory surveillance. For clozapine the estimates of severe neutropenia rates range from 0.38% to 2.0%, with a 2018 meta-analysis of 108 publications placing the incidence at 0.9% (95% CI 0.7–1.1%) [4]. These values are sufficiently high to demand routine blood count monitoring to decrease the risk of sepsis and fatality. The success of this approach was documented in early US data obtained shortly after the US Food and Drug Administration (FDA) approval on September 26, 1989. During the years 1990–1994, 99,502 individuals were started on clozapine and placed in the Novartis-maintained US registry. Based on rates derived from pre-registry data worldwide, the use of monitoring decreased the rate of severe neutropenia by over 60%, and of related deaths by nearly 92% [5]. The 2018 meta-analysis covering clozapine-related neutropenia concludes that the risk of death related to neutropenia from clozapine use is only 0.013% [4]. It is worth noting that the 0.38% incidence of severe neutropenia from the early US sample of 99,502 patients resulted in a change in CBC monitoring for weeks 26–52 from weekly to every 14 days.

In 2015 the FDA approved new clozapine hematologic monitoring guidelines based on findings from a quarter century of clozapine experience [6]. Embedded in these changes are several important insights (Box 6.1).

 Box 6.1 Concepts Underlying New US Clozapine Guidelines

1. Clozapine therapy is associated with neutropenia but not leukopenia. No additional safety benefit is conferred by having separate thresholds for total WBC. Only ANC monitoring is necessary.

2. The minimum starting ANC threshold of 2000/mm^3 and the thresholds for increased monitoring and treatment interruption were unnecessarily high.

3. Those of African descent had markedly lower rates of clozapine utilization and continuation, in part due to the presence of BEN. Moreover, patients with BEN are at lower risk for severe neutropenia than other individuals, and can safely be started on clozapine with an ANC threshold of 1000/mm^3.

Utilizing these revised US guidelines, a retrospective analysis of hematologic outcomes from a cohort of 246 US veterans with schizophrenia treated from 1999 to 2012 was performed to explore the implications of this policy change on clozapine interruptions. No episodes of severe neutropenia were observed during the study period, but under the revised recommendations the proportion of treatment interruptions among those starting clozapine would have decreased by 80% [6].

● Benign Ethnic Neutropenia

That individuals of African descent might have lower WBC values than norms derived from Caucasians was first noted in a 1941 US paper, but it was not until 1966 that an extensive analysis of samples from healthy African Americans referred to a St. Louis hematology department led the authors to develop a concept of racial variations in WBC [7]. Importantly, the authors noted that, despite subnormal leukocyte counts, these individuals did not appear to be at risk for infection. Over the next decade the term benign ethnic neutropenia (BEN) was elaborated, and its association with variations in Duffy blood group antigens described [8].

The Duffy group was recognized in 1950 as another set of red blood cell antigens that pose a risk for transfusion reactions, with proteins also expressed in various tissues (endothelium, brain, heart, kidney and pancreas). The two forms of the Duffy antigen were designated A and B, and the respective surface markers Fya, Fyb. In 1968, the gene that controls expression of what was now known as the Duffy antigen receptor for chemokines (DARC) was located to chromosome 1 (1q21–q22), and the two allele groups FY*A and FY*B were found to differ by only a single nucleotide polymorphism (SNP) 125G>A [8]. Although it was known in 1954 that a significant proportion of those with African descent did not present either DARC surface Fy antigens [designated as Fy (a–/b–) or null/null], not until 2008 was the SNP most strongly associated with null/null status identified. This SNP, rs2814778, is a functional T46C polymorphism located in the DARC gene promoter region, with the CC genotype present among 70–75% of black people. It is only in these individuals who are [Fy (a–/b–)] that DARC proteins are not expressed, and it is only these individuals who manifest lower ANC values than norms derived from predominantly Caucasian populations. Interestingly, the absence of RBC DARC surface antigens prevents invasion by the malarial organisms *Plasmodium vivax* and *Plasmodium knowlesi* [9].

African heritage has the strongest association with BEN, but it has been reported from groups in nearby Middle Eastern areas, particularly Yemenite Jews and certain Arab populations [10]. Despite these associations, 24% of children evaluated for BEN in an academic New York hematology clinic reported ethnicities other than African or

Middle Eastern [11]. As has been shown in a number of studies, it is DARC genetics and not self-identified race that determines whether an individual has BEN [12,13]. As seen in Table 6.2, only those who have the null/null variant [Fy (a–/b–)] will manifest low ANC.

Table 6.2 ANC values by DARC genotype in a cohort of 6005 self-identified African Americans [12].

DARC (a/b) genotype	N	Mean ANC (/mm³)
–/–	4111	2459
+/–	1647	3982
+/+	247	4013

The current definition of BEN in adults is recurrent ANC less than 1500/mm³ in the absence of other secondary causes of neutropenia, such as infections, drugs, cancer, autoimmune diseases, metabolic disturbances, and hematologic disorders. Those with BEN often have an ANC that at times exceeds 1500/mm³, but 2% may have values in the range of 500–1000/mm³ [14]. Consistent with the terminology, this is a benign variant and is not associated with increased risk of infection or infection-related complications. Moreover, those with BEN have normal bone marrow morphology, and other leukocyte counts are normal [10]. Individuals of African descent also appear to be at lower risk for the development of severe neutropenia during clozapine treatment [15].

Once the BEN diagnosis is established, the individual must be registered as such so that appropriate standards for initiation and management of ANC values are applied. Prior to the creation of BEN-specific ANC criteria, many of these patients were either deemed ineligible for clozapine, or had clozapine trials terminated due to ANC values that dipped below the threshold for continuation [15]. Whether due to poor record keeping or inaccurate understanding of nomenclature, some of these patients were deemed "not rechallengeable" or were recorded as having experienced "agranulocytosis" despite ANC values ≥ 500/mm³. When the records fail to reveal ANC counts < 500/mm³ these patients must be considered as candidates for clozapine treatment. As will be discussed below, the US has modified language in clozapine package inserts that permits individuals with severe neutropenia to be rechallenged under certain circumstance (see section B, US Monitoring).

Box 6.2 Considerations in Making the BEN Diagnosis

1. *Suspect* BEN in individuals with a pattern of ANC values < 1500/mm³, particularly when one of the following have been present:

   a. Low ANC during periods when not exposed to medications associated with neutropenia (especially valproate and antipsychotics).

   b. Low ANC values despite varying classes of antipsychotics.

   c. Absence of other conditions associated with *persistent* neutropenia.

   d. African or Middle Eastern heritage is suggestive, but it can occur in those of mixed heritage.

2. *Confirming* the BEN diagnosis:

   a. In many countries a hematology consultant must see the patient and attest to the BEN diagnosis. This typically will involve genetic testing, but the consultant is responsible for establishing the diagnosis.

   b. Where a hematology consultation is not required, the gold standard is genetic testing for DARC polymorphisms. Only those who are null/null [Fy (a–/b–)] have BEN. Presence of either antigen [(Fy a+/b–) or [Fy (a–/b+)] is not associated with low ANC values and BEN.

   c. In some countries (e.g. US) a clinician who is not a hematologist (i.e. psychiatrist) may designate the individual as having BEN due to overwhelming clinical evidence (e.g. meeting all criteria 1a–1d) without genetic testing. In those circumstances it is incumbent on the clinician to eliminate all other possible causes, particularly ongoing exposure to valproate.

● **Addressing Low Baseline ANC**

In those without genetic evidence of BEN yet who do not meet the ANC threshold for starting clozapine, or for those with BEN but whose ANC at times is < 1000/mm³, other sources of neutropenia must be sought. Certain syndromes such as cyclic neutropenia are exceedingly rare (1 in 1 million persons), but autoimmune neutropenia and viral illnesses are included in the differential, along with exposure to xenobiotics in the form of medications. For many patients, medication-related neutropenia will be the primary cause of persistently low ANC. Medications other than clozapine have been associated with severe neutropenia, and a few have Level 1 evidence based on findings of a definite causal relationship (Table 6.3).

Unfortunately, the list of medications that induce milder forms of neutropenia is quite extensive, so a review of CBC records during periods of exposure to various

Table 6.3 Nonchemotherapy medications with either Level 1 (definite) or Level 2 (probable) evidence for severe neutropenia [29].

Class	Level 1 Medications (# of definite cases as of 2007)	Level 2 Medications (# of probable cases as of 2007)
Analgesic/ nonsteroidal anti-inflammatory	Aminopyrine (2), diclofenac (1), diflunisal (1), dipyrone (6), ibuprofen (1)	Acetaminophen (1), bucillamine (1), fenoprofen (1), mefenamic acid (1), naproxen (2), pentazocine (2), phenylbutazone (1), piroxicam (1), sulindac (1)
Antiarrhythmics	Disopyramide (1), procainamide (3), quinidine (3)	Ajmaline (4), amiodarone (1), aprindine (1)
Antibiotics/HIV	Ampicillin (1), carbenicillin (1), cefotaxime (1), cefuroxime (1), flucytosine (1), fusidic acid (1), imipenem-cilastatin (1), nafcillin (1), oxacillin (2), penicillin G (4), quinine (2), ticarcillin (1)	Abacavir (2), amodiaquine (10), amoxicillin-clavulanic acid (1), cefamandole (1), cefepime (2), ceftriaxone (6), cephalexin (1), cephalothin (3), cephapirin (4), cephradine (1), chloroguanide (1), clarithromycin (1), cloxacillin (1), dapsone (17), hydroxychloroquine (2), indinavir (1), isoniazid (1), mebendazole (1), nifuroxazide (1), nitrofurantoin (1), norfloxacin (1), penicillin-G procaine (1), piperacillin (1), terbinafine (5), trimethoprim-sulfamethoxazole (3), vancomycin (5), zidovudine (2)
Anticonvulsants	Phenytoin (1)	Carbamazepine (3), lamotrigine (4)
Antihelminthic	Levamisole (2)	
Antithyroid	Propylthiouracil (1)	Carbimazole (21), methimazole (55)
Cardiovascular	Clopidogrel (1), methyldopa (1), ramipril (1), spironolactone (1)	Bepridil (1), bezafibrate (1), captopril (9), metolazone (1), ticlopidine (15), vesnarinone (2)
Gastrointestinal	Cimetidine (1), metoclopramide (1)	Famotidine (3), mesalazine (1), metiamide (4), omeprazole (2), pirenzepine (2), ranitidine (4)
Immune modulator/ rheumatologic	Infliximab (1)	Gold (5), penicillamine (2), sulfasalazine (12)
Psychotropics	Chlorpromazine (2), fluoxetine (1)	Amoxapine (1), clomipramine (1), cyanamide (1), desipramine (1), dothiepin (1), doxepin (1), imipramine (1), indalpine (1), maprotiline (1), meprobamate (1), methotrimeprazine (1), mianserin (9), olanzapine (1), thioridazine (1), ziprasidone (1)

6

medications, and during periods of no treatment, can shed light on whether low ANC is a persistent issue or developed subsequent to a specific agent. Among patients with severe mental illness, the more likely offenders are other antipsychotics or anticonvulsants, especially valproic acid or divalproex. While valproate is known to induce concentration-dependent thrombocytopenia in 5–40% of patients, the reported neutropenia rate ranges from 5% to 26% [16]. Table 6.4 provides a comparison with phenytoin from a group managed in an epilepsy clinic in Utrecht.

Table 6.4 WBC and ANC counts in patients on valproate or phenytoin [16].

	Valproate	Phenytoin
WBC (/mm³)	7.94	7.85
ANC (/mm³)	4.36	5.23

Linear regression analyses of these data revealed a significant correlation between valproic acid serum concentration and the ANC ($r_p = -0.26$; $p < 0.001$) [16]. This finding has been replicated in studies examining neutropenia during clozapine treatment: use of valproate was associated with twofold increased neutropenia risk (OR 2.28, 95% CI 1.27–4.11, $p = 0.006$), with greater associations for higher valproate doses [17].

Box 6.3 Suggested Approach to those with Low Baseline ANC (< 1500/mm³ For the General Population, Or < 1000/mm³ For Those With BEN)

1. DARC genetic testing ought to be performed in any individual when there is suspicion of BEN.

2. Scour all available laboratory records for ANC values obtained during periods without exposure to medications associated with neutropenia (especially valproate and antipsychotics, but nonpsychiatric medications must also be considered).

3. If there are periods with ANC values above the clozapine initiation threshold and a pattern suggestive of drug-induced neutropenia, systematically transition the patient away from possible offending agents one at a time, allowing 4 weeks to establish new ANC values after each agent is discontinued and before another change is made.

4. If steps 1–3 do not resolve the issue, consider hematology consultation to look for other conditions associated with *persistent* neutropenia.

When the above fail to satisfactorily achieve ANC values consistently above the appropriate initiation threshold (BEN or non-BEN), then adjunctive strategies using lithium or filgrastim to support ANC counts must be considered. These are discussed below in the subsection **Managing Frequent Treatment Interruption Due to Low WBC/ANC**.

● **Time Course of Severe Neutropenia**

Data amassed from 11,555 US patients treated from February 1990 to April 1991 documented that the highest period of severe neutropenia risk occurred during the first 6 months of treatment, with a marked decline in cases reported after 12 months (Figure 6.1).

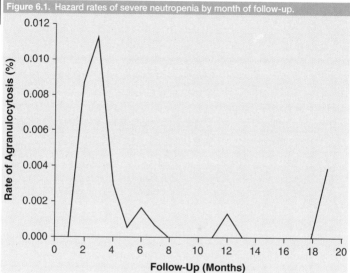

Figure 6.1. Hazard rates of severe neutropenia by month of follow-up.

(Adapted from: Alvir, J. M., Lieberman, J. A., Safferman, A. Z., et al. (1993). Clozapine-induced agranulocytosis. Incidence and risk factors in the United States. *New England Journal of Medicine*, 329, 162–167 [30].)

The cumulative 12-month rate was 0.80% (95% CI 0.61–0.99%) and the 18-month rate was 0.91% (95% CI 0.62–1.20%). These early data are nearly identical to those found in a 2018 meta-analysis of 108 studies covering clozapine-related neutropenia which calculated a severe neutropenia incidence of 0.9% (95% CI 0.7–1.1%) [4]. The peak incidence of severe neutropenia occurs at 1 month of exposure and declines to negligible levels after 1 year of treatment. Consistent with these data, routine monitoring schemes mandate higher frequency during the first

4–6 months of treatment (weekly), decreasing to every 2 weeks for the remainder of the first year of treatment, and monthly after week 52. Due to case reports of severe neutropenia occurring after years of clozapine exposure, monthly monitoring continues indefinitely. When patients have extended treatment interruptions, or interruption due to CBC abnormalities, the clock may be "reset" to a higher monitoring frequency as mandated by local guidelines (see discussion below).

The unpredictable timing of severe neutropenia episodes has not precluded manufacturers from including warnings about "downward trends," "single drops" or "substantial drops" in total WBC and/or ANC for the past two decades. The recently updated US prescribing guidelines have removed all mention of trend data or drops as these changes did not prove predictive of severe neutropenia events and resulted in unnecessary concern and additional monitoring. Nonetheless, these are still commonly found worldwide, and clinicians must be mindful of the necessary response to these events. For example, the 2015 UK Zaponex® Treatment Access System manual states:

> If a Single Drop or Downward Trend is detected in a patient's blood result history and the WBC count value falls below 7.0×10^9/l, a Single Drop/ Downward Trend Warning will be faxed to the patient's healthcare providers. The consultant is then advised by ZTAS to assess the patient's general health and determine whether or not an increase of the monitoring frequency to twice weekly is necessary until the blood results have stabilized.

Associations between older age and female gender appeared during the early analysis of severe neutropenia cases, but none of these are significant enough to alter routine monitoring schemes, and recent data have cast doubt on the gender association [18]. Certain genetic polymorphisms have been associated with clozapine-induced severe neutropenia, especially the human leukocyte antigen (HLA) markers HLA-DQB1 and HLA-B [19]. The largest genetic study to date examined 66 severe neutropenia cases and 5583 clozapine-treated controls, and then combined their results with findings from the Clozapine-Induced Agranulocytosis Consortium (163 cases and 7970 controls) [20]. In addition to replicating the previously identified variant in HLA-DQB1 (OR = 15.6, $p = 0.015$, positive predictive value = 35.1%), this analysis found an association with a SNP (rs149104283) located on the intron of hepatic transporter genes (OR = 4.32, $p = 1.79 \times 10^{-8}$), loci previously implicated in simvastatin-induced myopathy and docetaxel-induced neutropenia. Two other markers of interest were also identified. At the present time, the presence of these genetic markers is not robust enough to alter monitoring frequency or preclude initiating clozapine treatment.

While demographic and genetic risk factors are neither modifiable nor actionable, the ongoing use of valproate preparations has been confirmed as a risk factor for forms of neutropenia that lead to discontinuation of clozapine treatment. Clinical records of 136 patients who discontinued clozapine due to a neutropenic event were matched 1:1 with clozapine-treated controls by duration of treatment. In the multivariable analysis, the concurrent use of valproate doubled the risk of discontinuation due to neutropenia (OR 2.28, 95% CI 1.27–4.11, $p = 0.006$), and this risk was positively correlated with higher valproate dose [17]. Although the purpose of this analysis was not to specifically examine severe neutropenia cases, it highlights concerns about valproate-induced neutropenia, especially for those exposed to higher doses and serum levels [16]. While valproate or divalproex are the medications of choice for clozapine-associated seizure phenomena (see Chapter 10), alternative mood stabilizers, particularly lithium, need to be considered when starting clozapine, especially for patients whose ANC values might hover slightly above the threshold for treatment interruption or increased monitoring frequency.

● Hypothesized Mechanism for Neutropenia

Despite multiple *in vivo* and *in vitro* studies, the exact mechanism of clozapine-associated severe neutropenia has not been definitively identified, although immune hypotheses carry greater weight than those centering on direct bone marrow toxicity [21]. Different mechanisms might underlie milder forms of neutropenia seen during clozapine therapy [22], but the significant association with certain HLA haplotypes combined with *in vitro* assay results from patients who have experienced severe neutropenia point strongly to an immune basis for severe neutropenia. It is for this reason that patients who developed severe neutropenia during clozapine treatment were not to be rechallenged, and this precept is generally applied in most countries. Two recent developments have modified this position: (a) Revised US prescribing guidelines now state that, in patients who have had severe neutropenia: "For some patients who experience severe CLOZARIL related neutropenia, the risk of serious psychiatric illness from discontinuing CLOZARIL treatment may be greater than the risk of rechallenge (e.g., patients with severe schizophrenic illness who have no treatment options other than CLOZARIL). A hematology consultation may be useful in deciding to rechallenge a patient. In general, however, do not rechallenge patients who develop severe neutropenia with CLOZARIL or a clozapine product." (b) There is now a literature comprising 30 cases (as of 2017) in which patients with a history of neutropenia were rechallenged with clozapine while simultaneously receiving filgrastim to stimulate neutrophil production. After a median follow-up of 12 months, 76% of cases were able to continue clozapine (see section below, Rechallenging Severe Neutropenia Patients and Filgrastim Support).

Basic Hematologic Monitoring Guidelines and Response

● US Monitoring

As noted previously, the recently revised US monitoring guidelines differ from others worldwide in several major areas: the use of ANC only without total WBC; lower thresholds for starting clozapine for general population and BEN patients; removal of language about responding to sudden drops or other changes in ANC values aside from changes in ANC levels that coincide with degrees of neutropenia; removal of guidelines for platelet or eosinophil counts. Tables 6.5 and 6.6 present treatment recommendations based on ANC levels for the general patient population and BEN patients, respectively.

Table 6.5 US treatment recommendations based on ANC monitoring for the general patient population.

ANC level	Treatment recommendations	ANC monitoring
Normal range (≥ 1500/mm³)	• Initiate treatment • If treatment interrupted for < 30 days, continue monitoring as before • If treatment interrupted for ≥ 30 days, monitor as if new patient	• Weekly from initiation to 6 months • Every 2 weeks from 6 to 12 months • Monthly after 12 months
Mild neutropenia* (1000–1499/mm³)	• Continue treatment	• Three times weekly until ANC ≥ 1500/mm³ • Once ANC ≥ 1500/mm³, return to patient's last "normal range" ANC monitoring interval**
Moderate neutropenia* (500–999/mm³)	• Interrupt treatment for suspected clozapine-induced neutropenia • Recommend hematology consultation	• Daily ANC until ≥ 1000/mm³ **THEN** • Three times weekly until ANC ≥ 1500/mm³ • Once ANC ≥ 1500/mm³, check ANC weekly for 4 weeks, then return to patient's last "normal range" ANC monitoring interval**

continued overleaf

Table 6.5 continued

ANC level	Treatment recommendations	ANC monitoring
Severe neutropenia* (< 500/mm³)	• Interrupt treatment for suspected clozapine-induced neutropenia • Recommend hematology consultation • Do not rechallenge *unless prescriber determines benefits outweigh risks*	• Daily ANC until ≥ 1000/mm³ **THEN** • Three times weekly until ANC ≥ 1500/mm³ • If patient is rechallenged, resume treatment as a new patient under "normal range" monitoring once ANC ≥ 1500/mm³

* Confirm all initial reports of ANC < 1500/mm³ with a repeat ANC measurement within 24 hours.
** If clinically appropriate.

Table 6.6 US treatment recommendations based on ANC monitoring for patients with benign ethnic neutropenia.

ANC level	Treatment recommendations	ANC monitoring
Normal BEN range (established ANC baseline ≥ 1000/mm³)	• Obtain at least two baseline ANC levels before initiating treatment • If treatment interrupted for < 30 days, continue monitoring as before • If treatment interrupted for ≥ 30 days, monitor as if new patient	• Weekly from initiation to 6 months • Every 2 weeks from 6 to 12 months • Monthly after 12 months
BEN neutropenia* (500–999/mm³)	• Continue treatment • Recommend hematology consultation	• Three times weekly until ANC ≥ 1000/mm³ or ≥ patient's known baseline • Once ANC ≥ 1000/mm³, or is above the patient's known baseline, check the ANC weekly for 4 weeks, then return to patient's last "normal BEN range" ANC monitoring interval**
BEN severe neutropenia* (< 500/mm³)	• Interrupt treatment for suspected clozapine-induced neutropenia • Recommend hematology consultation • Do not rechallenge *unless prescriber determines benefits outweigh risks*	• Daily ANC until ≥ 500/mm³ **THEN** • Three times weekly until ANC ≥ patient's baseline • If patient is rechallenged, resume treatment as a new patient under "normal BEN range" monitoring once ANC ≥ 1000/mm³ or at patient's baseline

* The package insert recommends confirming all initial reports of ANC < 1500/mm³ with a repeat ANC measurement within 24 hours for the general patient population. For BEN patients, values < 1000/mm³ should be confirmed with a repeat ANC measurement within 24 hours.
** If clinically appropriate.

127

The US guidelines do not contain specific information about responding to late results, but failure to obtain ANC values at the designated interval prevents pharmacies from dispensing the next scheduled quantity of clozapine. If treatment is interrupted for 2–29 days or more, the patient must be titrated to the prior tolerated dose starting at no more than 12.5 mg BID the first day. No guidance is provided on the rapidity of titration, but shorter interruptions might allow very rapid resumption of the prior dose, while those of 2–4 weeks might require more gradual increases as the patient may have lost tolerance to the sedating and orthostatic properties of clozapine. Interruptions of 30 days or more necessitate treating the patient as a new start, with weekly ANC monitoring for the first 6 months.

● UK Monitoring

The UK monitoring scheme uses both total WBC and ANC values, and this is typical of most countries worldwide. Tables are provided for initiation (Table 6.7), and routine monitoring once on treatment (Table 6.8). The UK also has separate thresholds for those identified as having BEN (Table 6.9). To simplify clinical decisions, results are

Table 6.7 UK reference values for new patients or those who experience an interruption in treatment.

Blood counts × 10⁹/l	Classification	Action
WBC ≥ 4.0 AND neutrophils ≥ 2.5	Green	• Treatment may be initiated at the discretion of the treating consultant • Clozapine may be prescribed and dispensed for 7 days
WBC ≥ 3.5 and < 4.0 AND/OR neutrophils ≥ 2.0 and < 2.5	Amber	• Treatment with clozapine may be initiated when the treating consultant considers the patient eligible • Additional blood sampling is advised to ensure blood counts are not dropping
WBC ≥ 3.0 and < 3.5 AND/OR neutrophils ≥ 1.5 and < 2.0	Amber	• The blood result is not valid to initiate clozapine treatment • Additional blood sampling is required • Treatment may only be initiated on a Green result or intermediate Amber as described above
WBC < 3.0 AND/OR neutrophils < 1.5	Red	• The blood result is not valid to initiate clozapine treatment • Investigate the cause of the abnormal blood result

Table 6.8 UK reference values for routine results.

Blood counts × 10⁹/l	Classification	Action
WBC ≥ 3.5 AND neutrophils ≥ 2.0	Green	• Continue clozapine treatment
WBC ≥ 3.0 and < 3.5 AND/OR neutrophils ≥ 1.5 and < 2.0	Amber	• Increase monitoring frequency (twice-weekly) until results have stabilized in the Green range • Assess the clinical status of the patient
WBC < 3.0 AND/OR neutrophils < 1.5	Red	• Stop clozapine treatment immediately • Daily blood tests until results are in the Green range • Additional Red alert procedures (immediate clinical evaluation for infection, retrieving patient's clozapine supply, consultation with hematologist) • Patient is not rechallengeable and their details are placed into the Central Non-Rechallengeable Database (CNRD)

Table 6.9 UK reference values for patients with benign ethnic neutropenia.

Blood counts × 10⁹/l	Classification	Action
WBC ≥ 3.0 AND neutrophils ≥ 1.5	Green	• Continue clozapine treatment
WBC ≥ 2.5 and < 3.0 AND/OR neutrophils ≥ 1.0 and < 1.5	Amber	• Increase monitoring frequency (twice-weekly) until results have stabilized in the Green range • Assess the clinical status of the patient
WBC < 2.5 AND/OR neutrophils < 1.0	Red	• Stop clozapine treatment immediately • Daily blood tests until results are in the Green range • Additional Red alert procedures (immediate clinical evaluation for infection, retrieving patient's clozapine supply, consultation with hematologist) • Patient is not rechallengeable and their details are placed into the Central Non-Rechallengeable Database (CNRD)

Table 6.10 UK follow-up actions for missing results.

A blood test result is not in the system	Action
At the "expected next test date"	• The late flag **L** is displayed with the patient's record until a new blood result has been entered.
7 days after the expected test date	• Courtesy reminder – Late Results is sent to health-care providers. • For weekly and fortnightly monitored patients the previous result is no longer valid for dispensing clozapine to the patient. • The registry may contact health-care providers by telephone to discuss missing follow-up information and/or change the patient status to Interrupted.
14–28 days after the expected test date	• Additional weekly Reminders – Late Results are sent to health-care providers. • The previous result is no longer valid for dispensing clozapine to the patient. • The registry contacts health-care providers by telephone to discuss missing follow-up information. • Change of patient status to Interrupted.

Table 6.11 UK monitoring frequency after treatment break.

Monitoring frequency	Duration of treatment break	Monitoring frequency after treatment break
Weekly	≤ 3 days	Weekly, continue 18 weeks period
Weekly	> 3 days but ≤ 1 week	Weekly, continuing the 18 weeks period; patient must have at least 6 weeks of weekly monitoring prior to a decrease of the monitoring frequency to fortnightly
Weekly	> 1 week	Weekly, restart 18 weeks period
Fortnightly	≤ 3 days	Fortnightly, continue
Fortnightly	> 3 days but ≤ 4 weeks	Weekly monitoring for 6 weeks, then continue fortnightly
Fortnightly	> 4 weeks	Weekly, restart 18 weeks period
Monthly	≤ 3 days	4-Weekly, continue
Monthly	> 3 days but ≤ 4 weeks	Weekly monitoring for 6 weeks, then continue 4-weekly
Monthly	> 4 weeks	Weekly, restart 18 weeks period, after 18 weeks, switch to 4-weekly

classified in a color-coded manner as Green, Amber or Red as noted in Tables 6.7–6.9. UK guidelines specify certain responses for late or missing CBC results (Table 6.10) and provide detailed instructions on the CBC monitoring frequency after treatment interruptions (Table 6.11).

● Eosinophilia and Thrombocytopenia

As will be discussed in Chapter 12 there is concern about eosinophilia due to the association with myocarditis; moreover, eosinophilia may also occur as part of other drug hypersensitivity syndromes. As noted in Table 6.12, the UK has specific guidance about increasing the monitoring frequency to twice-weekly for high eosinophil counts (> 3000/mm³) or for low platelet counts (< 50 K). (The occurrence of eosinophilia, thrombocytopenia, thrombocytosis and leukocytosis will be discussed in Chapter 14.)

Table 6.12 UK reference ranges for eosinophils and platelets.

	Value	Action
High eosinophils	> 1000/mm³ – pretreatment > 3000/mm³ – on-treatment	Initiation/continuation of clozapine treatment is not recommended
		Increase monitoring frequency
		Clozapine therapy should be started only after blood results have stabilized under 1000/mm³
Low platelets	< 50 K	Initiation/continuation of clozapine treatment is not recommended
		Increase monitoring frequency
		Clozapine therapy should be started only after blood results have stabilized at or above 50 K

C Managing Frequent Treatment Interruption Due to Low WBC/ANC

The need to increase monitoring frequency or interrupt clozapine treatment imposes an enormous burden on clinicians and patients, and increases the risk that the patient may refuse to continue with treatment. Even with the lower US BEN thresholds, there are subsets of patients with BEN whose routine ANC naturally dips below 1000/mm³ and thus must be subjected to ANC checks three times per week until their values return to 1000/mm³ or above. In patients where removal of offending medications, especially valproate, and even hematology consultation has failed to find a reversible cause for ANC/WBC values that trigger increased monitoring or interruption, there are two off-label strategies documented in the literature to increase ANC values: lithium and filgrastim.

Box 6.4 Considerations in Using Lithium Augmentation for Low ANC/WBC

1. **Goal:** The goal of lithium therapy is to completely prevent low ANC/WBC values that trigger increased monitoring frequency or interruption.

2. **Eligible patients:** Indefinite use of lithium at full therapeutic serum levels might be needed to achieve the desired goal, so only patients who do not possess medical contraindications to long-term lithium use are candidates. This analysis involves consideration of estimated glomerular filtration rate (eGFR) and other medical issues. Certain medications that present unique hazards during lithium treatment (hydrochlorothiazide, lisinopril) will also have to be changed to alternative agents. The typical lithium monitoring requirements must be performed at a minimum every 6 months including (but not limited to): lithium levels, thyroid stimulating hormone, eGFR and serum calcium. (For further details on lithium prescribing see [31].)

3. **Dosing and adjustment:** Regardless of indication, lithium has a 24-hour brain half-life and should only be prescribed once per day, typically at bedtime. Importantly, use of lithium more than once per day significantly increases the risk of renal insufficiency [32]. Because the hematopoietic effect may take 2–3 weeks, there is no need for aggressive early dosing, especially where the tolerability of lithium is unknown. In some instances 300 mg QHS may achieve satisfactory results, but higher doses are commonly employed. Trough serum levels are obtained 1 week after each dosage change and a repeat CBC approximately 3 weeks after each dosage change. There is no nomogram to calculate lithium requirements based on nadir ANC values, but the failure to achieve the goal as stated above must prompt further dose increases up to a maximum serum level 1.0 meq/l (1.0 mmol/l). No greater hematopoietic effect is seen for higher serum levels.

While the association between lithium and granulocytosis has been recognized for decades, it was not proven until 1978 that lithium-induced granulocytosis is not merely a redistribution of neutrophils that are marginated or are in bone marrow reserves [23]. Lithium enhances the production of granulocyte colony-stimulating factor (G-CSF), and directly stimulates the proliferation of pluripotential stem cells [23]. During lithium exposure there are significant increases in bone

1. **Goal:** The goal of filgrastim therapy is to completely prevent low ANC/WBC values that trigger increased monitoring frequency or interruption.

2. **Eligible patients:** The only contraindication to the use of filgrastim is a history of serious allergic reactions to human granulocyte colony-stimulating factors such as filgrastim or pegfilgrastim. Consultation with a hematologist might be necessary to prescribe filgrastim, and local regulations might vary on who can prescribe filgrastim depending on inpatient vs. outpatient status.

3. **Dosing and adjustment:** The hematopoietic effect of filgrastim is seen within 24–48 hours, but the duration of effect is quite variable between patients. Filgrastim is available in vials or prefilled syringes containing 300 or 480 µg. A test dose of 300 µg subcutaneously is typically given and the ANC values tracked 2 times per week for the next 2 weeks and then weekly through week 4 to determine whether the ANC remains above the necessary thresholds, and that ANC values do not stay above 10,000/mm^3 for excessive periods. There is no nomogram to calculate filgrastim requirements based on nadir ANC values, but the failure to achieve the goal as stated above must prompt further dose increases. In some instances the literature reports thrice weekly doses of 300 µg might be necessary to achieve ANC/WBC values that do not fall below triggering thresholds, but dosing for some patients might be weekly [25]. Filgrastim must not be given when ANC values exceed 10,000/mm^3.

marrow colony-forming units and bone marrow organ cellularity. This effect occurs reproducibly in animal and human studies, and exhibits a dose dependency within the serum range of 0.30–1.0 meq/l (0.30–1.0 mmol/l) [23]. Higher serum levels in animal models did not generate greater effects, and very high levels that would be toxic in humans (5.0 meq/l or 5.0 mmol/l) cause bone marrow toxicity. At therapeutic doses of 900–1200 mg/day, the mean increase in ANC averaged 88% in one small trial, and the effect was seen in the first week after lithium was initiated, although peak ANC values may not occur until week 2 or 3 [24].

In patients who cannot take lithium or for whom lithium's effect is insufficient to prevent low ANC/WBC values that trigger increased monitoring frequency or treatment interruption, the recombinant granulocyte colony-stimulating factor filgrastim must be used. While the use of filgrastim has long been considered a standard part of severe neutropenia management, only since 1998 have there been cases of extended use to support patients with varying levels of clozapine-associated neutropenia [25]. Weekly exposures of up to 4 years have been documented without complications. Nonetheless, the package insert contains warnings about a number of potentially serious and fatal adverse effects that clinicians must be aware, of including: allergic reactions, splenic rupture, acute respiratory distress syndrome, exacerbation of sickle cell disorders, glomerulonephritis, alveolar hemorrhage and hemoptysis, capillary leak syndrome, thrombocytopenia, cutaneous vasculitis and leukocytosis.

 Response to Severe Neutropenia

Severe neutropenia (referred to in older literature as agranulocytosis) occurs when ANC values are $< 500/mm^3$. This represents a medical emergency due to the risk of sepsis, and must be managed appropriately from both the hematologic and psychiatric perspectives. Nonetheless, with modern monitoring schemes and treatment, the incidence of death related to neutropenia during clozapine use is estimated to be 0.013% (95% CI 0.01–0.017%) [4]. Importantly, the case fatality rate for severe neutropenia once diagnosed is only 2.1% (95% CI 1.6–2.8%) [4].

There are three primary considerations when severe neutropenia occurs: minimization of infection risk, management of cholinergic rebound from abrupt discontinuation of clozapine, and provision of appropriate antipsychotic therapy based on the patient's history of response (even if limited) and tolerability. (Chapter 4 provides an extensive discussion of strategies for managing cholinergic rebound, and considerations for antipsychotic therapy after clozapine discontinuation.)

● **Rechallenging Severe Neutropenia Patients With Filgrastim Support**

For patients who have demonstrably failed other antipsychotics, the removal of clozapine treatment implies a lifetime of unremitting psychosis, suicidality, aggression, or intolerable adverse effects. In this context, the revised US prescribing guidelines acknowledge this reality, and contain a statement quoted previously, but which is worth reiterating:

> For some patients who experience severe CLOZARIL related neutropenia, the risk of serious psychiatric illness from discontinuing CLOZARIL treatment may be greater than the risk of rechallenge (e.g., patients with severe schizophrenic illness who have no treatment options other than CLOZARIL).

Box 6.6 Response to Severe Neutropenia

Minimization of infection risk: The median duration of severe neutropenia from clozapine is 12 days, and at times may extend to 21 days, so patients may be at extended risk for infection and related complications [29]. For all patients, the following steps are important.

1. **Patient notification:** If outpatient, immediately contact the individual and have them transported to the clinic (or emergency department if after hours) for physical examination and repeat CBC. All supplies of clozapine must be removed from their control and they must be informed that their use of clozapine must be abruptly stopped. Until the ANC is safely above 500/mm^3 all severe neutropenia patients require close clinical surveillance to monitor for signs of infection and daily blood monitoring. For most outpatients this is best accomplished through hospital admission, with possible use of isolation precautions, and oversight by a hematologist. Inpatients on a psychiatric unit may best be served by transfer to a medical unit to minimize contact with large numbers of other people that can present a source of transmissible infection, and also to remove a source of risk due to acts of aggression by other patients (e.g. scratching, biting). The hematologist will also help manage any fever work-up and infectious complications should they occur.

2. **Use of filgrastim:** An extensive review of the literature on neutropenia not related to chemotherapy noted that the use of filgrastim at a mean dose of 300 μg is useful in shortening the duration of ANC recovery time without inducing any major adverse effects [33]. For more prolonged episodes of severe neutropenia repeated doses may be used at the discretion of the treating hematologist.

In addition to hematology consultation, extensive discussions with the patient, caregivers, family and possibly ethicists ought to be considered as part of the decision to rechallenge an individual who has previously experienced severe neutropenia. In some instances, another cause of neutropenia was identified (e.g. use of ribavirin as part of a hepatitis C treatment regimen in a patient on clozapine for 5 years), and the causal link to clozapine lessened. Nonetheless, all parties involved must understand the risks and what is at stake, including the fact that very frequent CBC monitoring (2–3 times per week) may continue for an extended period of time before a more routine schedule can be considered.

When the benefits of rechallenge are deemed to outweigh the risks, the literature now supports the use of filgrastim when clozapine is commenced. This will generally be performed in conjunction with a hematologist, and a prespecified CBC monitoring plan created to ensure that ANC counts remain above thresholds for treatment interruption or discontinuation, or do not persistently exceed 10,000/mm^3 due to the effects of filgrastim. A 2017 review documented 30 cases of extended filgrastim treatment in patients with varying levels of clozapine-associated neutropenia at doses ranging from 300 μg once weekly up to 300 μg three times per week [25]. Given the immune hypothesis for severe neutropenia, one must anticipate that the use of filgrastim may need to continue indefinitely, yet there is at least one published case in which filgrastim was able to be tapered off after many months [26].

 ## Use of Point-of-Care CBC Monitoring

Another option is the use of point-of-care (POC) blood monitoring devices in the psychiatric clinic or deployed to the patient's residence, obviating the need for a laboratory visit [27, 28]. As of 2019 there is one POC CBC device in the US (www.athelas.com). This device was approved only after rigorous testing at multiple sites and in multiple patient types (i.e. normal, medical conditions) had demonstrated coefficients of variation for ANC and WBC values equivalent to that from an automated hematology analyzer. The device can be operated by personnel in point of care settings, thereby providing maximum flexibility in the time and place of ANC testing. This device also uses a small 28 gauge lancet to obtain results from a finger-prick, a feature rated as being less painful than venipuncture. The results are available in 6 minutes, and the manufacturer has created an integrated network so that results are simultaneously transmitted to the clozapine monitoring registry, the prescriber and the pharmacy. If ANC results are within range, the pharmacy delivers medication directly to the patient within 24 hours. The Athelas device will likely be followed by approval of other POC devices, and the increasing adoption of this new technology, and its integrated system, will become commonplace due to the convenience of testing, rapidity of results, and decreased patient discomfort.

Summary Points

a. Monitoring and patient registry details vary considerably between countries, and are occasionally updated, so clinicians must be attentive to local regulations and developments.

b. Valproate is associated with neutropenia in a dose-dependent manner, and may interfere with treatment initiation or continuation.

c. Benign ethnic neutropenia is now recognized in many countries, and must be identified. Genetic testing for DARC null/null status (Fy (a–/b–)) is confirmatory.

d. Clinicians need to be expert at the use of lithium to forestall repeated increased monitoring or treatment interruption, and understand the literature on use of filgrastim.

e. Management of severe neutropenia requires minimization of infection risk, prevention of cholinergic rebound, and provision of antipsychotic therapy.

f. While patients with clozapine-induced severe neutropenia have been deemed not rechallengeable, updated US regulations now acknowledge that for select patients the benefits might outweigh the risks. Hematology consultation and use of filgrastim are important parts of this process.

6

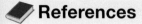

References

1. Curtis, B. R. (2017). Non-chemotherapy drug-induced neutropenia: Key points to manage the challenges. *ASH Hematology, The Education Program*, 2017, 187–193.

2. Amsler, H. A., Teerenhovi, L., Barth, E., et al. (1977). Agranulocytosis in patients treated with clozapine. A study of the Finnish epidemic. *Acta Psychiatrica Scandinavica*, 56, 241–248.

3. Nielsen, J., Young, C., Ifteni, P., et al. (2016). Worldwide differences in regulations of clozapine use. *CNS Drugs*, 30, 149–161.

4. Myles, N., Myles, H., Xia, S., et al. (2018). Meta-analysis examining the epidemiology of clozapine-associated neutropenia. *Acta Psychiatrica Scandinavica*, 138, 101–109.

5. Honigfeld, G., Arellano, F., Sethi, J., et al. (1998). Reducing clozapine-related morbidity and mortality: 5 years of experience with the Clozaril National Registry. *Journal of Clinical Psychiatry*, 59(Suppl 3), 3–7.

6. Sultan, R. S., Olfson, M., Correll, C. U., et al. (2017). Evaluating the effect of the changes in FDA guidelines for clozapine monitoring. *Journal of Clinical Psychiatry*, 78, e933–e939.

7. Broun, G. O., Herbig, F. K. and Hamilton, J. R. (1966). Leukopenia in Negroes. *New England Journal of Medicine*, 275, 1410–1413.

8. Paz, E., Bouzas, L., Hermida, J., et al. (2008). Evaluation of three dosing models for the prediction of steady-state trough clozapine concentrations. *Clinical Biochemistry*, 41, 603–606.

9. Schmid, P., Ravenell, K. R., Sheldon, S. L., et al. (2012). DARC alleles and Duffy phenotypes in African Americans. *Transfusion*, 52, 1260–1267.

10. Paz, Z., Nails, M. and Ziv, E. (2011). The genetics of benign neutropenia. *Israel Medical Association Journal*, 13, 625–629.

11. Ortiz, M. V., Meier, E. R. and Hsieh, M. M. (2016). Identification and clinical characterization of children with benign ethnic neutropenia. *Journal of Pediatric Hematology and Oncology*, 38, e140–143.

12. Reich, D., Nalls, M. A., Kao, W. H., et al. (2009). Reduced neutrophil count in people of African descent is due to a regulatory variant in the Duffy antigen receptor for chemokines gene. *PLoS Genetics*, 5, e1000360.

13. Dinardo, C. L., Kerbauy, M. N., Santos, T. C., et al. (2017). Duffy null genotype or Fy(a–b–) phenotype are more accurate than self-declared race for diagnosing benign ethnic neutropenia in Brazilian population. *International Journal of Laboratory Hematology*, 39, e144–e146.

14. Denic, S., Showqi, S., Klein, C., et al. (2009). Prevalence, phenotype and inheritance of benign neutropenia in Arabs. *BMC Blood Disorders*, 9, 3.

15. Kelly, D. L., Kreyenbuhl, J., Dixon, L., et al. (2007). Clozapine underutilization and discontinuation in African Americans due to leucopenia. *Schizophrenia Bulletin*, 33, 1221–1224.

16. Bartels, M., van Solinge, W. W., den Breeijen, H. J., et al. (2012). Valproic acid treatment is associated with altered leukocyte subset development. *Journal of Clinical Psychopharmacology*, 32, 832–834.

17. Malik, S., Lally, J., Ajnakina, O., et al. (2018). Sodium valproate and clozapine induced neutropenia: A case control study using register data. *Schizophrenia Research*, 195, 267–273.

18. Demler, T. L., Morabito, N. E., Meyer, C. E., et al. (2016). Maximizing clozapine utilization while minimizing blood dyscrasias: Evaluation of patient demographics and severity of events. *International Clinical Psychopharmacology*, 31, 76–83.

19. Goldstein, J. I., Jarskog, L. F., Hilliard, C., et al. (2014). Clozapine-induced agranulocytosis is associated with rare HLA-DQB1 and HLA-B alleles. *Nature Communications*, 5, 4757.

20. Legge, S. E., Hamshere, M. L., Ripke, S., et al. (2017). Genome-wide common and rare variant analysis provides novel insights into clozapine-associated neutropenia. *Molecular Psychiatry*, 22, 1502–1508.

21. Regen, F., Herzog, I., Hahn, E., et al. (2017). Clozapine-induced agranulocytosis: evidence for an immune-mediated mechanism from a patient-specific in-vitro approach. *Toxicology and Applied Pharmacology*, 316, 10–16.

22. Wicinski, M. and Weclewicz, M. M. (2018). Clozapine-induced agranulocytosis/granulocytopenia: Mechanisms and monitoring. *Current Opinion in Hematology*, 25, 22–28.

23. Focosi, D., Azzara, A., Kast, R. E., et al. (2009). Lithium and hematology: Established and proposed uses. *Journal of Leukocyte Biology*, 85, 20–28.

24. Ballin, A., Lehman, D., Sirota, P., et al. (1998). Increased number of peripheral blood CD34+ cells in lithium-treated patients. *British Journal of Haematology*, 100, 219–221.

25. Myles, N., Myles, H., Clark, S. R., et al. (2017). Use of granulocyte-colony stimulating factor to prevent recurrent clozapine-induced neutropenia on drug rechallenge: A systematic review of the literature and clinical recommendations. *Australian & New Zealand Journal of Psychiatry*, 51, 980–989.

26. Gopalakrishnan, R., Subhalakshmi, T. P., Kuruvilla, A., et al. (2013). Clozapine re-challenge under the cover of filgrastim. *Journal of Postgraduate Medicine*, 59, 54–55.

27. Kelly, D. L., Ben-Yoav, H., Payne, G. F., et al. (2018). Blood draw barriers for treatment with clozapine and development of point-of-care monitoring device. *Clinical Schizophrenia & Related Psychoses*, 12, 23–30.

28. Bui, H. N., Bogers, J. P., Cohen, D., et al. (2016). Evaluation of the performance of a point-of-care method for total and differential white blood cell count in clozapine users. *International Journal of Laboratory Hematology*, 38, 703–709.

29. Andersohn, F., Konzen, C. and Garbe, E. (2007). Systematic review: Agranulocytosis induced by nonchemotherapy drugs. *Annals of Internal Medicine*, 146, 657–665.

30. Alvir, J. M., Lieberman, J. A., Safferman, A. Z., et al. (1993). Clozapine-induced agranulocytosis. Incidence and risk factors in the United States. *New England Journal of Medicine*, 329, 162–167.

31. Meyer, J. M. (2018). Pharmacotherapy of psychosis and mania. In L. L. Brunton, R. Hilal-Dandan and B. C. Knollmann (Eds.), *Goodman & Gilman's The Pharmacological Basis of Therapeutics*, 13th Edition (pp. 279–302). Chicago, IL: McGraw-Hill.

32. Castro, V. M., Roberson, A. M., McCoy, T. H., et al. (2016). Stratifying risk for renal insufficiency among lithium-treated patients: An electronic health record study. *Neuropsychopharmacology*, 41, 1138–1143.

33. Andres, E. and Mourot-Cottet, R. (2017). Clozapine-associated neutropenia and agranulocytosis. *Journal of Clinical Psychopharmacology*, 37, 749–750.

6

7 Managing Constipation

INTRODUCTION

Constipation is a common problem in western societies, but gastrointestinal hypomotility (GIH) assumes greater significance during clozapine therapy for several reasons: GIH is highly prevalent; GIH accounts for 36% of all medically related causes of treatment discontinuation [1]; and in its most severe form, paralytic ileus, there is a fatality rate of 15.0–27.5% [2]. Gastrointestinal illness accounted for 20% of all medically related hospital admissions for clozapine-treated patients at one major US medical center, of which 61% were for hypomotility-related problems [3]. The magnitude of clozapine's effect on motility is dramatic: the median colonic transit time (CTT) in one study was 23 hours among inpatients on nonclozapine antipsychotics, compared to 104 hours for those on clozapine [4]. Moreover, 80% of the clozapine-treated patients had

PRINCIPLES

- Due to high rates of gastrointestinal hypomotility, including constipation and ileus, other strongly anticholinergic medications, or medications that induce constipation by other mechanisms (e.g. opioids, iron supplements) should be avoided if at all possible in clozapine-treated patients.

- The reported fatality rates from ileus of 15.0–27.5% are far greater than those seen with severe neutropenia (2.2–4.2%).

- Medications for constipation must commence with the first prescription for clozapine, initially starting with docusate, then polyethylene glycol (PEG)-3350 and a stimulant added in succession.

- Bulk laxatives (e.g. psyllium preparations) are not to be used in clozapine-treated patients as very slow colonic transit times present a risk of inspissation and exacerbation of constipation.

- For individuals who fail to respond to a combination of the three first-line agents (docusate + PEG-3350 + stimulant), including those who have experienced ileus, there is extensive experience in certain hospital systems with secretogogues such as lubiprostone, and two cases of successful use of the motility agent prucalopride (available in the US since 2018).

evidence of GIH, and transit times in all colonic segments were abnormal. Importantly, clozapine-associated GIH occurred irrespective of gender, age, ethnicity, or length of clozapine treatment [4]. Only plasma clozapine level correlated with GIH severity as measured by transit time.

While neutropenia has extensive warnings and mandated monitoring protocols, mitigation of GIH must garner significant clinical attention, and treatment must start at the onset of clozapine titration. Clozapine discontinuation due to GIH or the development of ileus need to be viewed as preventable outcomes. With careful monitoring, aggressive use of inexpensive first-line agents, removal of other offending medications, and use of newer intestinal secretogogues (e.g. lubiprostone, linaclotide, plecanatide), or the motility medication prucalopride, clinicians have a number of management strategies available to address this prevalent problem.

Prevalence and Postulated Mechanisms

Based on a variety of clinical criteria the reported incidence of constipation for clozapine-treated patients ranges from 32% to 60%. The use of colonic transit time (CTT) provides a quantitative framework for understanding clozapine's impact on gastrointestinal motility. International data reveal a mean adult CTT of 28.79 ($\pm$ 18.07) hours [4]. By defining GIH as CTT more than 2 SD above the population mean, or $\geq$ 65 hours, 80% of clozapine-treated patients in a CTT study met criteria for GIH. In a Danish study of 26,597 schizophrenia patients treated from 1996 to 2007, the use of clozapine for schizophrenia was associated with a twofold increased risk for ileus (OR 1.99, 95% CI 1.21–3.29), and a sevenfold increased risk for fatal ileus (OR 6.73, 95% CI 1.55–29.17) [5]. While constipation begins early in clozapine treatment, the Danish data highlighted the fact that ileus tends to occur after more prolonged exposure and in a dose-dependent manner. Among the 123 clozapine-related ileus cases, the median time to developing ileus was 1528 days (interquartile range 1145–2039 days), and the odds ratio increased by a factor of 1.33 (95% CI 1.15–1.54) for each 100 mg of clozapine prescribed ($p < 0.0001$) [5].

Multiple mechanisms contribute to clozapine's high incidence of constipation. Despite norclozapine's muscarinic agonism, clozapine is a potent muscarinic antagonist across several receptor subtypes, and this appears to override the effect of norclozapine on GI motility. Clozapine also possesses weak antagonism at serotonin $5HT_3$ receptors (Ki = 241 nM at cloned human receptors), which is also associated with slower gastrointestinal motility. Not surprisingly, CTTs are positively correlated with plasma clozapine levels ($r = 0.451$, $p = 0.045$) [4]. Clozapine's high affinity for histamine H_1 receptors may also contribute to constipation risk due to decreased activity. A 2018 paper using data from 176 clozapine-treated Finnish patients found an association between the burden of genetic polymorphisms at receptors and other sites associated with constipation and clozapine-related gastrointestinal symptoms [6]. The other issue is the patient population who receives clozapine. These individuals are often severely mentally ill, and may have behavioral risk factors for constipation related to poor dietary habits, inactivity, and inadequate hydration. Moreover, some may be very poor reporters of somatic complaints, and thus will escape detection of significant GIH problems until a catastrophic event occurs. Given this confluence of medication-related and patient-related variables, and the known fatality rates from ileus, as much or greater attention must be paid to managing constipation as is devoted to assessment of neutrophil counts.

● Constipation Criteria and Stool Form Nomenclature

The Rome process is an international effort spanning the past 30 years to assist in the evidence-based diagnosis and treatment of functional gastrointestinal disorders such as irritable bowel syndrome and chronic constipation [7]. Because clozapine-associated GIH and constipation has a known cause, it would not be classified as a functional disorder, but does resemble the type of treatment-related constipation seen with chronic opioid use. The fourth edition of the Rome criteria (Rome IV) was published in May 2016, and, for the first time, criteria for Opioid-Induced Constipation (OIC) were elaborated. These criteria are essentially identical to those for functional constipation with rewording of the first criterion to emphasize the connection with medication use (Box 7.1).

Box 7.1 Rome IV Diagnostic Criteria for Opioid-Induced Constipation (C6) [7]

1. New, or worsening, symptoms of constipation when initiating, changing, or increasing opioid therapy that must include two or more of the following:

   a. Straining during more than one-fourth (25%) of defecations

   b. Lumpy or hard stools (Bristol Stool Form Scale 1–2) more than one-fourth (25%) of defecations

   c. Sensation of incomplete evacuation more than one-fourth (25%) of defecations

   d. Sensation of anorectal obstruction/blockage more than one-fourth (25%) of defecations

   e. Manual maneuvers to facilitate more than one-fourth (25%) of defecations (e.g. digital evacuation, support of the pelvic floor)

   f. Fewer than three spontaneous bowel movements per week

2. Loose stools are rarely present without the use of laxatives

As criteria 1a–1f are not medication-specific, and the parameters are exactly the same as for functional constipation, it is strongly suggested that hospital and clinical systems, as well as future research efforts, all use Rome IV criteria when making a diagnosis of clozapine-induced constipation. This standardization of diagnostic criteria based on elements arrived at by international experts in gastrointestinal motility disorders facilitates consistency in clinical and data-gathering activities. The term GIH is best applied in settings when CTT is directly measured, and where measured CTT values are ≥ 65 hours, or more than 2 SD greater than the population mean. To standardize the descriptive terminology of stool appearance in clinical and

Figure 7.1. Bristol Stool Form Scale.

Type 1	Separate hard lumps, like nuts	
Type 2	Sausage shaped but lumpy	
Type 3	Like a sausage but with cracks on its surface	
Type 4	Like a sausage or snake, smooth and soft	
Type 5	Soft blobs with clear-cut edges	
Type 6	Fluffy pieces with ragged edges, a mushy stool	
Type 7	Watery, no solid pieces	

(Adapted from: Lewis, S. J. and Heaton, K. W. (1997). Stool form scale as a useful guide to intestinal transit time. *Scandinavian Journal of Gastroenterology*, 32, 920–924 [8].)

research settings, the Bristol Stool Form Scale is also strongly recommended [8]. The Bristol Stool Form Scale (Figure 7.1) was developed over 25 years ago to provide an evidence-based method for assisting clinicians in estimating CTT. The simplicity of use even with children (using modified wording) has led to widespread application throughout the world and translation into numerous languages. Rome IV OIC criterion 1b references the Bristol Stool Form Scale in describing the types of stools that would qualify (category 1–2). Through the combined use of Rome IV medication-induced constipation criteria developed for opioids, and the Bristol Stool Form Scale, all members of the clinical team and outpatient caregivers can easily document that a patient meets constipation criteria, as well as the response to treatment.

 Treatment

Aside from clozapine, other medication classes are also independently associated with increased constipation risk in schizophrenia patients including tricyclic antidepressants (OR 2.29, 9% CI 1.29–4.09), anticholinergics (OR 1.48, 95% CI 1.00–2.19), and opioids (OR 2.14, 95% CI 1.36–3.36). The use of anticholinergics was also

Table 7.1 List of common strongly anticholinergic and constipating medications.

Psychotropics	Chlorpromazine, olanzapine, quetiapine (> 600 mg/day), amitriptyline, nortriptyline, clomipramine, imipramine, desipramine
Antiparkinsonian medications	Benztropine, diphenhydramine, trihexyphenidyl
Nonpsychiatric medications	Oxybutynin, tolterodine, darifenacin, solifenacin, trospium, glycopyrrolate
Other constipating medications	Iron (ferrous sulfate or gluconate), hydrocodone, oxycodone, codeine, hydromorphone, morphine, fentanyl, methadone, oxymorphone, tramadol

significantly associated with a nearly sixfold increase in ileus risk (OR 5.88, 95% CI 1.47–23.58) [5]. Given the additive pharmacodynamic effects on motility, management of clozapine-related constipation commences prior to the initiation of clozapine with the attempt to minimize exposure to constipating medications as noted in Table 7.1. It is important that clinicians are aware that a number of medications used for overactive bladder are potent antimuscarinic agents. If possible these too ought to be tapered off prior to or during the early initiation period of clozapine treatment to minimize the risk of constipation and ileus. The presence of other constipating agents such as oral iron supplements and opioids also should be diminished or eliminated completely prior to starting clozapine.

Chapter 3 provides an extensive discussion about transitioning patients from anticholinergic psychotropic medications or anticholinergic antiparkinsonian agents as clozapine is started. For the latter, there are well-defined relationships that can be employed to taper antiparkinsonian medications as clozapine is added (Box 7.2).

Box 7.2 Anticholinergic Equivalencies

Nonsmokers: 50 mg clozapine = 1 mg benztropine = 2.5 mg trihexyphenidyl = 25 mg diphenhydramine

Smokers: 100 mg clozapine = 1 mg benztropine = 2.5 mg trihexyphenidyl = 25 mg diphenhydramine

As noted in Chapter 3, an important part of the pretreatment evaluation is an assessment of current bowel function, seeking evidence for ongoing issues with constipation. During this process, one must gather appropriate history, including frequency and consistency of bowel movements (using the Bristol Stool Form Scale), supplemented with a relevant physical examination. In some hospital and clinic settings an abdominal X-ray is mandated, but even when not required may prove very useful when working with severely ill patients who are poor historians. If sufficient evidence exists for constipation, the patient can be managed with the usual strategies: minimization or discontinuation of offending agents when possible, and use of the three first-line medication classes to treat constipation as delineated below. Effective management of a pre-existing constipation problem may help forestall worse problems with clozapine that lead to treatment discontinuation or ileus.

Despite the prevalence and seriousness of the problem, the 2017 Cochrane systematic review of clozapine-induced constipation lamented: "There were no data comparing the common pharmacological interventions for constipation, such as lactulose, polyethylene glycol, stool softeners, lubricant laxatives, or of novel treatments such as linaclotide. Data available were very poor quality and the trials had a high risk of bias" [9]. Nonetheless, clinicians must treat patients using the limited evidence that exists, and most recommendations suggest using inexpensive first-line agents added sequentially before proceeding to the highly effective but more costly intestinal secretogogues, or the motility medication prucalopride. Table 7.2 summarizes the three classes of first-line agents used in managing constipation. With the exception of lactulose, all are extremely inexpensive and available without a prescription. Despite widespread use, the efficacy data for chronic constipation in the general population

Table 7.2 First-line agents for constipation.

	Mechanism	Starting dose	Maximum effective dose	Comments
Dioctyl sodium sulfosuccinate (docusate or DSS)	Anionic detergent that causes stool softening	250 mg QHS	250 mg BID	Commonly used despite a paucity of evidence supporting efficacy [18].
Polyethylene glycol 3350 (PEG-3350)	Osmotic agent	17 g qD	17 g BID	**Strong ACG recommendation. High quality of evidence.**
Lactulose	Osmotic agent	30 ml qD	30 ml BID	Strong ACG recommendation. Low quality of evidence.
Bisacodyl	Stimulant	5 mg QHS	15 mg BID	**Strong ACG recommendation. Moderate quality of evidence.**
Sennosides	Stimulant	8.6 mg QHS	17.2 mg BID	Absence of controlled data.

varies greatly. The comments in Table 7.2 reflect American College of Gastroenterology (ACG) recommendations and their assessment of the evidence quality based on standardized criteria for evaluation of clinical trial outcomes [10].

As indicated in Table 7.2, docusate theoretically acts to soften the stool but may be less effective than believed, so strong consideration must be given to starting docusate concurrently with a more effective medication. Osmotic agents draw water into the luminal cavity with the ACG evaluators finding polyethylene glycol (PEG-3350 or MiraLax) both effective and having high-quality evidence. Lactulose is costlier than PEG-3350, requires a prescription, and the quality of supporting data is low. In the past clinicians had been reluctant to prescribe stimulant laxatives due to (now disproved) concerns that these agents can damage the colon with long-term use, and a weak evidence base. As noted above, there is still limited data for sennosides, but convincing evidence for the efficacy of bisacodyl from well-designed randomized clinical trials published since 2010 [10].

Box 7.3 Principles for Managing Clozapine-Induced Constipation

1. Pretreatment assessment of the patient must occur for evidence of constipation prior to starting clozapine. Consider abdominal X-ray in unreliable patients (if not mandatory).

2. Remove other anticholinergic or other constipating medications as much as possible prior to starting clozapine, or taper off as clozapine is added.

3. Medications for constipation must commence with the first clozapine prescription for *every* patient even when constipation is not a current issue. Due to the limited efficacy data for docusate, consider simultaneously starting a second agent with docusate.

4. Many patients require one medication from each class of first-line agents simultaneously for adequate relief. No more than one agent from each class ought to be used.

5. Bulk-forming laxatives must not be used due to slow transit times presenting a risk of inspissation and worsening of the constipation problem.

6. Failure to relieve constipation for 48 hours must prompt a change in treatment (e.g. dose increase, additional agent of another class, use of enemas or manual disimpaction).

7. Magnesium can be used sparingly as a PRN medication (1 time per week or less), but not more often due to the risk of hypermagnesemia.

8. Signs of symptoms of ileus (see Box 7.4) must prompt immediate referral to a general hospital setting for further evaluation.

Unlike other patients with constipation, one important difference for managing clozapine-induced constipation is the avoidance of psyllium and other bulk-forming laxatives. Due to the markedly longer transit times in this patient population, these agents may undergo inspissation (dehydration), thereby exacerbating the problem. Multiple sources recommend against use of bulk-forming laxatives when managing clozapine-treated patients or other patients with prolonged CTT including the 2015 edition of the Maudsley Prescribing Guidelines in Psychiatry [11], and experts in colonic hypomotility [7] and GIH specific to clozapine therapy [12]. Neither mineral oil (liquid paraffin) nor magnesium is considered appropriate for routine use. Mineral oil (liquid paraffin) has limited efficacy data in adults and may be associated with unacceptable adverse effects such as soiling. In the pediatric population it has been largely replaced with PEG-3350. Excessive routine use of magnesium may result in hypermagnesemia, especially among those with reduced renal function, so these agents are best reserved for PRN use.

● **Efficacy of First-Line Agents**

Investigators in Porirua, New Zealand have performed the only prospective study of CTT changes utilizing a standardized treatment protocol. With a sample of 14 patients (10 male/4 female), median age 35 years, median plasma clozapine level 506 ng/ml (1547 mmol/l) and median treatment duration 2.5 years, changes in CTT and the proportion of patients with GIH (defined as ≥ 65 hours [> 2 SD from population norms]) or severe GIH (defined as > 101 hours [> 4 SD from population norms]) were tracked with radio-opaque markers while being treated with a regimen employing only the classes of first-line medications (see Table 7.3).

Table 7.3 The Porirua protocol for clozapine-induced gastrointestinal hypomotility and constipation [12].

Step 1	1. Start docusate 100 mg + senna 16 mg/night.
Step 2	2. *If still constipated after 48 hours*, increase docusate and senna every 2 days until no longer constipated or the maximum dose of docusate (100 mg BID) and senna (16 mg BID) have been reached.
Step 3	3. *If still constipated after another 48 hours*, perform digital rectal examination and consult with an expert about the need for enemas or disimpaction. If impacted stop docusate + senna. If not, then add PEG-3350 13.125 g BID.
Step 4	4. *If still constipated after another 48 hours*, consult with an expert about formulation of an individualized regimen.
General rules	If diarrhea develops after any step, gradually reduce and discontinue treatments in the reverse order that they were added.
	The Bristol Stool Form Chart is recommended as a monitoring tool.
	Medical evaluation for ileus if appropriate (see Box 7.4)

Using this protocol, the median CTT decreased from 110 hours at baseline to 62 hours ($p = 0.009$). Moreover, the prevalence of GIH decreased from 86% to 50%, and severe GIH from 64% to 21% [12]. These data echo naturalistic outcomes from the 6500 patient California Department of State Hospitals (Cal-DSH). Cal-DSH is the world's largest state hospital system, and at any time has over 700 clozapine-treated patients. Approximately 80% of patients on clozapine at Cal-DSH have constipation issues managed using only the three first-line classes routinely, with availability of PRN strategies (e.g. enemas).

Most aspects of the Porirua protocol are worth emulating, including: the avoidance of bulk-forming laxatives; use of a tracking form; the insistence on adding interventions every 48 hours if results are not seen. Many inpatients and outpatients may refuse digital rectal examination, and expert consultation may not be immediately available, so clinical judgement will need to be exercised when deciding on a course of action at Step 3. As noted below (PRN Medications), if there is sufficient concern about fecal impaction and the patient refuses digital examination, enemas are preferable to agents that stimulate motility (e.g. magnesium).

● Use of Secretogogues and Serotonergic Motility Agents

As data from the Porirua study and Cal-DSH indicate, even with assiduous application of medications from each class of first-line agents, 20–50% of patients may continue to have GIH or symptomatic constipation. A new class of agents, intestinal secretogogues, offer significant promise and are now extensively used in Cal-DSH for treatment-resistant constipation or in those patients with a history of ileus related to clozapine treatment.

The first of these agents, lubiprostone was approved by the United States Food and Drug Administration (FDA) in January 2006 for the treatment of chronic constipation in adults and for irritable bowel syndrome associated with constipation in women. In 2014, lubiprostone was subsequently recommended for use in the UK by the National Institute for Health and Care Excellence. Unlike stimulant or osmotic laxatives, lubiprostone is a prostaglandin E1 analogue that stimulates voltage-sensitive chloride channels on the luminal surface of gastrointestinal epithelial cells [13]. The net effect is an increase in chloride-rich luminal secretions that soften the stool and promote motility. There are no significant contraindications to its use aside from avoidance in those with mechanical intestinal obstruction. The first successful use of lubiprostone was reported in a Cal-DSH patient who developed ileus that required surgery without resection, but decompensated markedly when the treating clinicians attempted to find alternatives to clozapine.

The use of lubiprostone allowed this patient to resume clozapine therapy and he had continued on clozapine for several years at the time the case was published [14].

Based on Cal-DSH formulary criteria, patients are eligible to try lubiprostone after having failed the combination of maximum effective doses of docusate + an osmotic agent + a stimulant. Within the Cal-DSH system, lubiprostone has been recommended over the past 10 years for clozapine patients with treatment-resistant constipation, and in many instances achieved sufficient efficacy to the extent that other medications could be tapered off. As of March 1, 2018 there were 112 patients within Cal-DSH on lubiprostone. A detailed review of patients at one Cal-DSH site noted that 38 of the 182 clozapine-treated patients were on lubiprostone (21%) with mean daily dose of 36.2 μg, and modal dose of 24 μg BID. Lubiprostone was so effective that 17 of the 38 patients were able to have all osmotic and stimulant medications withdrawn.

Recently, two newer medications have become available: linaclotide and plecanatide. Linaclotide was approved by the FDA in August 2012 for constipation-predominant irritable bowel syndrome and chronic idiopathic constipation, and subsequently was also approved by the European Medicines Agency. It is an agonist at guanylate cyclase-C receptors on the luminal membrane resulting in two effects: increased luminal chloride and bicarbonate secretions, and inhibition of sodium ion absorption, thereby increasing the secretion of water into the lumen [15]. Linaclotide has minimal systemic absorption. Plecanatide is also a guanylate cyclase-C agonist and was approved in the US in January 2017 for chronic idiopathic constipation. Both linaclotide and plecanatide are contraindicated in patients who are suspected of having a mechanical gastrointestinal obstruction. As of May 1, 2019 there were 16 Cal-DSH patients on linaclotide, but none yet on plecanatide.

Clinicians should not be deterred from using secretogogues despite the absence of controlled data for clozapine-induced GIH. When managing serious and potentially fatal treatment outcomes, clinicians often must act without the gold standard of randomized, controlled studies. For example, there may never be controlled studies of filgrastim use to support ANC values in those with a history of clozapine-related neutropenia, but the accumulated case reports present a compelling picture of possible benefit and limited adverse effects. Similarly, the only source of data on secretogogues for clozapine-related GIH for the near future will likely be case-based. In addition to the extensive Cal-DSH experience, lubiprostone has demonstrated efficacy in randomized controlled studies of a related disorder, opioid-induced constipation, thus providing more rationale to support the use of secretogogues for clozapine-treated patients [16].

Recently available in the US, prucalopride is a selective serotonin $5HT_4$ agonist that stimulates colonic mass movements and lacks QTc concerns seen with the earlier compound cisapride. Prucalopride was initially approved in Europe in 2009 for treatment of chronic constipation in women who fail standard laxative therapy, was subsequently approved for men, and also approved in the UK, Canada and Australia. In addition to being highly selective for $5HT_4$ receptors, prucalopride was well tolerated in clinical trials, can be administered orally once daily (2 mg qD), and has low potential for drug–drug interactions. The only contraindications are intestinal perforation or obstruction, severe inflammatory conditions (e.g. Crohn's disease, ulcerative colitis or toxic megacolon), and severe renal impairment (eGFR < 30 ml/min). There is one publication that summarizes use of prucalopride in two patients with clozapine-induced GIH [17]. One patient went from a bowel movement every 5 days with a PRN enema every 6 days, to a bowel movement every 2.7 days with PRN enemas every 27 days. The second patient had a limited increase in bowel movement frequency from every 6 days to every 5.4 days, but no longer required PRN use of enemas (previously every 15 days).

Table 7.4 Intestinal secretogogues.

Name	Mechanism	Starting dose	Max. dose	Comments
Lubiprostone	Prostaglandin E1 analogue	8 µg BID	24 µg BID	Give with food and water No drug interactions
Linaclotide	Guanylate cyclase-C agonist	145 µg qD	290 µg qD	Give > 30 min before first meal No drug interactions
Plecanatide	Guanylate cyclase-C agonist	3 mg qD	3 mg qD	No drug interactions

At the time of their last review, the ACG gave the two available secretogogues (lubiprostone and linaclotide) strong recommendations based on high quality of evidence [10]. Prucalopride and plecanatide were not included in the review. The biggest barrier to treatment with any of these newer medications is the cost. However, given the system costs related to clozapine discontinuation (e.g. psychiatric hospitalization, legal consequences, etc.), and the lack of therapeutic alternatives to clozapine, the expense is justifiable in those who have failed less-costly regimens. Moreover, none of these newer medications have significant drug–drug interactions, so all are options in patients on complex medication regimens.

● PRN Medications

Many patients will have adequate control most weeks using various combinations of first-line agents, secretogogues, or prucalopride, but may have periods of exacerbation. The two most commonly used options are enemas and magnesium-containing preparations. Table 7.5 presents basic dosing facts and considerations in use of PRN laxatives.

Frequent need for PRN medications indicates that routine treatment is suboptimal. If the patient is on maximal doses of each class of first-line agents, a secretogogue must be started. In the uncommon event that constipation remains problematic despite routine agents + secretogogues or prucalopride, expert consultation is necessary.

● Decreasing Plasma Clozapine Levels for Difficult to Manage Constipation

As discussed in Chapter 5, tracking plasma clozapine levels is central to effective management. As CTTs are linearly correlated with plasma clozapine levels, clinicians should obtain a trough plasma level and review the course of treatment to determine

Table 7.5 Recommended PRN medications.

	Dose	Frequency	Comments
Magnesium hydroxide (5 ml contains 166.7 mg Mg = 400 mg magnesium hydroxide)	5 ml PO	Daily	Low magnesium exposure Avoid if impaction suspected
Magnesium citrate (300 ml contains 2800 mg Mg = 17.45 g magnesium citrate)	300 ml PO	Weekly	Limit use due to high magnesium load, especially in older individuals or patients with decreased renal function Avoid if impaction suspected
Enemas – mineral oil	One *per rectum*	Daily	Preferred agent if impaction suspected and patient refuses disimpaction
Enemas – water-based	One *per rectum*	Daily	Phosphate enemas may contribute to decline in eGFR

whether the patient requires the current plasma level for optimal psychiatric response. Often the patient has been carefully titrated to the present dose and level, so dose reduction invites risk of psychotic exacerbation. In some instances the current plasma level is not only in the upper end of the range (700–1000 ng/ml or 2140–3057 mmol/l) but prior titration was rapid, with insufficient time allowed to determine response before further dose escalation. Assuming that the patient is psychiatrically stable and minimally symptomatic, one might consider a modest dose reduction of no more than 5% every 4 weeks to determine whether psychiatric stability can be maintained at lower plasma levels, but with improved tolerability. Plasma levels are rechecked 1–2 weeks after each dose decrease. Any increase in symptoms requires an immediate end to the taper and resumption of the prior stable dose, with plasma level confirmation 1 week later.

C   Diagnosing Possible Ileus

Fatality rates from ileus vastly exceed those from severe neutropenia, so any signs or symptoms suggestive of severe ileus must be responded to urgently. Box 7.4 contains a list of clinical features that demand urgent evaluation irrespective of the time of day or day of the week. Outpatients must be urgently transported to a clinic or emergency department for examination. When ileus suspicion is high, inpatients and outpatients must be transferred to a general hospital (if not there already) for evaluation and admission. Delays in this process increase the risk of bowel ischemia, perforation and peritonitis.

When patients are admitted, they may be on NPO status for an extended time due to the use of nasogastric suction precluding oral administration of medications. Moreover, clozapine may be held to lower exposure and promote motility, especially if surgery is performed. Analogous to the severe neutropenia patient who has clozapine abruptly discontinued, there is a risk of cholinergic rebound and delirium. As the oral route will not be available, consider using parenteral benztropine to mitigate cholinergic rebound, administering small doses (e.g. 1 mg) intramuscularly as needed based on clinical evidence of cholinergic rebound symptoms such as confusion or frank delirium. The use of small doses and the parenteral route will hopefully minimize benztropine's impact on motility. Benztropine doses that provide equivalent anticholinergic activity to the prior clozapine dose and level need not be used. The goal is to prevent cholinergic rebound with the smallest possible exposure. (Chapter

4 provides an extensive discussion of strategies for managing cholinergic rebound, and considerations for antipsychotic therapy after clozapine discontinuation.)

1. Moderate to severe abdominal pain or discomfort lasting more than 1 hour

   OR

2. Abdominal pain/discomfort lasting more than 1 hour and at least one of the following:

   a. Vomiting (especially feculent vomitus)

   b. Distension

   c. Absent or high-pitched bowel sounds

   d. Diarrhea (especially bloody)

   e. Hemodynamic instability or other signs of sepsis

● **Rechallenging the Ileus Patient**

Despite a clinician's best efforts, some patients may develop ileus and require not only hospitalization for decompression, but surgical intervention with bowel resection. As ileus can prove life-threatening, clinicians are understandably reluctant to restart clozapine, especially when the patient has been gravely ill or required surgery. Nonetheless, most of these patients have no therapeutic alternatives and need to be approached with the same considerations as those who wish to rechallenge patients with prior severe neutropenia. The case for rechallenging a patient with a history of ileus, even with bowel resection, is strengthened when the patient was deprived of a trial of an intestinal secretogogue or perhaps prucalopride. The first case report of lubiprostone use was in a patient who developed poorly controlled psychosis when managed with nonclozapine antipsychotics after hospitalization and surgical exploration for clozapine-related ileus [14]. As most ileus patients have failed combinations of first-line agents, the treatment algorithm during rechallenge is inverted: secretogogues or prucalopride are started at the commencement of clozapine therapy, and other classes added sequentially as needed (see Box 7.5). Medication expense is often cited as a reason to prevent access to newer agents, but the cost of medical hospitalization for ileus can exceed the annual medication cost of a secretogogue or prucalopride by a factor of 100-fold or more.

Box 7.5 Constipation Medications During Clozapine Rechallenge After Ileus

1. Commence a secretogogue at the lowest available dose during the first week of clozapine treatment. If diarrhea occurs, hold the secretogogue and retry in 7–10 days.

2. As the clozapine titration proceeds, adjust the secretogogue dose so that the patient has no constipation complaints, and has very rare need for PRN medications (< 1 per fortnight). Consider switching to another secretogogue with a different mechanism of action (if available in the country) when maximum doses of the current agent are not sufficiently effective. Do not combine secretogogues.

3. If constipation management remains inadequate despite maximal secretogogue doses, sequentially add first-line agents starting with docusate, then a stimulant or osmotic, and then combining maximum doses of all three classes.

Summary Points

7

a. Treatment for constipation begins with the initiation of clozapine therapy, and includes minimizing exposure to other anticholinergic and constipating medications.

b. Even with combined use of first-line agents from each class, 20–50% of clozapine-treated patients will have persistent hypomotility and constipation.

c. Intestinal secretogogues and possibly prucalopride offer significant benefit for patients who fail maximal combined doses of docusate + an osmotic + a stimulant. Lubiprostone has been used for 10 years in the California Department of State Hospitals for treatment-resistant constipation. Experience is slowly accruing with the newest secretogogues linaclotide and plecanatide, and with the selective 5HT$_4$ agonist prucalopride.

d. Secretogogues or prucalopride must be used when rechallenging patients who have previously experienced ileus on first-line agents.

References

1. Pai, N. B. and Vella, S. C. (2012). Reason for clozapine cessation. *Acta Psychiatrica Scandinavica*, 125, 39–44.

2. Cohen, D. (2017). Clozapine and gastrointestinal hypomotility. *CNS Drugs*, 31, 1083–1091.

3. Leung, J. G., Hasassri, M. E., Barreto, J. N., et al. (2017). Characterization of admission types in medically hospitalized patients prescribed clozapine. *Psychosomatics*, 58, 164–172.

4. Every-Palmer, S., Nowitz, M., Stanley, J., et al. (2016). Clozapine-treated patients have marked gastrointestinal hypomotility, the probable basis of life-threatening gastrointestinal complications: A cross sectional study. *EBioMedicine*, 5, 125–134.

5. Nielsen, J. and Meyer, J. M. (2012). Risk factors for ileus in patients with schizophrenia. *Schizophrenia Bulletin*, 38, 592–598.

6. Solismaa, A., Kampman, O., Lyytikainen, L. P., et al. (2018). Genetic polymorphisms associated with constipation and anticholinergic symptoms in patients receiving clozapine. *Journal of Clinical Psychopharmacology*, 38, 193–199.

7. Lacy, B. E., Mearin, F., Chang, L., et al. (2016). Bowel disorders. *Gastroenterology*, 150, 1393–1407.

8. Lewis, S. J. and Heaton, K. W. (1997). Stool form scale as a useful guide to intestinal transit time. *Scandinavian Journal of Gastroenterology*, 32, 920–924.

9. Every-Palmer, S., Newton-Howes, G. and Clarke, M. J. (2017). Pharmacological treatment for antipsychotic-related constipation. *Cochrane Database of Systematic Reviews*, 1, Cd011128.

10. Wald, A. (2016). Constipation: Advances in diagnosis and treatment. *JAMA*, 315, 185–191.

11. Taylor, D., Paton, C. and Kapur, S. (2015). *The Maudsley Prescribing Guidelines in Psychiatry*, 12th Edition. Chichester: Wiley-Blackwell.

12. Every-Palmer, S., Ellis, P. M., Nowitz, M., et al. (2017). The Porirua Protocol in the treatment of clozapine-induced gastrointestinal hypomotility and constipation: A pre- and post-treatment study. *CNS Drugs*, 31, 75–85.

13. Lacy, B. E. and Levy, L. C. (2008). Lubiprostone: A novel treatment for chronic constipation. *Clinical Interventions in Aging*, 3, 357–364.

14. Meyer, J. M. and Cummings, M. A. (2014). Lubiprostone for treatment-resistant constipation associated with clozapine use. *Acta Psychiatrica Scandinavica*, 130, 71–72.

15. Love, B. L., Johnson, A. and Smith, L. S. (2014). Linaclotide: A novel agent for chronic constipation and irritable bowel syndrome. *American Journal of Health-System Pharmacy*, 71, 1081–1091.

16. Nee, J., Zakari, M., Sugarman, M. A., et al. (2018). Efficacy of treatments for opioid-induced constipation: A systematic review and meta-analysis. *Clinical Gastroenterology and Hepatology*, 16, 1569–1584.

17. Thomas, N., Jain, N., Connally, F., et al. (2018). Prucalopride in clozapine-induced constipation. *Australian & New Zealand Journal of Psychiatry*, 52, 804.

18. Canadian Agency for Drugs and Technologies in Health. (2014). *Dioctyl Sulfosuccinate or Docusate (Calcium or Sodium) for the Prevention or Management of Constipation: A Review of the Clinical Effectiveness*. Ottawa, ON: Canadian Agency for Drugs and Technologies in Health.

8

Managing Sedation, Orthostasis and Tachycardia

INTRODUCTION

In 2016 the United States Food and Drug Administration (FDA) added the category of *falls* as subsection 5.9 of the Warnings and Precautions listings for all antipsychotic package inserts. This mandated language reflected the concept that changes in blood pressure or alertness may not meet criteria for orthostatic hypotension or sedation as an adverse event during clinical trials, yet together they increase the risk of falling. Increased fall risk, especially among older patients, is one concern related to sedation and orthostasis when starting clozapine, but the other concern is that a patient will find tiredness or dizziness unacceptable when commencing treatment and refuse to continue with clozapine. Using case register data from the South London and Maudsley National Health Service Foundation Trust, it was found that 45% of 316 new clozapine starts from 2007 to 2011 discontinued clozapine within 2 years of initiation [1]. Moreover, 52% of the discontinuations were due to patient decision, and adverse drug reactions were 2.6 times more likely to be the cause than dislike of laboratory visits [1].

While there is a study of rapid clozapine titration for severely ill forensic inpatients [2], and a similar study for treatment-resistant schizophrenia inpatients [3], clinicians must be mindful that many patients may not be under compulsory treatment orders and will opt to terminate a clozapine trial when experiencing adverse effects. Sedation

PRINCIPLES

- Sedation must be addressed, as it is the most common adverse drug reaction cited by newly started patients as a reason for treatment discontinuation. Management strategies include administering all or most of the dose at bedtime, slowing the titration, and minimizing other sedating medications.

- For minimally symptomatic patients on stable clozapine doses who are still bothered by sedation, consider modest dose reductions if plasma clozapine levels are at the higher end of the therapeutic range (700–1000 ng/ml or 2140–3057 mmol/l).

- Adjunctive aripiprazole or modafinil can be considered for sedation when other methods have failed, but the supporting data are weak.

- Orthostasis occurs early in treatment and is initially managed by maintaining adequate fluid and salt intake, slowing the titration, minimizing other alpha$_1$-adrenergic antagonists and adjusting doses of antihypertensives. If those steps are not effective, the volume expanding mineralocorticoid fludrocortisone should be used.

- Tachycardia is first addressed by ruling out orthostasis. Tachycardia without orthostatic hypotension is never a reason to stop clozapine. When other causes have been eliminated, persistent tachycardia is managed using the selective beta$_1$-adrenergic antagonist atenolol.

8

and orthostasis are two commonly encountered issues when starting clozapine that may be exacerbated by rapid dose escalation, so prescribers must be adept at modifying titration schedules and swiftly responding to the occurrence of these side effects in order to maximize patient retention. Tachycardia may at times be due to untreated orthostasis, but is also frequently encountered in those without such problems. Although not a primary focus of patient complaints and easily treated in most instances, it is unfortunately still cited as a cause of treatment discontinuation by clinicians [1], despite expert recommendations that tachycardia should not be a reason to stop clozapine [4]. A recurring theme in this volume is that treatment-resistant schizophrenia spectrum patients have no viable options should clozapine therapy be terminated. Recognizing and managing burdensome adverse effects such as sedation and orthostasis, and appreciating that tachycardia is not a reason to stop clozapine, are all useful concepts in the successful implementation of clozapine therapy.

Sedation

Although sialorrhea and gastrointestinal hypomotility may be more prevalent, sedation is frequently cited as a reason for early treatment discontinuation. In the South London and Maudsley National Health Service Foundation Trust study of 316 patients commencing clozapine, sedation was the number one adverse drug reaction (ADR) cited as a reason for discontinuation by both clinicians and by patients; moreover, the risk of discontinuation was highest in the first few months of clozapine treatment [1]. A prevalence estimate of 44% was cited in a 2016 review of clozapine ADRs [5], and this is consistent with data from the Clinical Antipsychotic Trials of Intervention Effectiveness (CATIE) study, in which the prevalence of "hypersomnia/ sleepiness" in phases 2 and 3 were 45% and 32%, respectively [6,7]. Sedation is related to the combined effects of muscarinic and histamine H_1 antagonism, and thus might be expected to have a dose (or more accurately plasma level) relationship, but this is not easily proven from the clinical trials data. The 2017 Cochrane review on clozapine dosing noted that patients randomized to low-dose clozapine (150–300 mg/ day) had a lower risk of lethargy (RR 0.77, 95% CI 0.60 to 0.97) compared to standard doses (301–600 mg/day), but this conclusion is based on results from one trial [8]. Analysis of naturalistic data from 30 patients on clozapine monotherapy at the Institut de Neuropsiquiatria i Adiccions in Barcelona found that norclozapine levels correlated with hours slept ($r = 0.367$, $p = 0.03$) [9].

In clinical practice patients are titrated to the dose necessary to achieve the desired outcome (e.g. violence reduction, decrease in positive symptoms of schizophrenia) using clinical response, plasma-level data and tolerability as guides. While tolerance to sedation may develop over time, patients must agree to remain on clozapine for a sufficient time for this process to occur. As noted above, the greatest risk for stopping clozapine treatment due to an ADR is during the first few months of therapy. Below are some principles to help manage sedation risk in patients starting clozapine therapy. While there is a range of individual sensitivity to sedation, plasma levels can be very helpful to guide future treatment in those who appear exquisitely sensitive despite removing other offending medications and adjustment of the clozapine titration. Frequent communication with patients and caregivers is important to emphasize that excessive sedation is not acceptable and that every effort will be made to address this complaint. If a patient has significant complaints of daytime sedation and poor sleep quality prior to the clozapine trial, evaluation for obstructive sleep apnea may be needed prior to commencing clozapine, as these will likely be worse.

Box 8.1 Managing Sedation When Commencing Clozapine

1. Prior to starting treatment, minimize exposure to benzodiazepines and anticholinergics. The strategies for tapering these agents are outlined in Box 3.5.

2. Ask the patient to report problems with sedation as soon as they occur so that adjustments can be made to the doses of existing medications, or to the clozapine titration.

3. Clozapine is commonly prescribed as a single nightly QHS dose in North American without apparent loss of efficacy [27]. This should be considered for all patients during the early weeks of clozapine initiation. Single doses up to 500 mg QHS in nonsmokers appear to be well tolerated in clinical practice and should be considered for all patients unless dose-limiting adverse effects occur that can be alleviated through divided doses.

4. As noted in Chapter 3, titrations must be individualized based on the clinical scenario, demographic variables (e.g. age), the presence of CYP inducers (e.g. smoking, omeprazole, carbamazepine) or inhibitors and patient response to clozapine itself. The concept of a standard titration is a myth.

5. When sedating medications cannot be withdrawn (e.g. a patient transitioning from high-dose quetiapine or chlorpromazine to clozapine), these agents should be cross-tapered with clozapine, with careful attention paid to patient complaints of sedation.

6. If the patient complains of significant sedation, revert back to the last prior clozapine dose, and taper off any existing sedating medications to the extent possible, especially benzodiazepines, antiparkinsonian medications, antihistamines. Once the complaints abate after 3–7 days, the clozapine titration can proceed, but the rapidity of dose escalation may need to be moderated. If the complaints persist despite these measures, plasma clozapine levels may be very useful to determine whether the patient is a poor metabolizer with higher than expected levels for the dose (see Chapter 5), or just more sensitive to sedation.

8

At times, patients may not complain of sedation during the titration phase, but notice the problem once they are psychiatrically improved and working on functional goals. There are two options for these individuals once all other sedating medications have been discontinued (including anticholinergic agents with CNS effects used for overactive bladder): dose reduction (using plasma levels) or use of adjunctive medications to promote daytime alertness. When considering dose reduction the approach is very similar to that outlined in Chapter 7 (Decreasing Plasma Clozapine Levels for Difficult to Manage Constipation). Dose reduction may be a viable strategy when individuals are psychiatrically stable and minimally symptomatic, the plasma level is at the high end of the therapeutic range, and there is evidence that the patient may have been titrated rapidly to this plasma level without allowing sufficient time to respond before each dose increase. There are limited data to provide guidance on the extent to which decreasing the plasma clozapine level will improve complaints of sedation. Among 133 clozapine-treated patients at the Institut de Neuropsiquiatria i Adiccions in Barcelona who complained of excessive sedation, clozapine dose reduction decreased the time spent asleep in < 20% of patients [9]. Nonetheless, it may benefit selected patients, so the following approach is suggested.

1. Consider a dose reduction of no more than 5% every 4 weeks to determine whether psychiatric stability can be maintained at lower plasma levels, but with decreased sedation. Plasma levels are rechecked 1–2 weeks after each dose decrease.

2. Any increase in symptoms requires an immediate end to the clozapine taper and resumption of the prior stable dose, with plasma level confirmation 1 week later.

When dose reduction is not an option or is not effective, adjunctive medications can be considered. Among the available options, aripiprazole is somewhat compelling as it is unlikely to cause symptomatic exacerbation and there is no abuse liability. In the Barcelona cohort ($n = 133$) noted above, aripiprazole augmentation reduced hours slept in 26.1% [9]. There are also data on the use of aripiprazole to address residual schizophrenia symptoms, with four double-blind placebo-controlled trials as of 2014 [10]. In those studies the degree of psychiatric improvement did not reach statistical significance, although there was a trend towards benefit. At mean aripiprazole doses ranging from 11.1 to 15.5 mg/day in each study, aripiprazole was significantly more likely than placebo to induce akathisia or anxiety, so initial doses should be modest (e.g. 2.5 mg/day) and patients observed for these adverse effects. Aripiprazole should only be tried in patients on clozapine as antipsychotic monotherapy, and dose adjustments are needed for cytochrome P450 (CYP) 2D6 poor metabolizers, or those on 2D6 or 3A4 inhibitors, or 3A4 inducers. There are reports of symptomatic worsening when aripiprazole is added to nonclozapine antipsychotics, likely due to displacement of strong D_2 antagonists by the partial agonist aripiprazole [11]. Aripiprazole and its active metabolite reach steady state in 21 days, so if there is no benefit for sedation after 3 weeks at a given dose, higher doses ought to be tried. The adjunctive aripiprazole trial should be terminated for adverse effects (akathisia, anxiety, parkinsonism) or the maximum dose of 30 mg/day is reached (for those not on CYP inhibitors or inducers or 2D6 poor metabolizers).

In the stimulant class, modafinil was approved in the US on December 24, 1998 to promote wakefulness in those with excessive daytime sedation, and the active *R* enantiomer armodafinil was subsequently approved on June 15, 2007 for a similar indication. Although the mechanism was not completely understood at launch, modafinil has subsequently been characterized as a very weak but very selective inhibitor of dopamine reuptake. In addition to compelling *in vitro* and *in vivo* animal data, a human imaging study found that 200 mg of modafinil resulted in 51.4% dopamine transporter occupancy, and the 300 mg dose in 56.9% occupancy [12]. By way of comparison, clinically relevant doses of methylphenidate occupy 60–70% of dopamine transporters [13]. Although modafinil appears to have lower abuse risk than traditional stimulants, the abuse liability is not absent. There are also rare reports of drug reaction with eosinophilia and systemic symptoms or Stevens–Johnson syndrome. Nonetheless, modafinil is generally well tolerated and has been studied extensively for negative symptoms and cognitive dysfunction in schizophrenia and also for its impact on metabolic parameters [14–16]. It has not proven successful for those purposes, and unfortunately only one of four randomized, double-blind, placebo-controlled trials for sedation proved positive. It is worth noting that the dose range of 200–300 mg/day was well tolerated in those studies without apparent risk of symptomatic worsening [14], although there are rare case reports of symptom exacerbation [17]. The starting dose is 100 mg qam (each morning), and it can be advanced if needed by 100 mg/day each week to a maximum dose of 300 mg qam.

The use of methylphenidate and amphetamines is limited by their significant abuse potential and the risk for exacerbation of positive psychotic symptoms. Nonetheless, there are two early case reports from 1993 in which methylphenidate at doses of 5–30 mg/day was helpful when dose reduction was no longer possible [18]. In 2016, three cases were reported in which extended-release methylphenidate (Concerta®) was used to improve cognitive function with the specific goal of reducing persistent impulsive violence in clozapine-treated forensic inpatients [19]. At doses of 18 or 36 mg once daily there was a significant reduction in violence and no worsening of the underlying psychotic disorder. Although the medication was administered in a highly controlled setting, even in controlled inpatient units concerns about abuse need to be examined whenever a stimulant is prescribed. There are no data about use of

8

amphetamine preparations for sedation in clozapine-treated patients, and none for other purposes (e.g. cognitive enhancement).

B Orthostasis

Orthostatic hypotension is defined as sustained reduction in systolic blood pressure (SBP) of at least 20 mmHg or in diastolic blood pressure (DBP) of at least 10 mmHg within 3 min of standing. Although there are studies of rapid clozapine titration as noted previously [2,3], minimizing orthostasis is one reason clozapine is often titrated slowly. The US package insert contains multiple warnings about orthostasis in bold type to alert clinicians to the potential seriousness of this problem, and urges gradual titration as one mitigating strategy. Recent reviews cite a prevalence of 9%, but patients may report complaints of dizziness or faintness without meeting strict criteria for orthostatic hypotension [5]. In the CATIE trial, the prevalence of "orthostatic faintness" in phases 2 and 3 were 12% and 24%, respectively [6,7]. As with sedation, there is a relationship with dose to the extent that those exposed to low doses in clinical trials (150–300 mg/day) experienced less dizziness (RR 0.56, 95% CI 0.39 to 0.81) compared to standard doses (301–600 mg/day) [8]. While several strategies are available to manage clozapine-related orthostasis, and expert reviews recommend termination only for "continuous malignant syncope" despite countermeasures [4], dizziness was the fourth most common reason for clinicians to stop clozapine in the South London and Maudsley National Health Service Foundation sample of 316 new starts [1].

The underlying mechanism relates to the high affinity of clozapine and norclozapine for $alpha_1$-adrenergic receptors and subsequent reduction in peripheral vascular tone. Clozapine in particular is a nonselective antagonist at the $alpha_{1A}$-adrenergic and $alpha_{1B}$-adrenergic receptors, and thus differs from newer medications used for lower urinary tract symptoms in males that are selective $alpha_{1A}$-adrenergic antagonists (e.g. tamsulosin), and have lower rates of orthostasis. There is marked individual variation in sensitivity to $alpha_1$-adrenergic antagonism with older age, baseline blood pressure, concurrent use of other $alpha_1$-adrenergic antagonists or antihypertensives, and the clozapine dose all influencing the ability to tolerate a particular titration schedule. For patients not on medications that act

Box 8.2 Managing Orthostasis When Commencing Clozapine

1. Prior to starting treatment, minimize exposure to nonselective alpha$_1$-adrenergic antagonists associated with orthostasis. (The strategies for tapering these agents are outlined in Box 3.5.)

2. For older patients, those with a history of orthostasis, and patients on agents that lower blood pressure (antihypertensives, nonselective alpha$_1$-adrenergic antagonists), consider slower titration schedules until tolerability is established. As noted in Chapter 3, titrations must be individualized based on the clinical scenario, demographic variables (e.g. age), the presence of CYP inducers (e.g. smoking, omeprazole, carbamazepine) or inhibitors and patient response to clozapine itself.

3. Frequent measurement of orthostatic blood pressures during the first weeks of treatment as outlined in Chapter 3. Ask the patient to report problems with dizziness as soon as they occur so that it can be established that this is related to blood pressure changes (and not other causes, e.g. Meniere's disease), and so adjustments can be made to doses of existing medications, or to the clozapine titration. Advise patients to rise slowly when standing during the titration phase.

4. When nonselective alpha$_1$-adrenergic antagonist antipsychotics cannot be withdrawn (e.g. a patient transitioning from chlorpromazine to clozapine), these should be cross-tapered with clozapine, with frequent orthostatic vital sign measurements and attention to complaints of dizziness.

6. If the patient manifests orthostatic drops in blood pressure, *revert back to the last prior clozapine dose, encourage adequate oral fluid intake* and evaluate the role of existing medications.

    a. If there are psychotropics with nonselective alpha$_1$-adrenergic antagonism, attempt to taper these further. If antihypertensives need to be adjusted, consult with the primary care provider. For patients on terazosin or prazosin for benign prostatic hypertrophy, switching to selective alpha$_{1A}$-adrenergic antagonists such as tamsulosin is associated with markedly reduced blood pressure effects. Reassess blood pressure frequently over the ensuing 3–7 days after changes are made.

    b. If there are no offending medications besides clozapine, reassess blood pressure frequently over the ensuing 3–7 days to see if tolerance has developed.

7. If orthostasis persists despite these measures, the mineralocorticoid fludrocortisone is the medication of choice, starting at 0.1 mg PO qD. The main contraindication is presence of congestive heart failure. Doses can be increased every 7–10 days based on blood pressure results to a maximum of 0.3 mg qD. Patients on long-term therapy must have potassium levels monitored every 2–3 months.

8. Use of compression stockings can be considered, but may be of limited value and poorly tolerated in warmer climates.

as nonselective alpha$_1$ antagonists there is a phenomenon known as the first dose effect: marked sensitivity to the hypotensive effect is much greater with the first dose of an antagonist and is lower when the same medication is dosed 72 hours later [20]. This ongoing process of receptor desensitization and tolerance to the hypotensive effect develops over days to weeks, but in some patients orthostatic hypotension or dizziness complaints become dose-limiting and demand immediate action to prevent falls and injuries, and to prevent the patient from refusing to persist with clozapine.

The management of orthostasis very much parallels that of sedation with one major exception: when the removal of offending medications other than clozapine, adjustment of clozapine doses and increased fluid intake fail to yield meaningful results there is a specific treatment for orthostasis: the potent mineralocorticoid agonist fludrocortisone. Fludrocortisone has been available for over 60 years for the management of orthostatic hypotension and is the drug of choice for conditions such as postural orthostatic tachycardia syndrome [21]. Fludrocortisone acts on renal distal tubule cells to promote reabsorption of sodium and water, thereby expanding vascular volume. As some potassium wasting occurs, potassium levels must be monitored every 2–3 months to prevent hypokalemia. The primary contraindication is congestive heart failure. In addition to fludrocortisone one can try compression stockings, but the benefit is often limited, and the stockings poorly tolerated in warmer climates. Rare patients can be encountered who continue to have problematic orthostasis despite maximum efforts including fludrocortisone and extremely slow titrations, but for most patients orthostasis is not a reason to terminate clozapine treatment.

 Tachycardia

Sustained tachycardia is defined as heart rate > 100 beats per minute (BPM) in the resting state. For most medications with prominent alpha$_1$-adrenergic antagonist properties, reflex tachycardia would be the consequence of poor vasomotor tone, and this is the first consideration when tachycardia is detected for clozapine-treated patients; however, persistent tachycardia is reported at rates varying from 25% to

54%, suggesting that other autonomic mechanisms are contributing [5,22]. Akin to orthostasis, there is a dose relationship with rates on low-dose regimens (150–300 mg/day) 57% of that seen with standard doses (301–600 mg/day) [8]. Despite the fact that tachycardia management is straightforward, and expert reviews suggest that tachycardia should never be grounds for discontinuing clozapine [4], it was the third most common reason for clinicians to stop clozapine in the South London and Maudsley National Health Service Foundation sample of 316 new starts [1].

Before concluding that persistent tachycardia is due to clozapine itself, the clinician has a small number of considerations as outlined in Box 8.3. In addition to short-term concerns that tachycardia may be due to orthostasis, additive pharmacodynamic effects, infection, pain, drug reaction, systemic illness or myocarditis, there is a long-term consideration: persistent tachycardia is associated with increased mortality from cardiac and noncardiac causes [22]. Many clinicians are aware that sustained tachycardia increases risk for cardiomyopathy [23]; however, a meta-analysis of 45 prospective cohort studies found that for each increment of 10 BPM in resting heart rate there was an increased relative risk for the following (after adjusting for risk related variables): 1.12 (95% CI 1.09–1.14) for coronary artery disease, 1.05 (95% CI 1.01–1.08) for stroke, 1.12 (95% CI 1.02–1.24) for sudden death, 1.16 (95% CI 1.12–1.21) for noncardiovascular diseases, 1.09 (95% CI 1.06–1.12) for all types of cancer and 1.25 (95% CI 1.17–1.34) for noncardiovascular diseases excluding cancer [24]. As noted in Chapter 3 (see Box 3.1 and Table 3.4), another issue that arises from tachycardia is erroneous concerns about QT prolongation. Many ECG machines continue to use the older Bazett QT correction formula that was derived in 1920 from 39 healthy male controls and significantly overcorrects the QTc for faster heart rates [25]. For this reason, American Heart Association guidelines for ECG interpretation recommend against using Bazett's formula with high heart rates, as the "adjusted QT values may be substantially in error" [26]. Unfortunately, many clinicians are not aware of these guidelines or even what correction formula is used in their ECG machines, leading to unnecessary alarm and concern. For all of these reasons, the goal of treatment is a resting heart rate always under 100 BPM, and ideally closer to 80 BPM because each 10 BPM increment increases mortality risk.

Box 8.3 Decision Algorithm When Persistent Tachycardia is Detected

Step 1. Is it due to orthostasis? Strongly suspect when occurring shortly after a dose increase, or after changes to the regimen that would increase plasma clozapine levels.

    a. Yes: For patients initiating clozapine, hold the titration and treat the orthostasis.

    b. Yes: For patients on established therapy: if there is a suspected increase in the plasma level due to the addition of an inhibitor or removal of an inducer (e.g. smoking cessation), obtain a plasma clozapine level and reduce the dose based on the expected kinetic impact of the change (see Chapter 5). If this is not tolerated for psychiatric reasons, then treat the orthostasis.

    c. No: See if items 2, 3 or 4 are considerations. If not, go to step 5.

Step 2. Have anticholinergic or adrenergic agonist medications been added that promote tachycardia?

    a. Yes: Taper these off in lieu of other agents, with the sole exception of a patient with treatment-resistant sialorrhea who requires glycopyrrolate. For the latter, go to step 5.

    b. No: See if items 3 or 4 are considerations. If not, go to step 5.

Step 3. Is there infection, pain or systemic illness (including drug reactions and interstitial nephritis)?

    a. Yes: Treat the underlying condition. In some instances this may require stopping clozapine (drug reactions, interstitial nephritis). Once treated, go to step 5 if tachycardia persists.

    b. No: See if item 4 is a consideration. If not, go to step 5.

Step 4. If occurring during the first 6 weeks of clozapine treatment, are there signs or laboratory parameters suggestive of myocarditis (see Chapter 12)?

    a. Yes: Stop clozapine and provide supportive treatment.

    b. No: Go to step 5.

Step 5. When none of items 1–4 are present, the treatment of choice is atenolol, a selective beta$_1$-adrenergic antagonist that does not readily enter the CNS and is not hepatically metabolized.

    a. Starting dose: 12.5 mg PO qam. Monitor for orthostasis.

    b. Titration: If tachycardic with no signs of orthostasis, may increase in 12.5 mg increments every 7 days. Most patients respond to doses ≤ 50 mg/day, but doses up to 100 mg qam can be tried.

    c. Conversion from propranolol: If a patient was started on propranolol for tachycardia management, this can be converted to atenolol in the ratio of 40 mg/day propranolol = 25 mg qam atenolol. If the patient is on propranolol for akathisia or tremor, then employ propranolol for tachycardia management using this dose equivalence.

Summary Points

a. Sedation is a highly prevalent condition and affects 45% of clozapine-treated patients. It is the most common adverse drug reaction cited by patients as a reason for discontinuing treatment. Prompt recognition during the early phase of treatment, adjustment of clozapine titration and minimizing concurrent sedating agents are the core strategies for managing sedation. Careful dose reduction can be considered in select cases with plasma-level guidance. Adjunctive medications to promote wakefulness can be tried but may be disappointing.

b. Orthostasis should almost never be a reason to stop clozapine treatment. Encouragement of adequate fluid intake, prompt recognition during the early phase of treatment, adjustment of clozapine titration and minimizing concurrent offending agents are the initial strategies. When these are insufficient, the potent mineralocorticoid fludrocortisone is the treatment of choice.

c. Tachycardia should never be a reason to stop clozapine treatment. Persistent clozapine-related tachycardia is diagnosed after eliminating other possible causes including orthostasis, effects of other medications on heart rate, infection, pain, drug reactions and systemic conditions. When these are ruled out, the beta$_1$-adrenergic antagonist atenolol is the treatment of choice.

8

References

1. Legge, S. E., Hamshere, M., Hayes, R. D., et al. (2016). Reasons for discontinuing clozapine: A cohort study of patients commencing treatment. *Schizophrenia Research*, 174, 113–119.

2. Ifteni, P., Nielsen, J., Burtea, V., et al. (2014). Effectiveness and safety of rapid clozapine titration in schizophrenia. *Acta Psychiatrica Scandinavica*, 130, 25–29.

3. Poyraz, C. A., Ozdemir, A., Saglam, N. G., et al. (2016). Rapid clozapine titration in patients with treatment refractory schizophrenia. *Psychiatry Quarterly*, 87, 315–322.

4. Nielsen, J., Correll, C. U., Manu, P., et al. (2013). Termination of clozapine treatment due to medical reasons: When is it warranted and how can it be avoided? *Journal of Clinical Psychiatry*, 74, 603–613.

5. Citrome, L., McEvoy, J. P. and Saklad, S. R. (2016). Guide to the management of clozapine-related tolerability and safety concerns. *Clinical Schizophrenia & Related Psychoses*, 10, 163–177.

6. McEvoy, J. P., Lieberman, J. A., Stroup, T. S., et al. (2006). Effectiveness of clozapine versus olanzapine, quetiapine, and risperidone in patients with chronic schizophrenia who did not respond to prior atypical antipsychotic treatment. *American Journal of Psychiatry*, 163, 600–610.

7. Stroup, T. S., Lieberman, J. A., McEvoy, J. P., et al. (2009). Results of phase 3 of the CATIE schizophrenia trial. *Schizophrenia Research*, 107, 1–12.

8. Subramanian, S., Vollm, B. A. and Huband, N. (2017). Clozapine dose for schizophrenia. *Cochrane Database of Systematic Reviews*, 6, Cd009555.

9. Perdigues, S. R., Quecuti, R. S., Mane, A., et al. (2016). An observational study of clozapine induced sedation and its pharmacological management. *European Neuropsychopharmacology*, 26, 156–161.

10. Srisurapanont, M., Suttajit, S., Maneeton, N., et al. (2015). Efficacy and safety of aripiprazole augmentation of clozapine in schizophrenia: A systematic review and meta-analysis of randomized-controlled trials. *Journal of Psychiatric Research*, 62, 38–47.

11. Takeuchi, H. and Remington, G. (2013). A systematic review of reported cases involving psychotic symptoms worsened by aripiprazole in schizophrenia or schizoaffective disorder. *Psychopharmacology (Berlin)*, 228, 175–185.

12. Kim, W., Tateno, A., Arakawa, R., et al. (2014). In vivo activity of modafinil on dopamine transporter measured with positron emission tomography and [(1)(8)F]FE-PE2I. *International Journal of Neuropsychopharmacology*, 17, 697–703.

13. Hannestad, J., Gallezot, J. D., Planeta-Wilson, B., et al. (2010). Clinically relevant doses of methylphenidate significantly occupy norepinephrine transporters in humans in vivo. *Biological Psychiatry*, 68, 854–860.

14. Saavedra-Velez, C., Yusim, A., Anbarasan, D., et al. (2009). Modafinil as an adjunctive treatment of sedation, negative symptoms, and cognition in schizophrenia: A critical review. *Journal of Clinical Psychiatry*, 70, 104–112.

15. Henderson, D. C., Freudenreich, O., Borba, C. P., et al. (2011). Effects of modafinil on weight, glucose and lipid metabolism in clozapine-treated patients with schizophrenia. *Schizophrenia Research*, 130, 53–56.

16. Andrade, C., Kisely, S., Monteiro, I., et al. (2015). Antipsychotic augmentation with modafinil or armodafinil for negative symptoms of schizophrenia: Systematic review and meta-analysis of randomized controlled trials. *Journal of Psychiatric Research*, 60, 14–21.

17. Neto, D., Spinola, C. and Gago, J. (2017). Modafinil in schizophrenia: Is the risk worth taking? *BMJ Case Reports*, 2017,

18. Burke, M. and Sebastian, C. S. (1993). Treatment of clozapine sedation. *American Journal of Psychiatry*, 150, 1900–1901.

19. Skoretz, P. and Tang, C. (2016). Stimulants for impulsive violence in schizophrenia spectrum disordered women: A case series and brief review. *CNS Spectrums*, 21, 445–449.

20. von Bahr, C., Lindstrom, B. and Seideman, P. (1982). Alpha-receptor function changes after the first dose of prazosin. *Clinical Pharmacology and Therapeutics*, 32, 41–47.

21. Testani, M., Jr. (1994). Clozapine-induced orthostatic hypotension treated with fludrocortisone. *Journal of Clinical Psychiatry*, 55, 497–498.

22. Ronaldson, K. J. (2017). Cardiovascular disease in clozapine-treated patients: Evidence, mechanisms and management. *CNS Drugs*, 31, 777–795.

23. Gupta, S. and Figueredo, V. M. (2014). Tachycardia mediated cardiomyopathy: Pathophysiology, mechanisms, clinical features and management. *International Journal of Cardiology*, 172, 40–46.

24. Zhang, D., Wang, W. and Li, F. (2016). Association between resting heart rate and coronary artery disease, stroke, sudden death and noncardiovascular diseases: A meta-analysis. *CMAJ*, 188, e384–e392.

25. Luo, S., Michler, K., Johnston, P., et al. (2004). A comparison of commonly used QT correction formulae: The effect of heart rate on the QTc of normal ECGs. *Journal of Electrocardiology*, 37(Suppl), 81–90.

26. Kim, D. D., White, R. F., Barr, A. M., et al. (2018). Clozapine, elevated heart rate and QTc prolongation. *Journal of Psychiatry and Neuroscience*, 43, 71–72.

27. Takeuchi, H., Powell, V., Geisler, S., et al. (2016). Clozapine administration in clinical practice: Once-daily versus divided dosing. *Acta Psychiatrica Scandinavica*, 134, 234–240.

8

9

Managing Sialorrhea

INTRODUCTION

Sialorrhea may be the most common adverse effect of clozapine treatment, with prevalence estimates ranging from 30% to 90%, yet it is often underreported, underrecognized, and undertreated, leading to treatment dissatisfaction and discontinuation, social consequences, and possible medical morbidity in the form of aspiration events. Recent data indicate that the prevalence is likely closer to the 90% figure based on a detailed 2016 study of 98 clozapine-treated patients who were assessed for hypersalivation using two rating scales: the Nocturnal Hypersalivation Rating Scale and the Drooling Severity and Frequency Scale [1]. Sialorrhea was experienced by 92% of subjects overall, more commonly at night (85% of subjects) than in the daytime (48%). Daytime symptoms were severe in 18%, and sialorrhea was considered frequent or occurring on a constant basis in 20%.

- A highly prevalent problem that causes social embarrassment, increases risk for treatment discontinuation, and may result in medical complications (e.g. aspiration pneumonia).

- Locally applied therapies must be tried first, as use of systemic anticholinergic medications will double the risk for ileus. Atropine 1% drops sublingually or ipratropium 0.06% spray intraorally are first-line agents.

- When patients fail first-line therapy, botulinum toxin-B injections into salivary glands is the preferred second-line therapy due to extensive double-blind, placebo-controlled trial data for sialorrhea due to medications or neurological causes.

- If botulinum toxin-B injections are not effective, other nonanticholinergic options to consider include alpha-adrenergic modulators (e.g. clonidine) and possibly amisulpride.

- A systemic anticholinergic medication should be considered the treatment of last resort due to the increased risk for ileus, and for fatal ileus. If a systemic anticholinergic must be used, glycopyrrolate is the preferred medication due to limited CNS penetration. The addition of glycopyrrolate must be accompanied by vigilant tracking of constipation, and aggressive management of gastrointestinal hypomotility should it occur.

Importantly, sialorrhea had at least a moderate impact on the quality of life in 15% of study subjects. While many studies of clozapine discontinuation focus on physician determined medical concerns, sialorrhea emerges as the third most common adverse drug reaction cited by *patients* as a reason for discontinuing treatment, behind sedation and nausea [2]. Importantly, sialorrhea during clozapine therapy has been associated with reports of aspiration pneumonia [3]. The extent of pneumonia risk from clozapine treatment has been quantified in three studies, with rates 1.99–3.18 times higher in clozapine-treated patients compared with other antipsychotics [3]. Supporting this concept is the finding that pulmonary illness was the most common cause (32%) of medically related hospital admissions for clozapine-treated patients at one major US medical center, of which 58% were for pneumonia [4]. Lastly, parotitis has also been reported and associated with hypersalivation [5].

Unfortunately, clinicians are forced to confront this problem with a virtual absence of well-designed clinical trials that focus specifically on clozapine and sialorrhea. The 2008 Cochrane review on clozapine-induced hypersalivation lamented: "The quality of reporting was poor with no studies clearly describing allocation concealment and much data were missing or unusable." They concluded: "There are currently insufficient data to confidently inform clinical practice. The limitations of these studies are plentiful and the risk of bias is high" [6]. Nonetheless, there are some insights and treatment principles that can be gleaned from these studies. Importantly, sialorrhea is not unique to clozapine treatment, and is seen in an array of neurological disorders (i.e. cerebral palsy, Parkinson's disease), or secondary to medications such as acetylcholinesterase inhibitors [7,8]. Fortunately, there are a large number of randomized, double-blind, placebo-controlled trials in this literature, including six studies alone utilizing botulinum toxin-B [9]. As the pathophysiology of hypersalivation during clozapine treatment is not distinct from other common etiologies, one can use this larger body of data from sialorrhea treatment studies to devise rational strategies for managing this vexing issue during clozapine therapy.

 ## Salivary Gland Innervation and Physiology

Humans have three main pairs of salivary glands: parotid, submandibular, and sublingual glands, along with hundreds of minor submucosal glands. In the resting state the majority of salivary fluid (68%) is provided by the submandibular and sublingual glands, and 28% comes from the parotid. However, when stimulated, 53% of salivary fluid comes from the parotid gland and 46% from the submandibular and sublingual glands [10]. The sublingual and minor salivary glands secrete mucus and are responsible for most of the protein content in saliva. Salivary secretion is controlled by brainstem salivary nuclei located in the medulla oblongata that receive diffuse inputs from the central nervous system (e.g. hypothalamus, frontal cortex, amygdala) and signals created by tactile, olfactory, temperature and taste stimuli (Figure 9.1). Both inhibitory GABA-ergic and excitatory glycinergic neurons form synapses with the salivary nuclei, but these cells also express muscarinic M_3 receptors, with central M_3 antagonists decreasing salivary flow. Reflex salivary secretion is centrally mediated via alpha$_2$-adrenergic receptors, with agonists (e.g.

Figure 9.1. Connections between central nervous system structures and salivary gland.

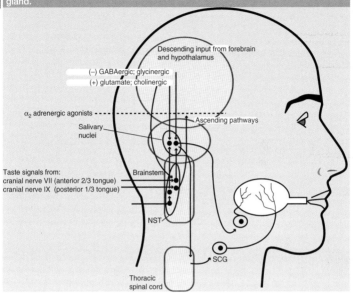

(Adapted from: Proctor, G. B. and Carpenter, G. H. (2014). Salivary secretion: Mechanism and neural regulation. *Monographs in Oral Science*, 24, 14–29 [10].)

clonidine) exerting an inhibitory effect of salivary flow. Salivary glands receive both parasympathetic and sympathetic innervation, with cholinergic response highly based on activity at muscarinic M_3 receptors, with evidence for involvement of M_1, M_4 and M_5 [10,11].

B Mechanism for Clozapine-Induced Sialorrhea and Risk Factors

As discussed in Chapter 7, muscarinic antagonism from clozapine is the primary cause of intestinal hypomotility, but it is the agonist effects of norclozapine that are hypothesized to induce sialorrhea. Although norclozapine has lower muscarinic affinity than clozapine across multiple receptor subtypes, norclozapine has higher intrinsic agonist activity, especially at M_1 (see Tables 9.1 and 9.2) [12]. That M_1 agonism may be the predominant mechanism for clozapine-induced sialorrhea is based on the efficacy of pirenzepine, a relatively selective M_1 antagonist, for clozapine-induced sialorrhea [13].

Table 9.1 Binding profile at cloned human receptors (Ki nM) [34] and PDSP Ki database (pdsp.med.unc.edu/pdsp.php).

	D_2	$5HT_{2A}$	$5HT_{2C}$	$5HT_{1A}$	M_1	M_3	α_{1A}	α_{1D}	H_1	Brain/ plasma ratio in PGP KO VS. WT
Clozapine	20	5.0	39.8	123.7	6.17	6.31	7.9	7.0	0.32	1.6 [35]
Norclozapine	63	5.0	15.9	13.9	67.6	158	5.0	85.2	6.3	?

Table 9.2 Muscarinic intrinsic activity relative to the full agonist carbachol [34].

	M_1	M_2	M_3	M_4	M_5
Clozapine	24 ± 3%	65 ± 8%	NR	57 ± 5%	NR
Norclozapine	72 ± 5%	106 ± 9%	27 ± 4%	87 ± 8%	48 ± 6%
Carbachol	101 ± 2%	101 ± 5%	102 ± 3%	96 ± 3%	105 ± 3%

Among patient variables, there is no obvious relationship with demographic characteristics, and no studies examining the association with plasma levels and sialorrhea. A 2017 Cochrane review on clozapine dosing did note a lower risk for hypersalivation among those prescribed doses of 300 mg/day or less (RR 0.70, 95% CI 0.57 to 0.84) [14], but there are no studies to suggest that decreasing clozapine doses results in a meaningful reduction in sialorrhea. Chapter 7 contains a section entitled "Decreasing Plasma Clozapine Levels for Difficult to Manage Constipation" that presents a discussion of important considerations when deciding to lower clozapine plasma levels to manage an adverse effect. In select patients this may be a viable strategy when they are psychiatrically stable and minimally symptomatic, the plasma level is at the high end of the therapeutic range, and there is evidence that the patient may have been titrated very rapidly to this plasma level without allowing sufficient time to respond before each dose increase. Unlike constipation, there are no data to provide guidance on the extent to which decreasing the plasma clozapine level will improve sialorrhea severity. There is one potential genetic marker of interest that was found during a study of M_1, M_3 and alpha$_{2A}$-adrenergic receptor polymorphisms in 237 clozapine-treated Finnish patients. While no association was found between muscarinic subtype variants and sialorrhea, there was an association with an alpha$_{2A}$-adrenergic receptor single nucleotide polymorphism [15]. Although this finding requires replication, it supports the use of clonidine, an alpha$_{2A}$-adrenergic agonist, as a third-line treatment option due to the role that alpha$_{2A}$-adrenergic signaling plays in reflex salivary secretion.

 Treatment Principles

There are two overarching principles in managing sialorrhea: (a) recognize that this is a problem with potentially life-threatening medical consequences due to aspiration events; and (b) reserve systemic anticholinergic medications as treatments of last resort due to the doubling of ileus risk, which itself can be fatal. The choice of treatments proceeds from less-costly, locally applied anticholinergic preparations with limited systemic exposure, to more effective but costlier botulinum toxin-B injections. For patients who fail these strategies, one should always consider nonanticholinergic options before proceeding to glycopyrrolate, the systemic anticholinergic of choice due to its limited CNS penetration.

● Rating Scales

Rating scales must be used to track treatment response, with the goal of having no or minimal symptoms throughout the day, including while sleeping. While nocturnal sialorrhea presents a risk of aspiration, it is daytime sialorrhea that is the most socially disabling aspect of the problem, and may further contribute to the isolation of a severely mentally ill individual. Unfortunately, there are no comprehensive rating scales for sialorrhea that incorporate severity, frequency and social impact, although attempts have been made to create such a scale for Parkinson's disease patients [16]. Among the instruments commonly used in clinical trials, the two-item Drooling Severity and Frequency Scale (DSFS) was initially created in 1988 to

1. Track hypersalivation with rating scales. The two-item Drooling Severity and Frequency Scale is among the most commonly used instruments in sialorrhea trials. This can be supplemented with the subject-rated single-item Nocturnal Hypersalivation Rating Scale (see Table 9.3).

2. Use locally acting anticholinergic medications first: (a) atropine 1% drops sublingually starting at bedtime (1–3 drops) and increasing to a maximum dose of 3 drops TID; or (b) ipratropium 0.06% spray intraorally starting at bedtime (1–3 sprays) and increasing to a maximum dose of 3 sprays TID.

3. Given the extensive clinical trials for sialorrhea of various causes (medication induced, secondary to neurological disorders), botulinum toxin-B salivary gland injections should be pursued as a second-line agent due to the efficacy, tolerability and extended duration of benefit (up to 20 weeks).

4. If botulinum toxin-B injections are not effective, other nonanticholinergic options to consider include alpha-adrenergic modulators (e.g. clonidine) and amisulpride.

5. Systemic anticholinergic medication should be considered the treatment of last resort due to the twofold increased risk for ileus. If a systemic anticholinergic must be used, glycopyrrolate is the preferred medication due to limited CNS penetration. Antiparkinsonian medications and tricyclic antidepressants should not be used. The addition of glycopyrrolate must be accompanied by vigilant tracking of constipation, and aggressive management of gastrointestinal hypomotility should it occur.

quantify sialorrhea in cerebral palsy patients, and has been used extensively since [17]. Moreover, the DSFS was suggested by an expert panel exploring rating scale options for dysautonomia symptoms in Parkinson's disease patients [16]. The DSFS has good face validity and is comprised of two items: severity, rated on a 1–5-point scale, and frequency on a 1–4-point scale (Table 9.3), The Nocturnal Hypersalivation Rating Scale (NHS) is a validated single-item self-report instrument created in 1997 that rates severity on a 5-point scale (scored as 0–4) [18]. The combined use of both instruments requires very little clinician time and provides both objective and subjective measures that all members of the clinical team, patients and caregivers can readily understand. Given the simplicity of use, outpatient caregivers can easily provide ratings to the treating clinician between appointments so that dosage adjustments of locally applied medications can be made when symptoms are not

Table 9.3 Sialorrhea rating scales.

Scale	Clinician or self-rated	Measures	Items
Drooling Severity and Frequency Scale (DSFS) [17]	Clinician	Severity	*Drooling Severity Scale* 1 = Never drools, dry 2 = Mild – drooling, only lips wet 3 = Moderate – drool reaches the lips and chin 4 = Severe – drool drips off chin and onto clothing 5 = Profuse – drooling off the body and onto objects (furniture, books)
		Frequency	*Drooling Frequency Scale* 1 = No drooling 2 = Occasionally drools 3 = Frequently drools 4 = Constant drooling
Nocturnal Hypersalivation Rating Scale NHS [18]	Self	Severity	0 = Absent 1 = Minimal (signs of saliva on the pillow in the morning) 2 = Mild (hypersalivation wakes the patient up once during night) 3 = Moderate (hypersalivation wakes the patient up twice during night) 4 = Severe (hypersalivation wakes the patient up at least 3 times during night)

adequately controlled. The goal of treatment is to have DSFS frequency and severity scores of 2 or lower, and an NHS score of 0 or 1.

● Atropine Drops and Ipratropium Spray

Avoidance of systemic anticholinergics led clinicians to try orally applied existing products. Atropine is a potent nonselective muscarinic antagonist with a variety of uses and modes of delivery, while ipratropium is a quaternary amine derivative of atropine designed not to cross the blood–brain barrier when administered in larger doses as an inhaled medication for asthma or nasal congestion. The first reports of atropine 1% ophthalmic drops placed sublingually and ipratropium bromide 0.03% nasal spray appeared in 2001, and by 2005 these had come to be viewed as accepted and effective alternatives to systemic anticholinergics [19]. In subsequent case reports the higher strength of ipratropium bromide (0.06%) was recommended more commonly. As with many medications used to manage clozapine-related sialorrhea, there are virtually no adequately designed and reported clinical trials, although the accumulated case-based data provide compelling evidence for efficacy and tolerability to the extent that these agents are considered first-line therapies for this purpose. They are also readily available, inexpensive, and for the doses employed, lacking in systemic adverse effects. The biggest barriers to effective use are twofold: (a) need for multiple applications throughout the day; (b) decreased efficacy if the patient can't swish around the medication with a very small amount of water (< 5 ml). The latter is often problematic, as the patient themselves, staff or caregivers may use too much water for this step, diluting the medication and resulting in large amounts being rinsed out. If a patient fails one agent, try the other before proceeding to botulinum toxin. Despite the issues with atropine drops and ipratropium spray, these can be very effective options for some patients (see Table 9.4). The goals of treatment are minimal symptom ratings on the DSFS and NHS as noted previously. A DSFS score of 2 or more on frequency or severity, or NHS rating > 1 despite maximal doses of each agent should prompt consultation for botulinum toxin salivary gland injections.

● Botulinum Toxin-B

Botulinum toxin exerts its activity by binding to the presynaptic terminal of cholinergic neurons and subsequently entering the cytoplasm where it interferes with SNARE proteins that mediate vesicle fusion. The activated form of the toxin protein consists of two polypeptides: a 100-kDa heavy polypeptide joined via disulfide bonds to a 50-kDa lighter chain. The heavy chain contains binding regions for the presynaptic nerve terminals, and binding results in uptake of the toxin protein into a presynaptic vacuole [20]. The heavy chain then facilitates translocation of the separate light chain from the vacuole into the cytoplasm of the presynaptic neuron. The light chain is a protease that cleaves one of two SNARE proteins (SNAP-25, synaptobrevin) needed for vesicle fusion and release of synaptic acetylcholine. The net effect is loss of cholinergic neurotransmission and the classical symptoms of botulism: muscle weakness. As will be discussed below, when administered into nonmuscular areas (e.g. sweat or salivary glands), cholinergic activity is also diminished [21]. The

Table 9.4 Using atropine 1% solution and ipratropium bromide 0.06% spray for sialorrhea.

	Initial dose	Maximum dose	Comments on use
Atropine 1% ophthalmic drops	1–2 drops sublingually QHS	3 drops sublingually TID	• Swish with a very small amount of water (< 5 ml) and then spit • Using even a slightly larger volume of water will dilute the effect greatly • If a patient cannot swish and spit reliably, then simply have the drops placed under the tongue
Ipratropium bromide 0.06% nasal spray	1–3 sprays intraorally QHS	3 sprays intraorally TID	• Swish with a very small amount of water (< 5 ml) and then spit • Using even a slightly larger volume of water will dilute the effect greatly • If a patient cannot swish and spit reliably, then omit this step • If preferred, can spray under the tongue

physiologic effect slowly reverses over weeks and months as new SNARE proteins are slowly regenerated. As depicted in Figure 9.2, there are multiple botulinum toxin types that vary slightly in sequence and structure, and consequently act at different sites among the SNARE proteins. Only two forms are commercially used: botulinum toxin-A (BTX-A), which exists in several formulations with different potency, and botulinum toxin-B (BTX-B).

BTX-A was approved in 1989 to treat blepharospasm and strabismus, but has been widely used since for dystonia, spasticity, chronic pain, and cosmetic applications. Although the neuromuscular effects of BTX-A were the primary focus of drug development, it was known from animal studies that natural or pharmacologically delivered botulinum toxin induces parasympathetic abnormalities, especially when directly injected into postganglionic locations. Recognition that BTX-A might be useful for autonomic purposes was first reported in 1994 when clinicians treating three hemifacial spasm patients documented decreased localized sweating in a specific facial area that persisted over several months [21]. This led to expanded uses for patients with hyperhidrosis, and for sialorrhea via injections into the parotid and submandibular glands [22]. Botulinum toxin B (BTX-B), also known as rimabotulinumtoxinB, was first approved in December 2000 for cervical dystonia, but clinical experience revealed that for autonomic purposes it possessed earlier onset than BTX-A, perhaps related to the fact that BTX-B cleaves a site on the SNARE protein synaptobrevin, while BTX-A acts on

Figure 9.2. Specific locations where forms of botulinum toxin act on SNARE proteins.

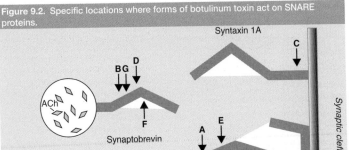

A-G: cleavage sites for various types of botulinum toxin

(Adapted from: Barr, J. R., Moura, H., Boyer, A. E., et al. (2005). Botulinum neurotoxin detection and differentiation by mass spectrometry. *Emerging Infectious Diseases*, 11, 1578–1583 [20].)

SNAP-25. In crossover trials for sialorrhea associated with amyotrophic lateral sclerosis or Parkinson's disease, the mean duration of benefit was comparable between the two agents (75 days BTX-A vs. 90 days for BTX-B), but the onset was 3 days sooner for BTX-B (mean 3.2 days) than for BTX-A (mean 6.6 days) [23].

As of 2017 there were six randomized, double-blind, placebo-controlled trials of BTX-B for sialorrhea of varying etiologies, with a mean duration of effect in larger studies of 19.2 weeks [9]. BTX-B treatment was well tolerated with no serious adverse events. The rates of presumed treatment-related adverse effects (dry mouth, change in saliva thickness, mild transient dysphagia, mild weakness of chewing) occurred in less than 10% of subjects. The studies varied in doses used and whether parotid and submandibular glands were both injected. The lowest dose was 1000 U into each parotid and 250 U into each submandibular gland, and the highest dose 4000 U into the parotid. Only one study used ultrasound guidance, as later studies found this unnecessary.

The first case report of BTX-A use for clozapine-related sialorrhea was in 2004 [24], and subsequent case reports documenting efficacy and tolerability for this use led to botulinum toxin being endorsed for clozapine-related sialorrhea in reviews published in 2007 and 2011 [19,25]. Despite the abundant efficacy data spanning 20 years across a range of disorders associated with sialorrhea, as recently as 2018 an article touted the potential use of botulinum toxin as a "novel treatment" for clozapine-induced sialorrhea [26]. The advantages of BTX-B in patients who have failed locally applied atropine or ipratropium include the long duration of action, potentially up to 4–6 months, and the absence of CNS or peripheral anticholinergic effects that would be experienced from systemic medications. In experienced hands the injection procedure is relatively quick once landmarks are mapped out. Ultrasound is not commonly used or deemed necessary. The injections are administered with a very fine 30-gauge needle that minimizes patient discomfort.

In major metropolitan areas a variety of physicians are available to administer these injections, particularly neurologists, otorhinolaryngologists, and also some physical medicine specialists who may work with cerebral palsy patients. Given the severity of clozapine-induced sialorrhea, injection of both parotid and submandibular glands is likely necessary using higher dosages of BTX-B, but doses can always be adjusted depending on the extent and duration of treatment response or complaints of adverse effects (primarily dry mouth). As with locally applied anticholinergics, the goal of treatment is to have DSFS frequency and severity scores of 2 or lower, and an NHS score of 0 or 1. Although the initial cost is greater than inexpensive prescribed medications, much of the system-wide expense will be recouped by avoiding hospital fees from treating aspiration pneumonia in patients with poorly controlled sialorrhea, hospital fees from treating ileus in patients who received systemic anticholinergics to manage sialorrhea, or psychiatric hospitalization costs when patients refuse to continue with clozapine treatment.

● Adrenergic Modulators (Clonidine)

Reflex salivary secretion is centrally mediated via $alpha_2$-adrenergic receptors, and agonists (e.g. clonidine and guanfacine) exert an inhibitory effect on salivary flow. While norclozapine itself acts through cholinergic agonism, a polymorphism in the $alpha_{2A}$-adrenergic receptor was associated with risk for clozapine-induced sialorrhea [15]. If replicated, this may increase enthusiasm for $alpha_{2A}$-adrenergic agonists in individuals with the particular variant if they exhibit unexpected benefit from these agents in clinical studies.

The sum total of the world's literature for guanfacine management of clozapine-induced sialorrhea is a single case report in 2004 in which 1 mg/day was effective and tolerated, although there are data in intellectually disabled children [19]. There is a much larger body of case reports for clonidine dating back to 1992, although no randomized trials. Some studies used the weekly transdermal patch delivering doses of 0.1–0.2 mg/day, while others have used oral doses up to 0.1 mg/day [19]. At these doses there was reduction in subjective complaints and severity of nocturnal salivation as measured by the wet area on the pillow. While these doses were tolerated, there is a risk of orthostasis and complaints of tiredness with use of alpha$_2$-adrenergic agonists, so they must be used cautiously and only in those who do not have current evidence of orthostasis, tachycardia or sedation. The oral form of clonidine is preferable to insure tolerability, and this can later be converted to transdermal patch if sufficiently effective. If effective, the primary advantage is avoidance of systemic anticholinergic effects and increased ileus risk. There is one retrospective chart review of the alpha$_1$-adrenergic receptor antagonist terazosin 2 mg QHS that appeared to show effectiveness comparable to benztropine for clozapine-related hypersalivation, but this has never been replicated and no cases reported in the subsequent literature [27]. As terazosin and clonidine both carry orthostasis risks, the former offers no advantage.

● Amisulpride and Sulpiride

Starting approximately 10 years ago, cases started to appear for use of the substituted benzamides to manage clozapine-related hypersalivation [28]. Although unavailable in North America, sulpiride and amisulpride are antipsychotics with high affinity for both dopamine D$_2$ and D$_3$ receptors, and no appreciable binding to muscarinic or alpha-adrenergic pathways [29]. While they have marked effects on prolactin secretion, there is a relatively lower risk for parkinsonism and akathisia than with typical antipsychotics, along with greater efficacy in some studies. Interestingly, and by unknown mechanisms, the addition of these agents at low doses has been reported to reduce the severity of hypersalivation, a fortuitous finding from an early trial of amisulpride augmentation for inadequate responders to clozapine [19]. In addition to case reports, the utility of this option is supported by a prospective randomized study of amisulpride 400 mg/day added to clozapine specifically for symptomatic sialorrhea ($n = 53$). During the 2 weeks of treatment with amisulpride, the mean NHS score dropped from 3.45 to 2.55 ($p < 0.0001$) [28]. While this is encouraging, the final NHS rating of 2.55 implies that patients are awakened on average of 1.5 times per night due to sialorrhea. Nonetheless, amisulpride was well tolerated, and thus provides another inexpensive nonanticholinergic strategy that could be sufficiently effective in some patients. Although 400 mg/day was used in the prospective amisulpride trial, there are case reports of efficacy at doses of

50–100 mg/day, and this is the recommended starting dose for this purpose [30]. The amisulpride dose can be advanced every 2 weeks based on response using the DSFS and NHS scores. In clozapine augmentation studies for schizophrenia symptoms doses up to 800 mg/day have been used, but these higher amisulpride doses may incur risks of QT prolongation and might offer no greater benefit for sialorrhea [31].

● Glycopyrrolate

While the use of systemic anticholinergics will increase the risk of ileus, at times they must be used when patients have failed other treatment modalities. For these patients the medication of choice is glycopyrrolate, a potent antagonist across all muscarinic receptor subtypes that does not cross the blood–brain barrier. For this reason it is preferable to any medication that has CNS effects, such as anticholinergic antiparkinsonian agents or tricyclic antidepressants [32]. Clozapine itself presents a significant CNS anticholinergic burden, so there is no compelling reason to add to this effect, particularly when glycopyrrolate has demonstrable efficacy for sialorrhea of varying etiologies in numerous randomized clinical trials [33]. Moreover, when directly compared to biperiden in a randomized, double-blind, crossover study, glycopyrrolate did not adversely impact cognition in a manner seen with biperiden [32].

Glycopyrrolate has erratic oral absorption with a reported T_{Max} of 5 hours. The duration of clinical effect is not well quantified in the literature, but most studies use BID dosing unless the target is only nocturnal sialorrhea. Box 9.2 presents the principles involved when adding a potent anticholinergic medication to existing clozapine therapy, and the need for vigilance in managing the expected worsening of constipation.

Box 9.2 Considerations During Use of Glycopyrrolate for Sialorrhea

1. Glycopyrrolate should be considered the treatment of last resort after patients have failed botulinum toxin-B. As a potent nonselective muscarinic antagonist, it will increase risk of ileus twofold.

2. Constipation must be tracked aggressively when added to clozapine-treated patients. Consider increasing the doses of laxative agents when starting glycopyrrolate, or adding another class of medication if at maximal daily doses of current agents.

3. The starting dose is 1 mg BID, and this can be advanced every 1–2 weeks based on DSFS and NHS ratings, assuming that constipation is adequately managed.

4. The maximum daily dose is 8 mg/day.

Summary Points

a. Sialorrhea is a highly prevalent condition that may affect nearly 90% of clozapine-treated patients, and has medical and social consequences.

b. Orally applied anticholinergics (atropine 1% solution, ipratropium bromide 0.06% spray) are the first-line treatments due to low cost and limited systemic absorption.

c. Botulinum toxin-B (BTX-B) injection into the parotid and submandibular glands has proven effective for sialorrhea from numerous etiologies (e.g. medications, neurological disorders) with six double-blind, placebo-controlled trials through 2017. It is the second-line agent of choice. BTX-B has onset within 4 days of the injection, duration of action that lasts 3–6 months, and no systemic effects.

d. Clonidine or amisulpride can be considered if the clinician wants to avoid using a systemic anticholinergic due to the increased ileus risk.

e. Systemic anticholinergic medications are the treatments of last resort after patients have failed orally applied medications (atropine, ipratropium) and botulinum toxin-B injections, due to increased ileus risk. Agents with CNS penetration (e.g. antiparkinsonian medications, tricyclic antidepressants) should not be used due to the adverse impact on cognition. Glycopyrrolate is the systemic anticholinergic of choice.

References

1. Maher, S., Cunningham, A., O'Callaghan, N., et al. (2016). Clozapine-induced hypersalivation: An estimate of prevalence, severity and impact on quality of life. *Therapeutic Advances in Psychopharmacology*, 6, 178–184.

2. Legge, S. E., Hamshere, M., Hayes, R. D., et al. (2016). Reasons for discontinuing clozapine: A cohort study of patients commencing treatment. *Schizophrenia Research*, 174, 113–119.

3. Kaplan, J., Schwartz, A. C. and Ward, M. C. (2018). Clozapine-associated aspiration pneumonia: Case series and review of the literature. *Psychosomatics*, 59, 199–203.

4. Leung, J. G., Hasassri, M. E., Barreto, J. N., et al. (2017). Characterization of admission types in medically hospitalized patients prescribed clozapine. *Psychosomatics*, 58, 164–172.

5. De Fazio, P., Gaetano, R., Caroleo, M., et al. (2015). Rare and very rare adverse effects of clozapine. *Neuropsychiatric Disease and Treatment*, 11, 1995–2003.

6. Syed, R., Au, K., Cahill, C., et al. (2008). Pharmacological interventions for clozapine-induced hypersalivation. *Cochrane Database of Systematic Reviews*, 3, Cd005579.

7. Freudenreich, O. (2005). Drug-induced sialorrhea. *Drugs Today (Barcelona)*, 41, 411–418.

8. Restivo, D. A., Panebianco, M., Casabona, A., et al. (2018). Botulinum toxin A for sialorrhoea associated with neurological disorders: Evaluation of the relationship between effect of treatment and the number of glands treated. *Toxins (Basel)*, 10, E55–63.

9. Dashtipour, K., Bhidayasiri, R., Chen, J. J., et al. (2017). RimabotulinumtoxinB in sialorrhea: Systematic review of clinical trials. *Journal of Clinical Movement Disorders*, 4, 9–17.

10. Proctor, G. B. and Carpenter, G. H. (2014). Salivary secretion: mechanism and neural regulation. *Monographs in Oral Sciences*, 24, 14–29.

11. Ryberg, A. T., Warfvinge, G., Axelsson, L., et al. (2008). Expression of muscarinic receptor subtypes in salivary glands of rats, sheep and man. *Archives of Oral Biology*, 53, 66–74.

12. Sugawara, Y., Kikuchi, Y., Yoneda, M., et al. (2016). Electrophysiological evidence showing muscarinic agonist-antagonist activities of N-desmethylclozapine using hippocampal excitatory and inhibitory neurons. *Brain Research*, 1642, 255–262.

13. Schneider, B., Weigmann, H., Hiemke, C., et al. (2004). Reduction of clozapine-induced hypersalivation by pirenzepine is safe. *Pharmacopsychiatry*, 37, 43–45.

14. Subramanian, S., Vollm, B. A. and Huband, N. (2017). Clozapine dose for schizophrenia. *Cochrane Database of Systematic Reviews*, 6, Cd009555.

15. Solismaa, A., Kampman, O., Seppälä, N., et al. (2014). Polymorphism in alpha 2A adrenergic receptor gene is associated with sialorrhea in schizophrenia patients on clozapine treatment. *Human Psychopharmacology Clinical and Experimental*, 29, 336–341.

16. Evatt, M. L., Chaudhuri, K. R., Chou, K. L., et al. (2009). Dysautonomia rating scales in Parkinson's disease: Sialorrhea, dysphagia, and constipation – Critique and recommendations by movement disorders task force on rating scales for Parkinson's disease. *Movement Disorders*, 24, 635–646.

17. Thomas-Stonell, N. and Greenberg, J. (1988). Three treatment approaches and clinical factors in the reduction of drooling. *Dysphagia*, 3, 73–78.

9

18. Spivak, B., Adlersberg, S., Rosen, L., et al. (1997). Trihexyphenidyl treatment of clozapine-induced hypersalivation. *International Clinical Psychopharmacology*, 12, 213–215.

19. Sockalingam, S., Shammi, C. and Remington, G. (2007). Clozapine-induced hypersalivation: A review of treatment strategies. *Canadian Journal of Psychiatry*, 52, 377–384.

20. Barr, J. R., Moura, H., Boyer, A. E., et al. (2005). Botulinum neurotoxin detection and differentiation by mass spectrometry. *Emerging Infectious Diseases*, 11, 1578–1583.

21. Bushara, K. O. and Park, D. M. (1994). Botulinum toxin and sweating. *Journal of Neurology, Neurosurgery, and Psychiatry*, 57, 1437–1438.

22. Petracca, M., Guidubaldi, A., Ricciardi, L., et al. (2015). Botulinum Toxin A and B in sialorrhea: Long-term data and literature overview. *Toxicon*, 107, 129–140.

23. Guidubaldi, A., Fasano, A., Ialongo, T., et al. (2011). Botulinum toxin A versus B in sialorrhea: A prospective, randomized, double-blind, crossover pilot study in patients with amyotrophic lateral sclerosis or Parkinson's disease. *Movement Disorders*, 26, 313–319.

24. Kahl, K. G., Hagenah, J., Zapf, S., et al. (2004). Botulinum toxin as an effective treatment of clozapine-induced hypersalivation. *Psychopharmacology (Berlin)*, 173, 229–230.

25. Bird, A. M., Smith, T. L. and Walton, A. E. (2011). Current treatment strategies for clozapine-induced sialorrhea. *Annals of Pharmacotherapy*, 45, 667–675.

26. Verma, R. and Anand, K. S. (2018). Botulinum toxin: A novel therapy for clozapine-induced sialorrhoea. *Psychopharmacology (Berlin)*, 235, 369–371.

27. Reinstein, M., Sirotovskya, L. and Chasonov, M. (1999). Comparative efficacy and tolerability of benzatropine and terazosin in the treatment of hypersalivation secondary to clozapine. *Clinical Drug Investigation*, 17, 97–102.

28. Kreinin, A., Miodownik, C., Sokolik, S., et al. (2011). Amisulpride versus moclobemide in treatment of clozapine-induced hypersalivation. *World Journal of Biological Psychiatry*, 12, 620–626.

29. Loy, F., Isola, M., Isola, R., et al. (2014). The antipsychotic amisulpride: Ultrastructural evidence of its secretory activity in salivary glands. *Oral Diseases*, 20, 796–802.

30. Kulkarni, R. R. (2015). Low-dose amisulpride for debilitating clozapine-induced sialorrhea: Case series and review of literature. *Indian Journal of Psychological Medicine*, 37, 446–448.

31. Barnes, T. R., Leeson, V. C., Paton, C., et al. (2017). Amisulpride augmentation in clozapine-unresponsive schizophrenia (AMICUS): A double-blind, placebo-controlled, randomised trial of clinical effectiveness and cost-effectiveness. *Health Technology Assessment*, 21, 1–56.

32. Liang, C. S., Ho, P. S., Shen, L. J., et al. (2010). Comparison of the efficacy and impact on cognition of glycopyrrolate and biperiden for clozapine-induced sialorrhea in schizophrenic patients: A randomized, double-blind, crossover study. *Schizophrenia Research*, 119, 138–144.

33. Man, W. H., Colen-de Koning, J. C., Schulte, P. F., et al. (2017). The effect of glycopyrrolate on nocturnal sialorrhea in patients using clozapine: A randomized, crossover, double-blind, placebo-controlled trial. *Journal of Clinical Psychopharmacology*, 37, 155–161.

34. Weiner, D. M., Meltzer, H. Y., Veinbergs, I., et al. (2004). The role of M1 muscarinic receptor agonism of *N*-desmethylclozapine in the unique clinical effects of clozapine. *Psychopharmacology*, 177, 207–216.

35. Doran, A., Obach, R. S., Smith, B. J., et al. (2005). The impact of P-glycoprotein on the disposition of drugs targeted for indications of the central nervous system: Evaluation using the MDR1A/1B knockout mouse model. *Drug Metabolism and Disposition*, 33, 165–174.

10 Managing Seizure Risk and Stuttering

INTRODUCTION

While weight gain and other adverse effects can be challenging to treat, seizure management is extremely successful to the extent that recent reviews comment that it should never be a reason to discontinue clozapine treatment [1]. Evidence suggests that psychiatric providers may have adopted this position, as case data on 316 new clozapine starts from 2007 to 2011 at the South London and Maudsley National Health Service Foundation Trust did not list seizures among reasons for clozapine cessation, although 20 other types of adverse drug reactions were cited [2]. Seizures are not unique to clozapine, and antipsychotic package insert warnings in the United States consider this a class effect, although the mechanisms for this common property remain unknown. Recent reviews note rates ranging from 0.2% to 0.5% with other antipsychotics, and a 9% incidence with high-dose chlorpromazine ($\geq$ 1000 mg/day) [3]. Experience during clinical trials led Novartis to include the following package insert warning:

PRINCIPLES

- Seizures are not uncommon but easily managed in most patients. It should never be a reason to discontinue clozapine treatment.

- Routine EEG screening is not warranted due to the high prevalence of minor findings, and should not be used in asymptomatic patients. Seizure treatment is based on clinically evident seizure activity.

- The relationship between dose (or plasma level) and seizure induction is not clear as some develop seizures during the early titration at low doses.

- Seizures often occur shortly after a dose increase, or after a jump in plasma level due to addition of a cytochrome P450 inhibitor or removal of an inducer (e.g. smoking cessation). Patients who have tolerated stable high levels for months without seizure activity do not require additional measures.

- New-onset stuttering has been observed rarely during titration or after dose increases and is hypothesized to be related to subclinical epileptiform activity. Dose reduction and slower retitration resolve the problem.

- Due to the low prevalence of seizures, prophylactic anticonvulsants should not be used as these will be unnecessary in > 90% of patients.

- When an anticonvulsant is needed, divalproex is the medication of choice as it best covers the spectrum of tonic–clonic and myoclonic events and has modest kinetic interactions with clozapine.

10

Seizure has been estimated to occur in association with clozapine use at a cumulative incidence at one year of approximately 5%, based on the occurrence of one or more seizures in 61 of 1743 patients exposed to clozapine during its clinical testing prior to domestic marketing (i.e., a crude rate of 3.5%). The risk of seizure is dose related.

The first large data set covering 1481 clozapine-treated patients was published in 1991, and reported a seizure rate of 2.8% [4]. The data also indicated a dose-dependent relationship, with a rate of 1.0% at doses < 300 mg/day, 2.7% for 300–599 mg/day, and 4.4% at doses ≥ 600 mg/day [3]. Although the incidence in this group was 2.8%, the authors estimated the cumulative risk as high as 10% at 3.8 years. However, a subsequent 1994 analysis by these same authors of 5629 patients found only 71 cases of tonic–clonic seizures, or a rate of 1.3% [5]. Of relevance to the debate about dose and seizure risk, the 1994 review noted that seizures tended to occur in two patterns: at low doses (< 300 mg/day) during the titration phase, and at high doses (≥ 600 mg/day) during the maintenance phase [5]. The only other risk was a prior history of seizures or epilepsy, with seizures in those patients often occurring early in treatment at low doses. Of those who were rechallenged, 78.3% continued on clozapine.

Although the 1994 postmarketing incidence of 1.3% is closer to that seen with other antipsychotics, subsequent case series with variable periods of exposures reported incidence rates as high as 22% [3]. Given the greater scrutiny with clozapine treatment, and the lack of systematic tracking for other antipsychotics, the true incidence and the magnitude of risk difference compared to other antipsychotics may never be known. As noted in Box 10.1, this is one of several unresolved issues with regards to the association between clozapine treatment and seizure induction.

Box 10.1 Ongoing Debates Regarding Clozapine and Seizure Risk [3]

1. What is the relative risk of seizures for clozapine-treated patients compared to those on other antipsychotics?

2. Does rapid titration increase seizure risk?

3. Is there a well-defined dose (and plasma level) threshold for increased seizure risk?

A 2015 paper neatly sums up the issues after an extensive review of the relevant literature:

> Clinically, most practitioners have adopted a theoretical maximum of 600 mg/day, but the literature presents several cases of seizures occurring at lower doses. The same controversies and uncertainties exist for the ability to predict increased risk of seizure using clozapine serum concentrations. The utility of clozapine serum concentration for the purpose of seizure prevention is debated within the literature, mainly because of the lack of a well-established concentration threshold. It would be a safe assumption that seizure is more likely at higher concentrations (i.e. > 1000 ng/ml or > 3057 nmol/l), but similar to total oral dose, seizures still occur at lower concentrations (i.e. < 300 ng/ml or < 900 nmol/l). Based on conflicting evidence, clozapine-induced seizures are not solely based on total dose or serum concentration. [3]

While this lack of certainty may appear daunting, the unclear relationship between many of these variables and the appearance of clinically evident seizures implies that the titration of clozapine should be made primarily with regards to the usual tolerability concerns including orthostasis and sedation. Moreover, the absence of a well-defined plasma-level relationship supports the use of clozapine at levels up to 1000 ng/ml or 3057 nmol/l if lower levels are tolerated and there is a need for greater efficacy (see Table 5.8) [6].

Box 10.2 General Principles Governing Clozapine Treatment and Seizure Risk

1. Due to the absence of a clear relationship between seizure induction and the rapidity of titration or dose, early dose adjustments should be based on other tolerability concerns (e.g. orthostasis, sedation).

2. Electroencephalographic (EEG) abnormalities without clinical seizure activity are not uncommon in clozapine-treated patients. Routine EEG monitoring is not recommended and should be performed only when clinically evident actions raise the suspicion of a seizure.

3. Patients in need of greater efficacy should not be deprived of clozapine treatment with levels as high as 1000 ng/ml or 3057 nmol/l due to concerns about seizures.

4. Divalproex is the anticonvulsant of choice for clozapine-related tonic–clonic, myoclonic or atonic seizures. Due to the risks of divalproex treatment (e.g. neutropenia, thrombocytopenia, weight gain, hyperammonemia), and the low incidence of clozapine-related seizures even at higher plasma clozapine levels, patients should not be placed on routine prophylactic anticonvulsant therapy.

5. Seizures often occur after a recent dose increase (e.g. titration phase) or an increased plasma level due to kinetic factors (addition of a CYP inhibitor, removal of a CYP inducer, smoking cessation). Patients who tolerate high levels without seizure activity do not require additional measures.

6. If a seizure occurs:

   a. **Scenario 1: After a dose adjustment or due to mitigating kinetic factors.** Obtain a plasma clozapine level (ideally as a 12-hour trough), hold clozapine for 24 hours, and reduce back to the prior tolerated clozapine dose (if after a dose increase), or adjust the dose based on the expected kinetic effect. (See Chapter 5 for discussion of kinetic effects of various CYP 450 inhibitors and smoking cessation.) Recheck the plasma clozapine level at steady state. Presumably the patient will remain seizure-free at a plasma level previously tolerated. If a second seizure occurs, or higher plasma levels are anticipated due to the need for further titration, add divalproex.

   b. **Scenario 2: No recent dose adjustment or known kinetic factors.** Obtain a plasma clozapine level (ideally as a 12-hour trough), check renal and hepatic function, look at medication history, hold clozapine for 24 hours and reduce the dose by 25%. If no cause can be found (e.g. benzodiazepine or alcohol withdrawal), and the plasma level is consistent with prior stable levels, add divalproex. If levels are > 30% above prior stable levels, adjust the clozapine dose, and recheck the plasma clozapine level at steady state. Presumably the patient will remain seizure-free at a plasma level previously tolerated. If a second seizure occurs, add divalproex.

10

Table 10.1 Seizure types and frequency reported in literature reviews [3,7].		
	Wong and Delva (2007) (mean rates)	Williams and Park (2015) (range)
Generalized		
• Tonic–clonic	54%	17.5–70.0%
• Myoclonic and/or atonic	28%	25–42.8%
• Tonic–clonic with other seizure types	12%	
Partial		6%
• Simple	3%	
• Complex	3%	

 Types of Clozapine-Associated Seizure Activity

Two extensive reviews of clozapine-associated seizures are summarized in Table 10.1 [3,7]. The most common seizure is a generalized or tonic–clonic event. Although individual papers report a wide range of values, generalized seizures comprise more than half of reported events. Less obvious but equally important are myoclonic or atonic seizures. Myoclonic events without loss of consciousness may present as jerks or tic-like movements anywhere in the body, but more commonly in the limbs or facial region. The latter at times can be confused with tardive dyskinesia, but clinical context will usually help clarify the situation (e.g. occurrence during clozapine titration). Atonic attacks result in loss of muscle tone, with individuals falling when occurring in the lower limbs. These "drop attacks" may be mistaken for orthostasis or the consequence of sedation, but the patient will often provide a compelling history of an event occurring without dizziness, and due to abrupt loss of muscle tone. Absence of orthostasis can be confirmed with blood pressure measurements. Recognition of myoclonic and atonic events is important not only to prevent injury, but due to the possible risk of a secondary generalized seizure. Partial seizures (simple or complex) are very uncommon, and there is only one case report in the literature of absence seizures that occurred in a 15-year-old patient [3].

 Routine EEG Monitoring or Anticonvulsant Prophylaxis

Although the seizure incidence is under 5%, clinical interest spurred a number of electroencephalographic (EEG) studies in clinically asymptomatic clozapine-treated patients, some dating back to 1978. Two important conclusions emerged from this literature:

a. High rates of asymptomatic EEG abnormalities can be found in clozapine-treated patients, and the prevalence is linearly related to the plasma clozapine level [8–10].

b. While there is a relationship between clozapine dose/plasma level and clozapine-related EEG abnormalities, a relationship between dose/plasma level and occurrence of seizures is not evident [10].

The latter point is critical, as close to 70% of patients whose plasma clozapine level is 350 ng/ml or 1070 nmol/l, the typical threshold for clinical response, will manifest some form of EEG abnormality [10]. However, less than 5% of these patients might have clinical evidence of seizure activity. It is for this reason that routine EEG monitoring is not recommended: more than 95% of the asymptomatic patients administered prophylactic anticonvulsants based solely on EEG findings will not benefit, but may sustain adverse effects. As will be discussed below, divalproex is the anticonvulsant of choice for clozapine-related seizures, but its use increases the risk for neutropenia twofold [11]. Moreover, divalproex combined with clozapine will result in additional weight gain. For patients without a seizure history an EEG is best reserved for confirmation of an unwitnessed generalized seizure, or when a patient presents with myoclonic or atonic events without secondary generalization. For patients without a seizure history, anticonvulsant treatment should only be implemented when there is clinically evident seizure activity.

Patients with a known seizure disorder can be treated with clozapine, with multiple case reports of successful therapy [3]. The underlying seizure disorder should be managed with an anticonvulsant prior to commencing clozapine, and the patient ideally should be seizure-free. Nonetheless, there is one case report of a psychotic patient with treatment-resistant epilepsy (including episodes of status epilepticus) whose psychosis markedly improved on clozapine 300 mg/day without an increase in the seizure frequency [12]. The preferred anticonvulsant is divalproex as it best covers the spectrum of clozapine-associated seizures and has modest kinetic effects. In large kinetic modeling studies, valproic acid was estimated to increase clozapine levels in nonsmokers with effect size 16%, and reduce level in smokers with effect size 22% [13]. The issues with weight gain and neutropenia have been noted, but use of divalproex also doubles myocarditis risk, although this is only of relevance during the first 6 weeks of clozapine treatment [14]. Nonetheless, divalproex presents the best option for long-term treatment. As noted in Chapter 5, the anticonvulsants phenytoin and carbamazepine lower clozapine levels by 50% and are to be avoided; achieving therapeutic plasma clozapine levels with this kinetic effect might not be

possible with the dosing limit of 900 mg/day in most countries. If the patient has been
stabilized on other anticonvulsants that have limited kinetic interactions with clozapine
(e.g. lamotrigine, topiramate, gabapentin, levetiracetam) no action need be taken.
For asymptomatic patients, there is no value in routine EEG surveillance; however, a
treating neurologist might opt for periodic monitoring in select patients who have had
prior difficulty achieving seizure control.

C The Relationship of Seizures to Dose or Plasma Level

The data from the 1991 paper continue to be widely quoted as evidence that seizure
risk increases in a dose-dependent fashion, yet many fail to refer to the much lower
rates cited in the 1994 paper with a sample size four times greater. As the data in Box
10.3 illustrate, not only is the overall rate lower in the 1994 sample, but the absolute
risk in patients with no prior seizure history is 1.5% on doses ≥ 600 mg/day, compared
to 0.9% for patients on the lowest doses [5]. Based on this risk difference, the number
needed to harm for higher doses is 166, meaning that one would have to treat 166
patients with doses ≥ 600 mg/day to have one additional patient experience a seizure
compared to doses < 300 mg/day. Another finding that often escapes mention is that
the greatest risk occurs in the lower and higher dosage ranges for those with no prior
seizure history. This would imply that some degree of tolerance to the impact on seizure
threshold may develop during titration, but that higher doses may eventually exceed
this capacity in some patients. With the exception of overdose situations with levels
>> 1000 ng/ml or >> 3057 nmol/l, data from the past 25 years fail to substantiate a
robust relationship between dose or plasma level and clinically evident seizure activity
[3]. That the rates for patients at higher doses are under 2% also argues against routine
anticonvulsant prophylaxis for any patient without a prior seizure history. Moreover,
once patients have achieved steady state after a dose increase and shown no seizure
activity after weeks or months, one can be reassured that, for this patient, that plasma
level appears insufficient to induce a seizure. When a seizure occurs in a patient on a
stable dose, one must look for kinetic interactions that may have abruptly increased the

Box 10.3 Rates of Seizures by Dosing Groups During Early Clozapine Studies [4,5]

	< 300 mg/day	300–599 mg/day	≥ 600 mg/day
1991 (N = 1481)	1.0%	2.7%	4.4%
1994 (N = 5629)	1.6%	0.9%	1.9%
1994 (N = 5629)*	0.9%	0.8%	1.5%

*Excluding patients with prior seizure history.

plasma clozapine level (e.g. addition of a cytochrome P450 [CYP] inhibitor, withdrawal of a CYP inducer, smoking cessation, renal or hepatic failure) or other factors that lowered the seizure threshold (e.g. alcohol or benzodiazepine withdrawal).

Although the data indicate seizures can occur during the early titration phase, the overall rate is low in those without a seizure history (0.9%), and may not relate to the rapidity of titration, despite manufacturer warnings to the contrary. Recent data from two studies of rapid clozapine titration for treatment-resistant schizophrenia or bipolar patients found no seizures among 155 inpatients [3]. In the schizophrenia trial ($n = 111$), the mean dose of 409 mg/day was reached after an average of 7.1 days [15]. Given the idiosyncratic and unpredictable nature of seizure occurrence, dosage titrations should proceed based on other clinical considerations of tolerability and efficacy, as it is unclear to what extent any titration schedule may impact seizure risk.

 D **New-Onset Stuttering**

There are 18 cases of new-onset stuttering in clozapine-treated patients, with a survey study of 654 clozapine patients in west of Ireland noting six cases, or a prevalence slightly under 1.0% [16]. Although there is no evidence of generalized seizure activity, and several cases specifically report normal EEGs, myoclonic jerking has been noted in some instances, and all cases have emerged during titration or after dose increase, a pattern commonly seen with clozapine-induced seizures. For this reason, the authors have hypothesized about the relationship with abnormal electrical activity, although this remains speculative, particularly where the EEG was normal [16]. Dose reduction usually resolves the problem; however, when this is ineffective or results in psychotic exacerbation, there are multiple case reports supporting the efficacy of an anticonvulsant. Orobuccolingual dyskinesia has been present in some cases, although typically this causes problems with articulation and not language fluency. The approach to dyskinesia would be the same as for other patients with tardive dyskinesia (see Chapter 13).

10

E **Treatment of Seizures**

As with many aspects of clozapine-related care, there is an absence of systematic trials examining various initial approaches (i.e. dose reduction, dose division) or the comparative merits of anticonvulsants. The general principles outlined in Box 10.2 represent a synthesis of recommendations that generally agree on three points:

a. Reduce exposure to clozapine shortly after a seizure.

b. If not occurring during titration or after a dose increase, investigate possible causes.

c. If the patient is anticipated to require dose (and plasma levels) above that which induced the seizure, or if a second seizure occurs, divalproex is the preferred anticonvulsant.

As clozapine's greatest effect on seizure threshold occurs when brain concentrations are at their peak, some publications (and manufacturer recommendations) suggest

Table 10.2 Anticonvulsants for clozapine-related seizures.*

	Supporting data	Concerns
	Preferred options	
Divalproex/ valproate	• Effective for generalized seizures, is the medication of choice for myoclonic/atonic seizures • Very modest kinetic interactions with clozapine • Can be orally loaded at 30 mg/kg over 24 hours • Greatest number of published case reports with clozapine • Good tolerability	• Weight gain • Increased neutropenia risk, especially with higher serum valproate levels • Thrombocytopenia • Hyperammonemia
Lamotrigine	• Effective for generalized seizures and recommended for myoclonic epilepsy when divalproex/valproate cannot be used • Good tolerability when titrated appropriately, limited weight gain • No kinetic interactions with clozapine • One case report with clozapine	• Risk of Stevens–Johnson Syndrome/toxic epidermal necrolysis with rapid titration • Modified titration required when added to divalproex/ valproate due to kinetic interaction • Cannot be loaded. May require many weeks before therapeutic
Gabapentin	• No kinetic interactions with clozapine • Two case reports with clozapine	• Not effective for myoclonic seizures
Topiramate	• No kinetic interactions with clozapine • May induce weight loss • Two case reports with clozapine	• Not effective for myoclonic seizures • May cause cognitive dysfunction • Metabolic acidosis

continued overleaf

Table 10.2 continued

	Supporting data	Concerns
	Medications to avoid	
Phenytoin	• Report of combined use with clozapine (from nationwide surveillance data)	• Lowers plasma clozapine levels ≥ 50% • Lowers plasma levels of other antipsychotics • Not effective for myoclonic seizures • Risk of Stevens–Johnson syndrome/toxic epidermal necrolysis
Carbamazepine	• Report of combined use with clozapine (from nationwide surveillance data) • One case report of use for clozapine-related myoclonus	• Lowers plasma clozapine levels ≥ 50% • Lowers plasma levels of other antipsychotics • Hyponatremia • Risk of Stevens–Johnson syndrome/toxic epidermal necrolysis in certain Asian groups – mandatory genotyping for HLA-B*1502 in at-risk individuals • Rare aplastic anemia and agranulocytosis • Can exacerbate myoclonus in some patients
Levetiracetam	• No kinetic interactions with clozapine • Effective for myoclonic seizures	• Higher rates of neuropsychiatric adverse effects than other anticonvulsants • No data on use with clozapine
Clonazepam	• Adjunctive benefit for nonclozapine-related myoclonic epilepsy • Multiple case reports of combined use with clozapine in patients with tardive dystonia	• Cognitive dysfunction, sedation and fall risk • Potential for misuse and dependence • No data on use with clozapine as an anticonvulsant

* For patients who have become pregnant or are planning a pregnancy, immediate consultation with a neurologist is necessary due to the increased risk of physical anomalies and neurodevelopmental impairment posed by anticonvulsants [20].

converting QHS doses into divided dosing with the goal of reducing the C_{Max}. This may temporarily obviate the need for an anticonvulsant, but for patients who seize during the titration phase at subtherapeutic plasma levels, there is a significant likelihood that another seizure will occur as the dose is increased further. Moreover, dividing the dose incurs greater daytime sedation, and also may decrease outpatient medication adherence compared to QHS dosing. For these reasons, adding divalproex when patients have a seizure during dose titration may be prudent in most circumstances.

There are no controlled anticonvulsant trials for clozapine-related seizures, yet divalproex has emerged as the medication of choice based on several criteria noted in Table 10.2, including its spectrum of activity that covers myoclonic seizures [3]. Due to the association between higher serum valproate levels and neutropenia (see Chapter 6), the lowest effective dose should be used to achieve effective seizure control. If neutropenia does occur, it can be managed with the strategies outlined in Chapter 6. The additive weight gain risk must be acknowledged and addressed as quickly as possible using all the options mentioned in Chapter 11. There is a paucity of cases on other agents, but lamotrigine can be considered a second-line option for this purpose if the patient cannot tolerate divalproex. Lamotrigine must be titrated slowly to avoid risk of Stevens–Johnson Syndrome/toxic epidermal necrolysis, and if lamotrigine is added to existing divalproex therapy the modified titration dosing schedule must be followed due to the inhibition of lamotrigine metabolism by divalproex.

The older agents phenytoin and carbamazepine are avoided primarily for their significant kinetic interactions with clozapine (and numerous other medications), and carbamazepine's small risk of neutropenia, yet there are early case reports of carbamazepine–clozapine combination therapy [17,18]. Levetiracetam is a frequently used anticonvulsant in the general population due to its spectrum of activity and absence of kinetic interactions, but this medication should be avoided in those with severe mental illness due to the high prevalence of neuropsychiatric side effects, combined with the absence of any case data for use with clozapine [19]. If a patient is planning to become pregnant or a pregnancy occurs, immediate neurologist consultation must be sought due to the risk for developmental anomalies and long-term cognitive effects associated with anticonvulsant use [20].

 Clozapine and ECT

An estimated 40–50% of treatment-resistant schizophrenia patients may fail to adequately respond to clozapine. As discussed in Chapter 2, one evidence-based strategy is the use of adjunctive electroconvulsive therapy (ECT). The practical concern with combined clozapine and ECT is the induction of prolonged seizures, but this was recently addressed in a comprehensive review published in 2015 [21]. Utilizing data from case reports and a small number of open-label trials (40 total publications), data on 208 patients who underwent combined treatment with clozapine and ECT was amassed. Most were adults with treatment-resistant schizophrenia spectrum disorders to whom ECT was added to clozapine for inadequate response. Short-term response rates varying from 37.5% to 100% were reported, with a small number of cases documenting sustained improvement over periods ranging from 3 weeks to 24 months. Side effects were as follows: delirium $n = 5$, tachycardia $n = 5$, and prolonged seizures $n = 4$ [21]. Given the large number of cases and low rates of adverse effects the authors concluded that the combination was effective and safe, and should be used in patients with treatment-resistant schizophrenia and inadequate clozapine response.

Summary Points

a. The seizure incidence is much lower than most clinicians anticipate, and there are no compelling data to support a strong association with rapidity of titration or dose/plasma level.

b. Seizures are never a reason to discontinue clozapine treatment.

c. Generalized (tonic–clonic) seizures are the most common form in clozapine-treated patients, but clinicians should be alert for myoclonic or atonic events occurring without secondary generalization and address these in the same manner as generalized seizures.

d. The management strategy is straightforward and depends on whether the seizure was associated with a titration, dose increase or jump in plasma clozapine levels, or due to other factors (e.g. alcohol or benzodiazepine withdrawal).

e. Divalproex is the anticonvulsant of choice due to its spectrum of activity (generalized and myoclonic seizures), preponderance of case data for clozapine-related seizures, and modest kinetic interactions.

10

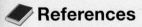

References

1. Nielsen, J., Correll, C. U., Manu, P., et al. (2013). Termination of clozapine treatment due to medical reasons: When is it warranted and how can it be avoided? *Journal of Clinical Psychiatry*, 74, 603–613.

2. Legge, S. E., Hamshere, M., Hayes, R. D., et al. (2016). Reasons for discontinuing clozapine: A cohort study of patients commencing treatment. *Schizophrenia Research*, 174, 113–119.

3. Williams, A. M. and Park, S. H. (2015). Seizure associated with clozapine: Incidence, etiology, and management. *CNS Drugs*, 29, 101–111.

4. Devinsky, O., Honigfeld, G. and Patin, J. (1991). Clozapine-related seizures. *Neurology*, 41, 369–371.

5. Pacia, S. V. and Devinsky, O. (1994). Clozapine-related seizures: Experience with 5,629 patients. *Neurology*, 44, 2247–2249.

6. Remington, G., Agid, O., Foussias, G., et al. (2013). Clozapine and therapeutic drug monitoring: Is there sufficient evidence for an upper threshold? *Psychopharmacology (Berlin)*, 225, 505–518.

7. Wong, J. and Delva, N. (2007). Clozapine-induced seizures: Recognition and treatment. *Canadian Journal of Psychiatry – Revue Canadienne de Psychiatrie*, 52, 457–463.

8. Spatz, R., Lorenzi, E., Kugler, J., et al. (1978). [The incidence of abnormal EEG patterns with clozapine therapy (Author's transl)]. *Arzneimittel-Forschung*, 28, 1499–1500.

9. Gunther, W., Baghai, T., Naber, D., et al. (1993). EEG alterations and seizures during treatment with clozapine. A retrospective study of 283 patients. *Pharmacopsychiatry*, 26, 69–74.

10. Varma, S., Bishara, D., Besag, F. M., et al. (2011). Clozapine-related EEG changes and seizures: Dose and plasma-level relationships. *Therapeutic Advances in Psychopharmacology*, 1, 47–66.

11. Malik, S., Lally, J., Ajnakina, O., et al. (2018). Sodium valproate and clozapine induced neutropenia: A case control study using register data. *Schizophrenia Research*, 195, 267–273.

12. Jette Pomerleau, V., Dubeau, F. and Ducharme, S. (2017). Clozapine safety and efficacy for interictal psychotic disorder in pharmacoresistant epilepsy. *Cognitive and Behaviorla Neurology*, 30, 73–76.

13. Diaz, F. J., Santoro, V., Spina, E., et al. (2008). Estimating the size of the effects of co-medications on plasma clozapine concentrations using a model that controls for clozapine doses and confounding variables. *Pharmacopsychiatry*, 41, 81–91.

14. Ronaldson, K. J., Fitzgerald, P. B., Taylor, A. J., et al. (2012). Rapid clozapine dose titration and concomitant sodium valproate increase the risk of myocarditis with clozapine: A case-control study. *Schizophrenia Research*, 141, 173–178.

15. Ifteni, P., Nielsen, J., Burtea, V., et al. (2014). Effectiveness and safety of rapid clozapine titration in schizophrenia. *Acta Psychiatrica Scandinavica*, 130, 25–29.

16. Murphy, R., Gallagher, A., Sharma, K., et al. (2015). Clozapine-induced stuttering: An estimate of prevalence in the west of Ireland. *Therapeutic Advances in Psychopharmacology*, 5, 232–236.

17. Peacock, L. and Gerlach, J. (1994). Clozapine treatment in Denmark: Concomitant psychotropic medication and hematologic monitoring in a system with liberal usage practices. *Journal of Clinical Psychiatry*, 55, 44–49.

18. Bak, T. H., Bauer, M., Schaub, R. T., et al. (1995). Myoclonus in patients treated with clozapine: A case series. *Journal of Clinical Psychiatry*, 56, 418–422.

19. Chen, B., Choi, H., Hirsch, L. J., et al. (2017). Psychiatric and behavioral side effects of antiepileptic drugs in adults with epilepsy. *Epilepsy & Behavior*, 76, 24–31.

20. Bromley, R., Weston, J., Adab, N., et al. (2014). Treatment for epilepsy in pregnancy: Neurodevelopmental outcomes in the child. *Cochrane Database of Systematic Reviews*, 10, Cd010236.

21. Grover, S., Hazari, N. and Kate, N. (2015). Combined use of clozapine and ECT: A review. *Acta Neuropsychiatrica*, 27, 131–142.

10

11

Managing Metabolic Adverse Effects

QUICK CHECK

INTRODUCTION

The primary use of clozapine is for schizophrenia spectrum patients with a history of suicidality or treatment-resistant psychosis. Although clozapine itself imposes significant metabolic burden, this is overlaid on the twofold higher rates of metabolic disorders (type 2 diabetes mellitus, metabolic syndrome) and twofold greater standardized mortality rates for cardiovascular disease in this patient population. Multiple factors contribute to this risk profile including lifestyle (e.g. smoking, dietary habits, sedentary behavior), metabolic effects of medications, and biological aspects of schizophrenia itself detectable in treatment-naive patients [1]. Given clozapine's metabolic impact, combined with the reality that patients may remain on clozapine throughout their lives, ongoing management of cardiometabolic risk is integral to the care of clozapine-treated individuals [2]. Despite this confluence of medication and disease-related risk, the use of clozapine is associated with lower mortality rates from unnatural and natural causes. Investigators

PRINCIPLES

- Nearly all clozapine-treated patients will manifest one or more metabolic adverse effects, with weight gain occurring very early in treatment.

- Given the high prevalence and early onset of weight gain, all patients are candidates for the two evidence-based treatments which must be started when clozapine is commenced: metformin and exercise (including dietary counseling).

- Laboratory monitoring of metabolic parameters can be adjusted based on known risks for diabetes. Physical activity must be tracked as a vital sign, along with smoking behavior.

- When they occur, diabetes and dyslipidemia are managed with usual medications.

- Metabolic adverse effects are generally never a reason to discontinue clozapine.

compared mortality trends in 14,754 individuals with schizophrenia, schizoaffective disorder or bipolar disorder followed in London from 2007 to 2011. There was a significant association between clozapine use ($n = 748$) and lower mortality even after controlling for confounders including clinical monitoring and disease severity (adjusted hazard ratio 0.4; 95% CI 0.2–0.7; $p = 0.001$) [3]. This adds to prior data from an 11-year Finnish study which showed that clozapine markedly reduces suicide-related mortality, while no pronounced differences for ischemic heart disease mortality were found between antipsychotics [4].

Nonetheless, substantial changes in cardiovascular risk are seen in long-term studies, and clozapine is considered in the highest risk group among all antipsychotics for weight gain, dyslipidemia and adverse impact on insulin resistance. Naturalistic data for 96 clozapine-treated patients spanning 21 years of follow-up (mean duration of clozapine use 13 years) noted elevated cardiovascular risk during the first 10 years of treatment, although there was a slight decline in risk after the first decade [2]. This sobering reality drives home the point that management of cardiometabolic issues is inherent to clozapine treatment, and that management strategies must be implemented at the time clozapine is commenced. In addition to the combined impact of the medication and the diagnosis of schizophrenia, many patients will possess one or more nonmodifiable factors that add to risk for weight gain or insulin resistance

Box 11.1 Principles in Managing Metabolic Adverse Effects of Clozapine

1. Clozapine is among the highest-risk antipsychotics for metabolic dysfunction. Nearly 100% of clozapine-exposed patients will manifest one of the common triad of metabolic adverse effects (weight gain, insulin resistance, dyslipidemia).

2. Nonmodifiable risk factors also contribute to increased risk for metabolic adverse effects:

   a. Weight gain: younger age, female gender, nonwhite race/ethnicity, family history.

   b. Insulin resistance: schizophrenia diagnosis, nonwhite race/ethnicity, family history.

3. Within the range of doses commonly used for schizophrenia spectrum disorders, there is *no evidence* of a dose relationship for metabolic disorders. Dose reduction is therefore not a strategy to mitigate or treat these issues.

4. Metformin has the greatest evidence base supporting benefit for weight gain, and should be started concurrently with clozapine.

   a. Metformin is safe with eGFR ≥ 30 ml/min, but use should be reviewed when eGFR falls below 45 ml/min [18]. Check B12 yearly.

   b. Metformin should be started at 500 mg PO qam. Higher initial doses cause gastrointestinal adverse effects (e.g. diarrhea, nausea). Use of extended release forms may improve tolerability.

   c. To reduce side effects metformin should titrated over a 3-week period with 500 mg qam the first week, 500 mg BID or 1000 mg XR qam the second week, and 1000 mg BID or 2000 mg XR qam starting week 3 if tolerated. If 2000 mg/day is not tolerated, try 1500 mg/day (metformin 750 mg BID or 1500 mg metformin XR qam).

   d. For patients with normal eGFR (e.g. ≥ 60 ml/min), yearly eGFR is sufficient. When eGFR falls below 60 ml/min, monitor every 3–6 months. When eGFR falls below 45 ml/min the metformin dose should be reduced by 50% and eGFR checked every 3 months. Metformin must be stopped when eGFR is < 30 ml/min.

5. All patients must be enrolled in a structured exercise program that should be maintained indefinitely unless the patient has shown ability to exercise independently.

6. Dietary counseling must be offered to all patients and caregivers starting with the beginning of clozapine therapy.

7. Routine periodic screening as noted in Table 11.3.

8. Physical activity should be tracked in the same manner as other vital signs (Table 11.3)

9. In stable patients, smoking status must be documented routinely and cessation medications and programs offered regularly.

during clozapine treatment. The principles outlined in Box 11.1 are thus based on the proposition that clozapine itself is a medication with significant metabolic burden, and that nearly 100% of clozapine-exposed patients will manifest one of the common triad of metabolic adverse effects (weight gain, insulin resistance, dyslipidemia). While numerous medications have been tried for clozapine-related obesity and metabolic disturbances (topiramate, sibutramine, phenylpropanolamine, modafinil, atomoxetine, rosiglitazone) these have not demonstrated benefit for patients on clozapine, although there might be positive data for use with other antipsychotics [5]. Metformin has repeatedly been proven effective for weight gain in numerous double-blind, placebo-controlled trials, and also significantly improves three of the five components of metabolic syndrome: waist circumference, fasting glucose and triglycerides [6]. As will be discussed below, all patients starting clozapine should be considered candidates for metformin at the outset of clozapine treatment, to which exercise and dietary counseling must be added. The longitudinal management of cardiometabolic risk represents an opportunity to integrate best practices from psychiatry, primary care and psychology into a concerted team effort to promote lifelong healthy behaviors and treat manageable medical conditions with the goal of keeping patients on clozapine and forestalling major cardiovascular events. With the exception of emergencies such as diabetic ketoacidosis (DKA), hyperosmolar hyperglycemic states (HHS), or out of control diabetes during which a temporary cessation of clozapine may be helpful, metabolic adverse effects should not be a reason for discontinuing clozapine treatment, as noted in recent reviews (Table 11.1) [7].

Table 11.1 Metabolic issues and discontinuing clozapine [7].

Complication	Grounds for discontinuation	Comments
Weight gain	Almost never	Try behavioral approaches, metformin
Hypertension	Almost never	Usual management
Dyslipidemia	Almost never	Usual management, especially agents that lower triglycerides
Metabolic syndrome	Almost never	Treat individual components
Diabetes mellitus	Out of control diabetes	Try usual management first and correct other diabetogenic causes. Generally manageable
Diabetic ketoacidosis or hyperosmolar hyperglycemic state	Acute episode	Hold clozapine during acute episode. Rechallenge after stabilization with tight monitoring

A Monitoring Metabolic Parameters

The key to managing metabolic risk is routine surveillance and early diagnosis based on the latest guidelines. The hypertension criteria in the US were significantly modified in late 2017, and thereby identified a new cohort of individuals as candidates for antihypertensive treatment [8]. Worldwide there are variations in the criteria listed in Table 11.2, so clinicians should be familiar with those employed locally, as well as recent updates. In ethnically diverse populations, appropriate BMI cutpoints should be used as indicators for increased efforts to manage weight gain. Although waist circumference is a criterion for the metabolic syndrome, abdominal obesity measurements are very inaccurate in the hands of most clinicians, so many institutions eschew this in lieu of tracking BMI, especially as BMI values in the obese category satisfy the waist circumference criterion [9]. Similarly, fasting laboratory values may be difficult to obtain from some outpatients, so hemoglobin A1C can also be used to track glycemic changes and diagnose diabetes mellitus. Table 11.3 outlines a basic approach to monitoring synthesized from published recommendations. While most concur on obtaining weight and blood pressure measures during monthly or bimonthly clinical visits, the frequency of fasting glucose and lipids must be tailored to inherent risk factors for cardiometabolic disease. In an individual with multiple diabetes risks (Box 11.2), monthly monitoring for the first 6 months of treatment is not unreasonable. As a general rule, metabolic laboratory measures are obtained more frequently in the first year, and adjusted based on the patient's needs. In the small cohort of patients on long-term clozapine treatment who manifest no cardiometabolic issues, fasting glucose and lipids must be obtained at least yearly.

Table 11.2 Criteria for hypertension, obesity, metabolic syndrome and diabetes mellitus.

		Measures		
		Europid individuals		Asian individuals[1]
Body mass index	Overweight	25.0–29.99 kg/m²		23.0–27.49 kg/m²
	Class I obesity	30.0–34.49 kg/m²		27.5–32.49 kg/m²
	Class II obesity	35.0–39.99 kg/m²		32.5–37.49 kg/m²
	Class III obesity	≥ 40.0 kg/m²		≥ 37.5 kg/m²
		Systolic		Diastolic
Adult blood pressure[2]	Normal	< 120 mmHg	and	< 80 mmHg
	Elevated	120–129 mmHg	and	< 80 mmHg
	Stage I hypertension	130–139 mmHg	or	80–89 mmHg
	Stage II hypertension	≥ 140 mmHg	or	≥ 90 mmHg

continued overleaf

Table 11.2 continued

	Measures		
	Blood Pressure	Systolic BP > 130 mmHg or diastolic BP > 85 mmHg, or treatment of previously diagnosed hypertension	
	Waist Circumference[4]		
	Europid[5]	Male	≥ 94 cm (37.0 in.)
		Female	≥ 80 cm (31.5 in.)
Metabolic syndrome (at least three criteria needed for diagnosis)[3]	*Asian*[5]	Male	≥ 90 cm (35.4 in.)
		Female	≥ 80 cm (31.5 in.)
	HDL	< 40 mg/dl (< 1.03 mmol/l) in males, < 50 mg/dl (< 1.29 mmol/l) in females, or specific treatment for this lipid abnormality	
	Triglycerides	Fasting values > 150 mg/dl (> 1.7 mmol/l), or specific treatment for this lipid abnormality	
	Glucose	Fasting plasma glucose > 100 mg/dl (> 5.6 mmol/l), or previously diagnosed type 2 diabetes	
Diabetes mellitus[6]	**Glucose**	Fasting values ≥ 126 mg/dl (≥ 7.0 mmol/l). Fasting is defined as no caloric intake for at least 8 hours[7]	
		OR	
		2-hour glucose ≥ 200 mg/dl (≥ 11.1 mmol/l) during 75 gram oral glucose tolerance test	
		OR	
		In a patient with classic symptoms of hyperglycemia or hyperglycemic crisis, a random plasma glucose ≥ 200 mg/dl (≥ 11.1 mmol/l)	
		OR	
		Hemoglobin A1C ≥ 6.5% (≥ 48 mmol/mol)	

Notes:

1. The BMI values for Asian individuals are suggested cutpoints for action, and may not directly correspond to obesity classifications for Europid individuals [47].

2. Based on the 2017 updated guideline from the American College of Cardiology/American Heart Association Task Force on Clinical Practice Guidelines [8].

3. Based on 2006 International Diabetes Federation criteria [1].

4. If BMI is > 30 kg/m² central obesity can be assumed and waist circumference does not need to be measured.

5. Europid values also apply to Subsaharan Africans, Mediterranean and Middle Eastern groups. Asian values apply to Chinese, Japanese, Korean, Malay, Filipino, Asian-Indian groups, and to Ethnic South and Central Americans.

6. Based on the 2018 American Diabetes Association criteria (American Diabetes Association 2018 [48]).

7. In the absence of unequivocal hyperglycemia, results should be confirmed by repeat testing.

Table 11.3 Routine monitoring.

	Measures
Body mass index	Monthly or every clinical visit (if less than monthly). (Given the significant variation between examiners in waist circumference measurements, this can be foregone in lieu of the more accurate weight.)
Blood pressure	Monthly or every clinical visit (if less than monthly).
Fasting glucose	a. Quarterly during first year, if normal then every 6–12 months. Consider monthly or bimonthly fasting glucose in the first 6 months if multiple DM risk factors are present. b. If fasting values are difficult to obtain, add hemoglobin A1C
Fasting lipids	Quarterly during first year, if normal then every 6–12 months.
Smoking status	a. Inquired at every visit and quantified. b. When psychiatrically stable, smoking cessation programs and medications should be offered quarterly.
Physical activity vital sign (PAVS)	Inquired at every monthly visit and recorded.

 Weight Gain

The most robust hypothesis for antipsychotic-associated weight gain involves histamine H_1 antagonism of hypothalamic sites that regulate food intake [10]. Weight gain is due to impaired satiety and not any direct impact on metabolic rate – patients simply eat more [1]. There may be an additional contribution from $5HT_{2C}$ antagonism as shown in animal models and some early studies of $5HT_{2C}$ polymorphisms with antipsychotic-related weight gain, although this association is not consistently found [11]. There are additional hypotheses focusing on how antipsychotics impact regulation of hormones related to appetite, adiposity and glycemic control (leptin, adiponectin, glucagon-like peptide-1) and changes in inflammatory markers, but this information has no direct clinical application at the present time aside from the compelling evidence that increased exercise reduces levels of systemic inflammation and improves the physical and psychological quality of life among the severely mentally ill (see section below on Exercise) [12].

Weight gain estimates vary widely depending on the time frame and population, but 60–75% of patients will gain ≥ 4.5 kg during the first year of treatment [13]. Naturalistic long-term data from an American sample noted a mean increase of 13.5 kg after 10 years, of which 4.5 kg occurred in the first 10 weeks of clozapine treatment [14]. Demographic factors that place patients at even higher weight gain risk include: younger age, low baseline BMI, nonwhite race, and concurrent use of divalproex [15]. As noted previously, genetic markers that predict weight gain are of great interest but lack robustness to be employed in routine clinical care [11]. As weight gain is an early complication of clozapine and carries long-term health risks, all patients starting clozapine must receive maximum combined efforts to mitigate this problem: dietary counseling and structured exercise (see below), and the antidiabetic agent metformin.

● Metformin

Metformin is a biguanide molecule synthesized in 1922 whose glucose-lowering properties in animals were noted in 1929 and promptly forgotten until human studies in 1957 [16]. Metformin's mechanisms are not completely understood, but it results in improved insulin sensitivity and reduced hepatic gluconeogenesis. Metformin increases the production of glucagon-like peptide-1 (GLP-1), a hormone whose levels may be adversely affected by clozapine, and thereby stimulates insulin release, inhibits glucagon secretion and possibly moderates appetite [17]. Unlike sulfonylureas, metformin has a low rate of hypoglycemia and has been used extensively in nondiabetic patients for management of prediabetic conditions and nonalcoholic fatty liver. Importantly, use of metformin in nondiabetics is associated with mild weight loss, possibly related to its GLP-1 effect, and decreased triglyceride levels due to greater insulin actions at lipoprotein lipase, the enzyme primarily responsible for hydrolyzing triglycerides [1,17]. Metformin also reduces risk of myocardial infarction and all-cause mortality in newly diagnosed diabetics in a manner not seen with sulfonylureas or insulin [18]. While older biguanide antidiabetics such as phenformin had unacceptable rates of lactic acidosis, recent guidelines indicate that metformin is safe for those with eGFR levels down to 30 ml/min, although ongoing use should be reviewed when the eGFR falls below 45 ml/min [18]. Also, check vitamin B12 levels yearly.

Metformin has been studied extensively for antipsychotic-related weight gain and metabolic adverse effects in adults and adolescents, primarily with agents of highest risk: olanzapine and clozapine. A 2016 review of the eight placebo-controlled trials specifically for clozapine-treated patients found that metformin was superior to placebo with a mean difference of -3.12 kg in weight and -1.18 kg/m^2 in BMI; metformin also significantly improved fasting glucose and triglycerides [6]. Metformin is generally well tolerated, but gastrointestinal (GI) adverse effects (diarrhea, nausea) can occur at high rates with aggressive titration. Box 11.1 provides a titration used in clinical trials that is designed to slowly advance the dose over several weeks, thereby lessening the risk of GI side effects. Unless eGFR is a limiting factor, all patients starting clozapine should commence metformin concurrently for the following reasons: (a) weight gain is a pervasive problem and occurs early in treatment; (b) metformin confers additional benefits beyond weight gain including triglyceride reduction and a delay in the rates of type 2 diabetes among prediabetic patients [1].

● Aripiprazole, Bariatric Surgery

As noted previously, numerous other medications have been studied for clozapine-related obesity and weight gain (topiramate, sibutramine, phenylpropanolamine, modafinil, atomoxetine) without significant results (although there might be data for use with other antipsychotics); however, there are two positive trials for adjunctive aripiprazole at doses of 5–15 mg/day [5]. Due to its mechanism of action, aripiprazole should only be tried in patients on clozapine as antipsychotic monotherapy as there are reports of symptomatic worsening when aripiprazole is added to nonclozapine antipsychotics, likely due to displacement of strong D_2 antagonists by the partial agonist aripiprazole [19]. Dose adjustments are needed for cytochrome P450 (CYP) 2D6 poor metabolizers, or those on 2D6 or 3A4 inhibitors, or 3A4 inducers. The adjunctive aripiprazole trial should be terminated for adverse effects (akathisia, anxiety, parkinsonism) or if no benefit is seen after 12–16 weeks.

Despite the best clinical efforts many patients will struggle with weight gain, obesity and related complications. In recent years there has been increased enthusiasm about considering the severely mentally ill as candidates for bariatric surgery, assuming clinical stability. Two 2017 reviews found that weight loss outcomes among schizophrenia patients were comparable to those with bipolar disorder or no mental illness, without significant deterioration of psychiatric symptoms [20,21]. It should be noted that those with schizophrenia spectrum disorders did have more postoperative emergency department visits and hospital days compared to patients with no mental illness [20]. If a clozapine-treated patient is deemed a bariatric surgery candidate, close monitoring of clozapine plasma levels, and the serum levels of other medications with narrow therapeutic indices (e.g. lithium valproate), is important so that dosage adjustments can be made to maintain preoperative drug levels.

Insulin Resistance and Type 2 Diabetes Mellitus

There are many hypotheses surrounding antipsychotic effects on glycemic control, with both weight and weight-independent mechanisms invoked [22]. Regardless of the etiology, clozapine is placed in the highest antipsychotic risk group for induction of metabolic syndrome and type 2 DM. Cross-sectional US data from 3123 clozapine-treated schizophrenia patients and matched schizophrenia patients on other antipsychotics noted that rates of DM were twofold higher on clozapine: 2.8% vs. 1.4% for standard antipsychotics (HR 1.63, 95% CI 0.98–2.70) [23]. In a US data set covering over 20 years of clozapine exposure, 42.7% of patients were diagnosed with DM [2]. Moreover, the prevalence of the metabolic syndrome is estimated to be as high as 61.6% [13]. Although there was early concern about abrupt onset of diabetic ketoacidosis (DKA) shortly after commencing clozapine, later studies demonstrated that these patients had untreated DM, with mean A1C of 13.3% at time of admission for DKA [24]. Pretreatment screening is thus critical so that undiagnosed DM can be addressed prior to starting clozapine. Table 11.1 presents criteria for DM and the related metabolic syndrome. The frequency of laboratory monitoring should be titrated to the number of traditional DM risk factors (Box 11.2). The same interventions used to manage weight gain (metformin, dietary advice, exercise) are also helpful in mitigating risk for DM and metabolic syndrome. It is important to emphasize that in prediabetic individuals enrolled in the long-term UK Diabetes Prevention Program trial, treatment with metformin resulted in modest weight loss and favorable changes in insulin sensitivity compared to placebo, all of which contributed to a reduction in the risk of diabetes independent from associated reductions in fasting glucose [25].

As with weight management, a number of medications other than metformin have been studied in prediabetic schizophrenia patients including pioglitazone and the injectable GLP-1 agonist exenatide. Short-term impact on metabolic parameters can be seen, but these agents lack the robustness of metformin's extensive benefits on weight and numerous metabolic and clinical parameters including mortality [26]. A 2017 meta-analysis of pharmacological and behavioral interventions for glycemic control in severely mentally ill adults found that behavioral interventions and metformin led to clinically important improvements in glycemic measurements [26]. (The only

1. First-degree relative with diabetes

2. High-risk race/ethnicity (e.g. African descent, Latino, Native American, Asian descent, Pacific Islander)

3. History of cardiovascular disease

4. Hypertension (≥ 140/90 mmHg or on therapy for hypertension)

5. Low HDL cholesterol (< 35 mg/dl (< 0.90 mmol/l) and/or elevated triglyceride level > 250 mg/dl (> 2.82 mmol/l)

6. Women with polycystic ovary syndrome

7. Physical inactivity

8. Other clinical conditions associated with insulin resistance (e.g. severe obesity, acanthosis nigricans)

other strategy that also showed benefit was antipsychotic switching, an option not typically available to patients on clozapine.) This preference for metformin is echoed by conclusions from a 2017 Cochrane review of newer DM medications that noted an absence of firm evidence that GLP-1 agonists (or dipeptidyl peptidase-4 inhibitors) substantially influence the risk of developing type 2 DM and its complications in those at increased risk for DM [27].

Clozapine-treated individuals who develop DM should be managed with the same protocols as other DM patients. Interestingly, a meta-analysis of 10 studies comprising 33,910 schizophrenia patients with DM showed that people with schizophrenia adhered to their DM medications on 4.6% more days per year than those without schizophrenia ($p < 0.01$, 95% CI 2.4–6.7%) [28]. The development of DM is not a reason to stop clozapine therapy, and there is no evidence to support dose reduction for managing glycemic control; however, during emergency situations when a patient has acute out of control DM, or is hospitalized for DKA or HHS, it is not unreasonable to consider temporarily holding clozapine for 24–48 hours if absolutely necessary while the patient is acutely ill, especially if there are issues with hypotension or mental status changes. The cholinergic rebound that can result from any abrupt cessation in clozapine treatment must also be adequately managed. (Chapter 4 provides an extensive discussion of strategies for managing cholinergic rebound, and considerations for antipsychotic therapy after clozapine discontinuation.) Once glycemic control has been reestablished, the patient can be rechallenged with clozapine, albeit with tight glucose monitoring [29]. Switching from clozapine is to be avoided given the absence of viable treatment options for most patients requiring clozapine.

Individuals who gain weight and become insulin-resistant are also at risk of developing nonalcoholic fatty liver disease (NAFLD). This can occur in the early years of antipsychotic therapy, and is associated with weight gain $\geq 7\%$ and deleterious changes in all of the five metabolic syndrome components [30]. Of clinical relevance, abnormalities in transaminases (AST, ALT) will insidiously develop in NAFLD patients who otherwise appear to lack risk factors for liver disease (e.g. nondrinkers, noncarriers of hepatitis B or C, nonusers of valproate), at times leading to misguided speculation that clozapine itself is causing hepatotoxicity. The diagnosis of NAFLD should be rapidly confirmed with hepatic ultrasound due to the low cost, accessibility and high sensitivity (80%) in patients with $> 30\%$ steatosis [31]. Treatment involves adjustment or addition of medications to manage insulin resistance, and exercise.

D Dyslipidemia

As with glycemic control, there are many hypotheses about weight and weight-independent mechanisms by which antipsychotics induce lipid abnormalities. The proportion of clozapine-treated patients with dyslipidemia varies greatly depending on the duration of treatment, with a 35% prevalence quoted in the literature [13]. Not surprisingly, those lipid abnormalities most closely tied with insulin resistance and the metabolic syndrome are seen in clozapine-treated patients, particularly hypertriglyceridemia and low high-density lipoprotein (HDL) cholesterol levels [1]. HDL levels are also further depressed by inactivity and smoking, stressing the importance of modifying these behaviors to raise HDL. The initial approach to managing modest levels of hypertriglyceridemia (< 500 mg/dl) involves lifestyle modification and improving insulin sensitivity, because the enzyme primarily responsible for hydrolyzing triglycerides (lipoprotein lipase) is responsive to the effects of insulin. Many clinicians use drugs to reduce triglyceride levels only when they exceed 500 mg/dl (5.65 mmol/l) and especially when values approach 1000 mg/dl (11.30 mmol/l), as these patients are at risk for pancreatitis. The initial choice of agents (statin, fibrate) is dictated by a variety of clinical concerns including the type of dyslipidemia and severity. Dyslipidemia is never a reason to discontinue clozapine, and even severe hypertriglyceridemia can be managed without the need to temporarily hold clozapine.

Exercise and Lifestyle Modification

One of the contributors to high rates of cardiovascular mortality in schizophrenia patients is sedentary behavior [32]. Exercise is one of the few evidence-based therapies proven to benefit patients with severe mental illness, and should be prescribed in the same manner as metformin at the outset of clozapine treatment. While most clinicians are familiar with the impact on cardiometabolic measures, a 2016 meta-analysis of 29 studies ($n = 1109$) found that exercise programs for schizophrenia patients were superior to control conditions for psychiatric and global outcomes including [33]:

- Total symptom severity ($n = 719$: Hedges' $g = 0.39$, $p < 0.001$)
- Positive symptoms ($n = 715$: Hedges' $g = 0.32$, $p < 0.01$)
- Negative symptoms ($n = 854$: Hedges' $g = 0.49$, $p < 0.001$)
- General psychopathology ($n = 475$: Hedges' $g = 0.27$, $p < 0.05$)
- Quality of life ($n = 770$: Hedges' $g = 0.55$, $p < 0.001$)
- Global functioning ($n = 342$: Hedges' $g = 0.32$, $p < 0.01$)
- Depressive symptoms ($n = 337$: Hedges' $g = 0.71$, $p < 0.001$).

The putative impact of exercise on psychiatric symptoms may relate to reductions in systemic inflammatory markers. Systemic inflammation occurs in concert with metabolic dysfunction and contributes to risk of cardiovascular events, but may also have adverse CNS consequences as noted in studies of patients with major depression or schizophrenia [34].

The first step in assessing the impact of any exercise intervention is to quantify the extent of a patient's activity, and recording this on a regular basis in a manner akin to other vital signs such as weight and blood pressure. The physical activity vital sign (PAVS) has been specifically developed for the purpose of tracking physical activity in primary care settings, and consists of a brief two-question assessment:

1. How many days during the past week have you performed physical activity where your heart beats faster and your breathing is harder than normal for 30 minutes or more?

2. How many days in a typical week do you perform activity such as this?

Responses are reported as a score for each item: x/y. The goal of PAVS tracking is to ascertain if patients meet the recommended 150 minutes per week of moderate physical activity. Investigators using the PAVS found that BMI decreased 0.91 kg/m^2

for every day of moderate intensity activity during a typical week in a general adult sample ($p < 0.001$) [35]. With its ease of use, the PAVS has also been studied in schizophrenia patients [36]. To assess fitness and metabolic status, a sample of 100 schizophrenia patients (mean age 38.1 years, 64% male, 64% smokers) completed the PAVS and other metabolic screening. Only 39% met the recommended activity levels (mean 187 ± 36 min/week). Moreover, less-active patients had 1.67 times greater risk for being overweight or obese, 4.65 times the risk for hypertension, and nearly threefold higher risk for metabolic syndrome [36].

A number of exercise and lifestyle intervention programs have been tailored for patients with severe mental illness, including the ACHIEVE [37] and STRIDE [38] protocols. The 18-month outcome data from ACHIEVE ($n = 279$) noted a mean between-group difference in weight of −3.2 kg favoring the intervention participant (−7.0 lb, $p = 0.002$) (see Figure 11.1). In addition, 37.8% of the participants in the intervention group lost 5% or more of their initial weight, as compared with 22.7% of those in the control group ($p = 0.009$) [37]. The 6-month data from STRIDE noted a −4.4 kg difference with the control group, with sustained differences 6 months after the program ended (−2.6 kg) [38]. These interventions are designed to be delivered by staff without specialized expertise and involve dietary advice and exercise starting at a level appropriate for sedentary persons, with gradual increases in duration and intensity [37]. Incentives and tracking tools for participants help reward progress, and recent data suggest that the use of telephone or internet-based reminders may be preferred by younger patients [39]. Although attendance at a weekly program may be challenging for patients, the results in the STRIDE study were achieved with participants attending on average 14.5 of 24 sessions over 6 months [38].

Providing dietary advice is a core component of these programs, given the data that schizophrenia patients have poor dietary habits in addition to sedentary lifestyle [40]. With individual support and group sessions in a Danish cohort of 54 schizophrenia patients, consumption of fast food was reduced from 1.2 to 0.8 times per week ($p = 0.016$), and consumption of soft drinks was reduced from 0.7 to 0.1 liters/day ($p = 0.006$) [41]. Dietary guidance should begin as early as possible in treatment as much of the weight gain occurs in the first months of clozapine treatment. Just as no patient should be deprived of metformin, exercise and related dietary counseling also confer pleiotropic benefits and must be considered standard of care for patients commencing clozapine therapy.

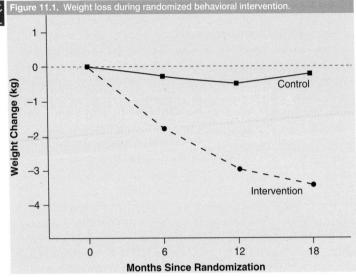

Figure 11.1. Weight loss during randomized behavioral intervention.

(Adapted from: Daumit, G. L., Dickerson, F. B., Wang, N. Y., et al. (2013). A behavioral weight-loss intervention in persons with serious mental illness. *New England Journal of Medicine*, 368, 1594–1602 [37].)

 Smoking

Genetic and neuroimaging studies indicate that high rates of smoking and other substance use disorders likely relate to the neurobiology of schizophrenia itself, and are not a consequence of treatment [42]. Unfortunately, prospective data (up to 16.9 years of follow-up) show that smoking increases mortality rates more than sixfold in patients with schizophrenia or bipolar disorder [43]. While smoking cessation is more difficult for patients with severe mental illnesses, smoking can and should be addressed, with compelling data for the safety and efficacy of bupropion [44] and also the nicotine partial agonist varenicline [45]. The leading experts suggest that smokers with schizophrenia spectrum disorders should not only be encouraged to quit smoking but should also receive varenicline, bupropion with or without nicotine replacement therapy (NRT), or NRT, all in combination with behavioral treatment for at least 12 weeks for the optimal chance at successful smoking cessation [46]. Discussions about smoking cessation are best commenced when patients are clinically stable and ready to tackle this issue, and are also on stable clozapine doses because changes in plasma clozapine levels must be monitored once the cytochrome P450 1A2-inducing properties of aryl hydrocarbons in smoke are removed. Like the PAVS, smoking should be quantified and tracked along with other vital signs, and cessation discussed during clinical encounters. While a patient may decline smoking cessation for years, he or she may suddenly change their mind due to rising costs or health reasons, hence the need for regular communication about this issue. It must be emphasized that switching to an electronic cigarette (i.e. vaping) might be considered to decrease exposure to harmful chemicals in cigarette smoke. While the health benefits of e-cigarettes are not yet proven, by not burning the tobacco leaf patients will lose exposure to the aryl hydrocarbons that induce cytochrome P450 (CYP) 1A2. Nicotine itself plays no role in CYP 1A2 induction. After switching to the e-cigarette, a patient will lose their CYP 1A2 induction over the next week, and clozapine levels may rise 50% or more [49]. For those who switch completely to an e-cigarette, close monitoring of plasma clozapine levels is important.

Summary Points

a. Weight gain is a highly prevalent condition and starts early in treatment. All patients are candidates for metformin and exercise/dietary counseling when clozapine therapy is commenced.

b. Aside from metformin, there are limited data supporting other adjunctive medications to mitigate weight gain and metabolic adverse effects, with the possible exception of aripiprazole for weight parameters. Metformin has robust data for reducing weight gain, improving indices of insulin resistance, delaying onset of type 2 diabetes mellitus, and reducing rates of cardiovascular events and mortality. Patients on metformin should have vitamin B12 levels checked yearly.

c. The physical activity vital sign (PAVS) and smoking behavior must be tracked along with weight, BMI and metabolic laboratory measures.

References

1. Meyer, J. M. and Stahl, S. M. (2009). The metabolic syndrome and schizophrenia. *Acta Psychiatrica Scandinavica*, 119, 4–14.

2. Nemani, K. L., Greene, M. C., Ulloa, M., et al. (2019). Clozapine, diabetes mellitus, cardiovascular risk and mortality: Results of a 21-year naturalistic study in patients with schizophrenia and schizoaffective disorder. *Clinical Schizophrenia & Related Psychoses*, 12, 168–176.

3. Hayes, R. D., Downs, J., Chang, C. K., et al. (2015). The effect of clozapine on premature mortality: An assessment of clinical monitoring and other potential confounders. *Schizophrenia Bulletin*, 41, 644–655.

4. Tiihonen, J., Lonnqvist, J., Wahlbeck, K., et al. (2009). 11-year follow-up of mortality in patients with schizophrenia: A population-based cohort study (FIN11 study). *Lancet*, 374, 620–627.

5. Zimbron, J., Khandaker, G. M., Toschi, C., et al. (2016). A systematic review and meta-analysis of randomised controlled trials of treatments for clozapine-induced obesity and metabolic syndrome. *European Neuropsychopharmacology*, 26, 1353–1365.

6. Siskind, D. J., Leung, J., Russell, A. W., et al. (2016). Metformin for clozapine associated obesity: A systematic review and meta-analysis. *PLoS ONE*, 11, e0156208.

7. Nielsen, J., Correll, C. U., Manu, P., et al. (2013). Termination of clozapine treatment due to medical reasons: When is it warranted and how can it be avoided? *Journal of Clinical Psychiatry*, 74, 603–613.

8. Whelton, P. K., Carey, R. M., Aronow, W. S., et al. (2018). 2017 ACC/AHA/AAPA/ABC/ACPM/AGS/APhA/ASH/ASPC/NMA/PCNA Guideline for the prevention, detection, evaluation, and management of high blood pressure in adults: Executive summary: A report of the American College of Cardiology/American Heart Association Task Force on Clinical Practice Guidelines. *Journal of the American Society for Hypertension*, 12, e1–579.

9. Sebo, P., Herrmann, F. R. and Haller, D. M. (2017). Accuracy of anthropometric measurements by general practitioners in overweight and obese patients. *BMC Obesity*, 4, 23–29.

10. Kim, S. F., Huang, A. S., Snowman, A. M., et al. (2007). Antipsychotic drug-induced weight gain mediated by histamine H1 receptor-linked activation of hypothalamic AMP-kinase. *Proceedings of the National Academy of Sciences of the United States of America*, 104, 3456–3459.

11. Suetani, R. J., Siskind, D., Reichhold, H., et al. (2017). Genetic variants impacting metabolic outcomes among people on clozapine: A systematic review and meta-analysis. *Psychopharmacology (Berlin)*, 234, 2989–3008.

12. Vancampfort, D., Van Damme, T., Probst, M., et al. (2017). Physical activity is associated with the physical, psychological, social and environmental quality of life in people with mental health problems in a low resource setting. *Psychiatry Research*, 258, 250–254.

13. Citrome, L., McEvoy, J. P. and Saklad, S. R. (2016). Guide to the management of clozapine-related tolerability and safety concerns. *Clinical Schizophrenia & Related Psychoses*, 10, 163–177.

14. Henderson, D. C., Nguyen, D. D., Copeland, P. M., et al. (2005). Clozapine, diabetes mellitus, hyperlipidemia, and cardiovascular risks and mortality: Results of a 10-year naturalistic study. *Journal of Clinical Psychiatry*, 66, 1116–1121.

15. Meyer, J. M. (2010). Antipsychotics and metabolics in the post-CATIE era. *Current Topics in Behavioral Neurosciences*, 4, 23–42.

16. Bailey, C. J. (2017). Metformin: Historical overview. *Diabetologia*, 60, 1566–1576.

17. Siskind, D., Friend, N., Russell, A., et al. (2018). CoMET: A protocol for a randomised controlled trial of co-commencement of METformin as an adjunctive treatment to attenuate weight gain and metabolic syndrome in patients with schizophrenia newly commenced on clozapine. *BMJ Open*, 8, e021000.

18. Lipska, K. J., Bailey, C. J. and Inzucchi, S. E. (2011). Use of metformin in the setting of mild-to-moderate renal insufficiency. *Diabetes Care*, 34, 1431–1437.

19. Takeuchi, H. and Remington, G. (2013). A systematic review of reported cases involving psychotic symptoms worsened by aripiprazole in schizophrenia or schizoaffective disorder. *Psychopharmacology (Berlin)*, 228, 175–185.

20. Fisher, D., Coleman, K. J., Arterburn, D. E., et al. (2017). Mental illness in bariatric surgery: A cohort study from the PORTAL network. *Obesity (Silver Spring)*, 25, 850–856.

21. Kouidrat, Y., Amad, A., Stubbs, B., et al. (2017). Surgical management of obesity among people with schizophrenia and bipolar disorder: A systematic review of outcomes and recommendations for future research. *Obesity Surgery*, 27, 1889–1895.

22. Johnson, D. E., Yamazaki, H., Ward, K. M., et al. (2005). Inhibitory effects of antipsychotics on carbachol-enhanced insulin secretion from perifused rat islets: role of muscarinic antagonism in antipsychotic-induced diabetes and hyperglycemia. *Diabetes*, 54, 1552–1558.

23. Stroup, T. S., Gerhard, T., Crystal, S., et al. (2016). Comparative effectiveness of clozapine and standard antipsychotic treatment in adults with schizophrenia. *American Journal of Psychiatry*, 173, 166–173.

24. Henderson, D. C., Cagliero, E., Copeland, P. M., et al. (2007). Elevated hemoglobin A1c as a possible indicator of diabetes mellitus and diabetic ketoacidosis in schizophrenia patients receiving atypical antipsychotics. *Journal of Clinical Psychiatry*, 68, 533–541.

25. Lachin, J. M., Christophi, C. A., Edelstein, S. L., et al. (2007). Factors associated with diabetes onset during metformin versus placebo therapy in the diabetes prevention program. *Diabetes*, 56, 1153–1159.

26. Taylor, J., Stubbs, B., Hewitt, C., et al. (2017). The effectiveness of pharmacological and non-pharmacological interventions for improving glycaemic control in adults with severe mental illness: A systematic review and meta-analysis. *PLoS ONE*, 12, e0168549.

27. Hemmingsen, B., Sonne, D. P., Metzendorf, M. I., et al. (2017). Dipeptidyl-peptidase (DPP)-4 inhibitors and glucagon-like peptide (GLP)-1 analogues for prevention or delay of type 2 diabetes mellitus and its associated complications in people at increased risk for the development of type 2 diabetes mellitus. *Cochrane Database of Systematic Reviews*, 5, Cd012204.

28. Gorczynski, P., Firth, J., Stubbs, B., et al. (2017). Are people with schizophrenia adherent to diabetes medication? A comparative meta-analysis. *Psychiatry Research*, 250, 17–24.

29. Vuk, A., Baretic, M., Osvatic, M. M., et al. (2017). Treatment of diabetic ketoacidosis associated with antipsychotic medication: Literature review. *Journal of Clinical Psychopharmacology*, 37, 584–589.

30. Morlan-Coarasa, M. J., Arias-Loste, M. T., Ortiz-Garcia de la Foz, V., et al. (2016). Incidence of non-alcoholic fatty liver disease and metabolic dysfunction in first episode schizophrenia and related psychotic disorders: A 3-year prospective randomized interventional study. *Psychopharmacology (Berlin)*, 233, 3947–3952.

31. Merrell, M. D. and Cherrington, N. J. (2011). Drug metabolism alterations in nonalcoholic fatty liver disease. *Drug Metabolism Reviews*, 43, 317–334.

32. Vancampfort, D., Firth, J., Schuch, F. B., et al. (2017). Sedentary behavior and physical activity levels in people with schizophrenia, bipolar disorder and major depressive disorder: A global systematic review and meta-analysis. *World Psychiatry*, 16, 308–315.

33. Dauwan, M., Begemann, M. J., Heringa, S. M., et al. (2016). Exercise improves clinical symptoms, quality of life, global functioning, and depression in schizophrenia: A systematic review and meta-analysis. *Schizophrenia Bulletin*, 42, 588–599.

34. Watkins, C. C. and Andrews, S. R. (2016). Clinical studies of neuroinflammatory mechanisms in schizophrenia. *Schizophrenia Research*, 176, 14–22.

35. Greenwood, J. L., Joy, E. A. and Stanford, J. B. (2010). The Physical Activity Vital Sign: A primary care tool to guide counseling for obesity. *Journal of Physical Activity and Health*, 7, 571–576.

36. Vancampfort, D., Stubbs, B., Probst, M., et al. (2016). Physical activity as a vital sign in patients with schizophrenia: Evidence and clinical recommendations. *Schizophrenia Research*, 170, 336–340.

37. Daumit, G. L., Dickerson, F. B., Wang, N. Y., et al. (2013). A behavioral weight-loss intervention in persons with serious mental illness. *New England Journal of Medicine*, 368, 1594–1602.

38. Green, C. A., Yarborough, B. J., Leo, M. C., et al. (2015). The STRIDE weight loss and lifestyle intervention for individuals taking antipsychotic medications: A randomized trial. *American Journal of Psychiatry*, 172, 71–81.

39. Nicol, G., Worsham, E., Haire-Joshu, D., et al. (2016). Getting to more effective weight management in antipsychotic-treated youth: A survey of barriers and preferences. *Child Obesity*, 12, 70–76.

40. Jakobsen, A. S., Speyer, H., Norgaard, H. C. B., et al. (2018). Dietary patterns and physical activity in people with schizophrenia and increased waist circumference. *Schizophrenia Research*, 199, 109–115.

41. Hjorth, P., Juel, A., Hansen, M. V., et al. (2017). Reducing the risk of cardiovascular diseases in non-selected outpatients with schizophrenia: A 30-month program conducted in a real-life setting. *Archives of Psychiatric Nursing*, 31, 602–609.

42. Khokhar, J. Y., Dwiel, L. L., Henricks, A. M., et al. (2018). The link between schizophrenia and substance use disorder: A unifying hypothesis. *Schizophrenia Research*, 194, 78–85.

43. Dickerson, F., Origoni, A., Schroeder, J., et al. (2018). Natural cause mortality in persons with serious mental illness. *Acta Psychiatrica Scandinavica*, 137, 371–379.

44. Stubbs, B., Vancampfort, D., Bobes, J., et al. (2015). How can we promote smoking cessation in people with schizophrenia in practice? A clinical overview. *Acta Psychiatrica Scandinavica*, 132, 122–130.

45. Evins, A. E., Cather, C., Pratt, S. A., et al. (2014). Maintenance treatment with varenicline for smoking cessation in patients with schizophrenia and bipolar disorder: A randomized clinical trial. *JAMA*, 311, 145–154.

46. Cather, C., Pachas, G. N., Cieslak, K. M., et al. (2017). Achieving smoking cessation in individuals with schizophrenia: Special considerations. *CNS Drugs*, 31, 471–481.

47. World Health Organization Expert Consultation.(2004). Appropriate body-mass index for Asian populations and its implications for policy and intervention strategies. *Lancet*, 363, 157–163.

48. American Diabetes Association. (2018). Classification and diagnosis of diabetes: Standards of medical care in diabetes – 2018. *Diabetes Care*, 41, S13–S27.

49. Khorassani, F., Kaufman, M., Lopez, L. V. (2018). Supratherapeutic serum clozapine concentration after transition from traditional to electronic cigarettes. *Journal of Clinical Psychopharmacology*, 38, 391–392.

12

Fever, Myocarditis, Interstitial Nephritis, DRESS, Serositis and Cardiomyopathy

QUICK CHECK

INTRODUCTION

Managing clozapine-treated patients requires clinicians to become familiar with specific medical concerns not typically seen with other antipsychotics. Among the many unique adverse events associated with clozapine treatment is a constellation of fever and immune-mediated pathologies including myocarditis, interstitial nephritis, serositis and drug reaction with eosinophilia and systemic symptoms (DRESS) [1]. While the onset of fever during the first weeks of clozapine treatment is a common and often benign occurrence, swift action is necessary with the goal of recognizing and addressing more serious issues or minimizing a treatment interruption when evidence for systemic problems is lacking. The latter concept is important, as fever during the first weeks of therapy may appear in approximately 20% of patients, and therefore is not a reason to permanently discontinue clozapine treatment when there is no evidence for myocarditis, interstitial nephritis, or other systemic drug reactions. Cardiomyopathy is another unusual clozapine-related syndrome that is typically a

- Onset of fever occurs in 20% of patients during the first 8 weeks of treatment, and commonly occurs without evidence of drug reaction, interstitial nephritis or myocarditis. In addition to routine fever work-up, troponin I/T levels, C-reactive protein (CRP), BUN/creatinine and urinalysis will help rule out myocarditis and interstitial nephritis. Benign fever is not a reason to permanently discontinue clozapine treatment, although it may be held temporarily during the fever work-up.

- Myocarditis occurs in up to 3.0% of patients, but is fatal if not recognized and clozapine discontinued. Onset is during the first 6 weeks (with rare exceptions), and should be considered in a patient experiencing fever without cause, or when a patient complains of malaise or flu-like symptoms, (particularly chest pain) without fever. Twenty per cent of cases may not experience fever.

- The troponin I/T level will be more than two times the upper limit of normal in over 90% of myocarditis cases. However, 7% of cases with left ventricular impairment by echocardiography will not have abnormal troponin levels, but will have CRP > 100 mg/l. Both troponin and CRP should be ordered when myocarditis is suspected. Other laboratory tests (e.g. eosinophil count) and ECG are less sensitive and less specific.

- Interstitial nephritis, serositis and drug reaction with eosinophilia and systemic symptoms (DRESS) are less common than myocarditis, but should also be suspected during the first 60 days of clozapine treatment when fever occurs without cause, or in patients reporting malaise or flu-like symptoms.

- Cardiomyopathy is an adverse effect occurring after many months or years of clozapine treatment. It should be suspected when patients complain of feeling tired (without recent medication changes), leg swelling, palpitations or shortness of breath.

later development, but presents a distinct group of clinical and ethical challenges when clozapine withdrawal fails to induce meaningful improvements in left ventricular ejection fraction (LVEF). Through a greater understanding of the time course and phenomenology of fever, myocarditis, interstitial nephritis, serositis, DRESS and cardiomyopathy clinicians can make evidence-based decisions about withholding clozapine treatment, and when resumption or rechallenge appears feasible.

A Fever

Fever can occur as a consequence of numerous medication- and nonmedication-related disorders, but the incidence of drug-related fever is substantially higher with clozapine than with other antipsychotics [2]. Rates as high as 55% are reported for clozapine, but the incidence of fever depends heavily on the temperature threshold of the particular study. When a temperature ≥ 37.5°C was used to define fever in one study the rate was 44%, but was only 19% with a threshold ≥ 38°C (Figure 12.1). As noted in Table 12.1, when fever is defined as a temperature ≥ 38°C, the incidence in multiple retrospective studies ranges from 14% to 20%, consistent with an early figure of 15.2% from 1983 [2]. As with many of clozapine's unusual properties, the mechanism is unknown, but the leading hypothesis, based on animal models, rests on altered cytokine levels [3]. The mean time to onset is approximately 2 weeks after starting clozapine and nearly all

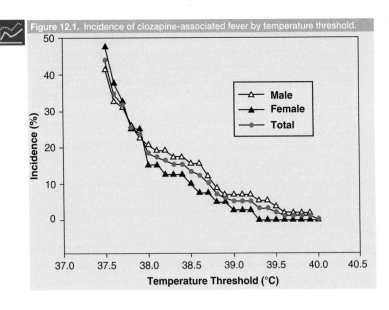

Figure 12.1. Incidence of clozapine-associated fever by temperature threshold.

(Adapted from: Jeong, S. H., Ahn, Y. M., Koo, Y. J., et al. (2002). The characteristics of clozapine-induced fever. *Schizophrenia Research*, 56, 191–193 [4].)

Table 12.1 Summary of detailed case series of clozapine-related fever.

Study	N	Mean age (SD)	Fever definition	% with fever	Mean time to onset of fever (SD)	Mean fever duration (SD)	Mean max. temp (SD)
Tham and Dickson 2002 [5]	93	33.9 ± 9.0 years	≥ 38°C (tympanic)	20.4	13.8 ± 5.1 days (range 3–26 days)	3.8 ± 2.6 days (range 1–12 days)	39.1 ± 0.74°C
Jeong et al., 2002 [4]	98	33.4 ± 11.2 years	≥ 37.5°C (axillary)	43.8[1]	67% had median time to onset of 11 days	3.1 ± 3.1 days	??
Pui-yin Chung et al., 2008 [3]	227	39.0 ± 12.2 years	≥ 38°C (tympanic)	13.7[2]	13.7 ± 7.1 days (range 5–47 days)	4.7 ± 3.0 days (range 1–12 days)	38.8 ± 0.5°C

Comments

[1] When the temperature threshold of 38°C was used, the rate was 19.4%.

[2] The incidence of all cases of fever was 18.1%, but 20% had identifiable nonclozapine-related causes of fever (pneumonia, influenza, postoperative fever, neuroleptic malignant syndrome from concurrent typical antipsychotic)

cases present in the first 6 weeks of treatment, with mean duration of the febrile episode 4.5 days (range of 1–12 days) [3–5]. Due to concerns about neutropenia-related infection, myocarditis, interstitial nephritis, and other drug reactions, an etiology must be sought in all cases of fever presenting during the first 2 months of clozapine treatment, but in 80% of instances no identifiable cause will be found [3]. Importantly, a 1-year retrospective study of patients experiencing benign fever during early clozapine treatment showed no evidence for unusual patterns of intolerability (e.g. neutropenia), with all patients able to continue clozapine during the first year of treatment [5].

Nonetheless, before concluding that any fever presenting during the first 2 months of clozapine exposure is benign, clinicians must exclude serious and potentially life-threatening conditions, and this evaluation is best performed in an emergency room setting where STAT test results and multiple test modalities are available. This sense of urgency will impact the care of < 20% of new clozapine starts, but the breadth of the approach outlined in Box 12.1 can often be performed in < 12 hours, and will help identify less-common syndromes (interstitial nephritis, DRESS and serositis) that might otherwise go overlooked when bacterial infection or myocarditis are not found.

Box 12.1 General Principles for the Approach to Fever

1. Any fever (temperature ≥ 38°C) emerging in the first 8 weeks of clozapine treatment should be evaluated immediately, as this is the period of greatest risk period for myocarditis (first 6 weeks), and for interstitial nephritis (first 8 weeks).

   a. The patient must be evaluated in an emergency department setting where a physical examination can be performed, and a complete blood count, chemistry panel (including liver function tests, amylase, BUN/creatinine, urinalysis, troponin I or T, and C-reactive protein) can be obtained in a timely manner. Additional tests (e.g. chest X-ray, blood and urine cultures, etc.) will often be performed as part of a routine fever work-up.

   b. Confirmatory studies such as echocardiography (myocarditis, pericarditis) or renal biopsy (interstitial nephritis) will be performed based on evidence from the symptoms, physical examination, and relevant abnormal laboratory findings.

   c. DRESS and serositis are diagnosed based primarily on history of new medication exposure, symptoms, physical examination, complete blood count and chemistry panel results.

   d. Clozapine should be held during the fever work-up. If more than 24 hours might elapse before resumption, coverage for cholinergic rebound will be necessary for patients on doses > 50 mg/day (see Chapter 4). If clozapine is held > 48 hours, retitration will be necessary.

2. The work-up when a fever occurs after more extended clozapine treatment (i.e. ≥ 90 days) should focus on common sources of infection (bacterial and viral) and evidence for severe neutropenia.

   a. The need for a physical examination and any testing beyond a complete blood count to rule out neutropenia will be determined based on usual clinical criteria (i.e. history, symptoms).

   b. Clozapine need not be held unless results confirm severe neutropenia.

 Myocarditis

The association between clozapine exposure and severe neutropenia was recognized in the mid-1970s and resulted in mandatory hematologic monitoring, but myocarditis is equally prevalent, and also presents a risk for fatal outcomes if not recognized. As with fever, the hypothesized mechanism is a hypersensitivity reaction involving increased cytokine levels, with eosinophilic infiltrates found in myocardial specimens during autopsy [6]. Although early case reports date back to 1980 [7], little attention was given to sporadic cases of sudden death after commencing clozapine until a 1999 review of 15 Australian cases appeared in *Lancet* [8]. This resulted in a warning added to the Novartis Australia Clozaril® package insert in December 1999, and created further interest in characterizing the phenomenon. There is little debate regarding the association between clozapine initiation and myocarditis, with the only question being the incidence of this condition. A range of values from 0.1% to 3.0% are quoted in the literature, with the higher figure provided by investigators in Australia who have led the way in analyzing local cases, and argue that the increased scrutiny within the country likely captures cases overlooked in other areas [6]. Another hypothesis, although untested, is that the Australian population might possess an enriched pool of certain genetic risks that increase myocarditis risk in a manner seen with neutropenia [9]. Until comparable analyses emerge from other localities, clinicians must proceed under the assumption that myocarditis is at least as common as severe neutropenia, so vigilance is required during the risk period.

Figure 12.2 presents the clinical features and laboratory tests that can help distinguish myocarditis cases from clozapine-treated controls without myocarditis. Detailed case-control analyses have pointed to an elevation in the level of the muscle

Figure 12.2. Features of 75 myocarditis cases compared to matched clozapine-treated controls.

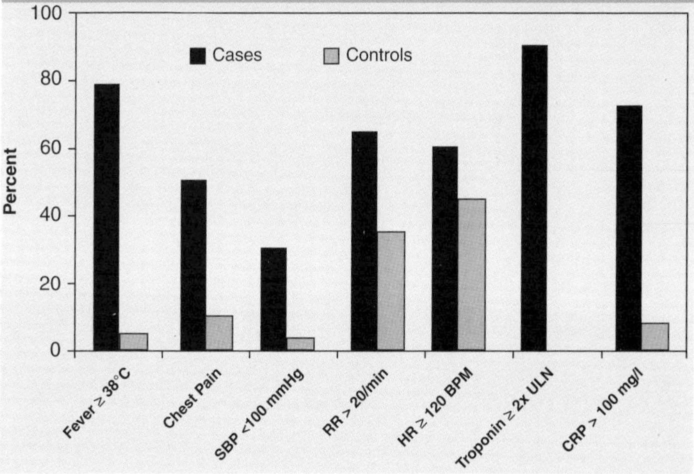

(Adapted from: Ronaldson, K. J., Fitzgerald, P. B., Taylor, A. J., et al. (2011). A new monitoring protocol for clozapine-induced myocarditis based on an analysis of 75 cases and 94 controls. *Australian & New Zealand Journal of Psychiatry*, 45, 458–465 [30].)

proteins troponin I or troponin T more than 2 times the upper limit of normal (ULN) or marked elevations of C-reactive protein (an acute-phase protein) as the initial tests of choice. Eosinophil counts are not predictive as these counts may peak up to 8 days after maximal troponin levels are recorded [6]. There are rare cases in which neither fever nor threshold elevations in troponin or CRP levels are present, yet the patient manifests other criteria of ventricular injury such as chest pain or a drop in cardiac output with systolic pressure falling below 100 mmHg. As with many of the hypersensitivity syndromes (e.g. interstitial nephritis, serositis), there may be respiratory, gastrointestinal or urinary tract complaints without evidence for infection. Although the presence of fever or systemic symptoms in the first 8 weeks of a clozapine trial should prompt the addition of troponin I or T and CRP to the battery of tests, echocardiography is recommended when other clinical data suggest myocarditis as a possibility, and certainly to confirm the degree of ventricular dysfunction once diagnosed. As is noted in Box 12.3, given the ease of laboratory monitoring using troponin and CRP, the addition of these tests to routine weekly blood counts for the first 6 weeks of treatment is both feasible and cost-effective.

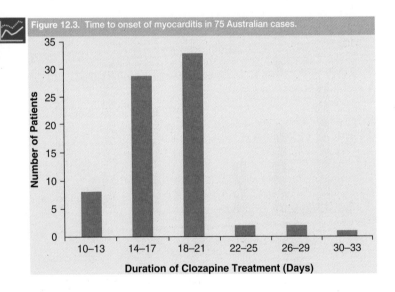

Figure 12.3. Time to onset of myocarditis in 75 Australian cases.

(Adapted from: Ronaldson, K. J., Fitzgerald, P. B., Taylor, A. J., et al. (2011). A new monitoring protocol for clozapine-induced myocarditis based on an analysis of 75 cases and 94 controls. *Australian & New Zealand Journal of Psychiatry*, 45, 458–465 [30].)

The onset in nearly all recently reported cases is in the first 5 weeks of clozapine treatment (Figure 12.3), but there is one reported case occurring on day 42, so the risk period is best thought of as the first 6 weeks of clozapine treatment. An analysis of 105 Australian cases found that a group of three factors accounted for up to 50% of the risk variance in that population. One of these, older age (especially $\geq$ 50 years old) is not modifiable, but rapid clozapine titration and the use of divalproex/valproate both increased risk (Box 12.2) [10]. As noted in other sections, there are other tolerability reasons to avoid rapid titration and the adverse effects of divalproex when possible.

Box 12.2 Essential Myocarditis Facts

1. The largest case-control series from Australia (n = 105) noted that all cases occurred by day 33, and 83% presented in the window of days 14–21. At least one case exists of onset on day 42, so the period of risk for myocarditis should be considered the first 6 weeks of treatment.

2. Eosinophil counts and EKG changes are neither sensitive nor specific enough to be diagnostic.

3. Among laboratory measures, an elevation of troponin I or T $\geq$ 2 times the upper limit of normal (ULN) is seen in nearly 90% of cases. In verified myocarditis cases where troponin levels were < 2× ULN, a C-reactive protein (CRP) level > 100 mg/l was found.

4. There are rare cases where troponin and CRP may fall short of these thresholds. Echocardiography must be obtained when there is suspicion of myocarditis based on clinical complaints occurring in the first 6 weeks of clozapine treatment (e.g. chest pain, drop in systolic blood pressure below 100 mmHg), and to confirm the extent of left ventricular dysfunction in those who meet criteria based on troponin or CRP levels.

5. Clozapine must be held during the work-up and discontinued immediately when the diagnosis is confirmed. Supportive treatment and continuous monitoring in an intensive care unit will be necessary. When promptly recognized, the prognosis is excellent with expectation of complete recovery of left ventricular function.

6. Among the modifiable factors, myocarditis risk increases by 26% for each 250 mg of cumulative clozapine exposure in the first 9 days of treatment, and concomitant divalproex/valproate use more than doubles risk (OR = 2.59; 95% CI 1.51–4.42). Age $\geq$ 50 years also doubles risk after controlling for other variables.

Once an individual has recovered from myocarditis, one is faced with the same dilemmas as the severe neutropenia patient: whether there is a need to rechallenge the patient if nonclozapine therapies prove woefully inadequate. Given the presumed immune-mediated mechanism, the concern is that myocarditis will recur, but perhaps with greater severity and decreased time to onset. A 2012 paper summarized the existing data and noted that in eight of 13 cases the rechallenge was successful. Among the unsuccessful challenges one patient had clozapine treatment terminated due to fever and EKG changes but without troponin elevation, and several cases had no troponin levels obtained, but had fever, systemic signs, tachycardia ≥ 130 BPM, hypotension (*n* = 2) and CRP levels > 100 mg/l occurring after only 1–7 doses [11]. As of 2018, there are 17 cases, of which 11 had successful rechallenges [12]. No obvious factor predicted successful rechallenge, but consultation with a cardiologist, diligent daily monitoring of temperature and blood pressure, and slow titration seem prudent as the time to recurrence tends to be quite swift when myocarditis occurs.

C Interstitial Nephritis

Although clozapine-related myocarditis was increasingly recognized in the 1980s, culminating with the 1999 review paper, the first case of acute interstitial nephritis with a strong causal relationship to clozapine initiation did not emerge until 1999 [13]. This underrecognition of interstitial nephritis is not surprising, as the sum total of the world's published literature amounts to 18 cases (Table 12.2), compared to 250 myocarditis cases covered in a comprehensive 2017 review [6]. The overlap in presenting features with myocarditis is quite significant: the majority of cases occur within weeks of starting clozapine, fever occurs in 80% of cases, and there may be

Table 12.2 Summary of interstitial nephritis cases.

Study	Age and gender	Time to onset	Fever	Proteinuria	Rash
Elias et al., 1999 [13]	38 F	11 days	No	Unknown	No
Fraser and Jibani 2000 [16]*	49 M	10 days	Yes	??	No
Southall 2000 [31]	24 F	8 days	Yes	Yes	No
Estebanez et al., 2002 [14]	69 M	≤ 90 days	No	Yes	No
Au et al., 2004 [32]	33 M	14 days	Yes	Yes	No
Hunter et al., 2009 [17]	57 F	2 days	Yes	Yes	No
Kanofsky et al., 2011 [33]	28 M	6 days	Yes	Yes	No
An et al., 2013 [34]	38 M	14 days	Yes	Yes	No
Mohan et al., 2013 [15]	53 F	60 days	Yes	Yes	No
Parekh et al., 2014 [35]	54 M	60 days	Yes	Yes	No
Chan et al., 2015 [36]	29 F	26 days	Yes	Yes	No

*These authors noted that seven cases of acute renal failure related to clozapine were reported to the UK Committee on the Safety of Medicines between December 1989 and February 2009. Fever was documented in three. One patient died, one remained dialysis-dependent, three recovered renal function, and outcomes in two were unknown.

systemic complaints. There is one case report in which a patient was not diagnosed until 90 days after commencing clozapine, but there is strong suspicion that symptoms were overlooked prior to the obvious presentation of acute renal failure [14]. The presence of two cases diagnosed 60 days from clozapine initiation establishes the period of risk at 8 weeks, slightly longer than that for myocarditis. The initial laboratory abnormalities can be detected with a urinalysis demonstrating proteinuria (and possibly red blood cells), often accompanied by significant decreases in estimated glomerular filtration rate (eGFR) as calculated from the serum creatinine [15]. As is noted in Box 12.3, given the ease of laboratory monitoring using serum creatinine the addition of this test to routine weekly blood counts for the first 8 weeks of treatment is both feasible and cost-effective. Importantly, both creatinine and urinalysis must be included in the work-up of any febrile episode presenting in the first 8 weeks of clozapine treatment. The definitive confirmation will come from renal biopsy, but the time course after starting clozapine, combined with the clinical features, abnormal urinalysis and declining renal function should identify all cases of interstitial nephritis.

 Box 12.3 Routine Laboratory Monitoring for Myocarditis and Interstitial Nephritis

1. The greatest period of risk for myocarditis is the first 6 weeks of treatment. A baseline troponin I/T and CRP prior to starting clozapine is feasible and cost-effective. Recommendations for baseline echocardiography in all clozapine-treated patients in the absence of clinical manifestations of cardiac dysfunction have not seen widespread adoption. The addition of routine troponin I/T and CRP to weekly CBC for the first 6 weeks of treatment is feasible and cost-effective.

2. The greatest period of risk for interstitial nephritis is the first 2 months of treatment. The addition of serum creatinine weekly for the first 8 weeks of treatment is feasible and cost-effective.

Rechallenging patients with a prior episode of interstitial nephritis involves the same concerns as for a prior episode of myocarditis: that this immune-mediated problem will reoccur and more quickly than with the first episode. There are only two papers that report outcomes in patients with a prior episode of interstitial nephritis. In one case, the patient developed nephritis within 2 days of resuming clozapine, and in the second case within 4 days despite the fact that the prior clozapine trial was 4 years earlier [16,17]. Unlike myocarditis, the absence of any successful rechallenges in the literature poses concerns for any attempts [12].

Drug Reaction with Eosinophilia and Systemic Symptoms (DRESS)

This is but one of a group of severe cutaneous adverse reactions (SCARs) that includes Stevens–Johnson syndrome/toxic epidermal necrolysis and acute generalized exanthematous pustulosis [18]. Although these disorders possess overlapping features, there are significant differences in prognosis and approach to the extent that a European consensus group created criteria for each SCAR and a registry (RegiSCAR). DRESS is an immune-mediated drug reaction resulting from T-cell stimulation that causes eosinophil activation and end-organ cytotoxicity (e.g. pancreatitis, hepatitis, nephritis, myocarditis). Although the general population incidence is 0.4 cases per 100,0000, the mortality rate can be as high as 10%, hence the need for early recognition [19]. While the incidence of eosinophilia (defined as an eosinophil count > 700/mm^3) was 1% in early clozapine clinical trials, this is but one component of DRESS criteria (Table 12.3) [18]. The onset is typically 2–6 weeks after drug initiation, and the variable manifestations may delay diagnosis when rash is absent. The pleiotropic presentation and high mortality rate appear daunting, yet this is an exceedingly rare adverse effect of clozapine treatment, with only five known cases [19–21]. The anticonvulsants divalproex ($n = 7$), carbamazepine ($n = 33$) and lamotrigine ($n = 17$) are reported more frequently as causes of DRESS in psychiatric patients [22]. Moreover, DRESS patients appear clinically ill, often with fever, rash, and a variety of somatic symptoms that demand attention. A 2016 review of all published psychotropic-related DRESS cases ($n = 55$) noted that fever was the most common symptom ($n = 38$), followed by maculopapular rash ($n = 32$), elevated liver enzymes ($n = 32$), lymphadenopathy ($n = 22$), facial edema ($n = 16$), and eosinophilia ($n = 16$) [22]. Using the RegiSCAR scoring system a "definite case" is defined by a total score ≥ 5 [18]. Immediate cessation of clozapine and supportive treatment in an intensive care unit are necessary, including use of corticosteroids and other immune modulators [23]. Measures to mitigate cholinergic rebound, and provision of appropriate antipsychotic therapy must also be instituted. (Chapter 4 provides an extensive discussion of strategies for managing cholinergic rebound, and considerations for antipsychotic therapy after clozapine discontinuation.) No specific surveillance measures need be taken, but the existence of these cases reinforces the need to obtain a physical examination and a set of basic laboratory measures when fever presents during the early 6–8 weeks of clozapine treatment. These patients are not candidates for rechallenge.

E Serositis

As part of a generalized immune-mediated reaction to clozapine, there are reports of serosal involvement (22 cases), including pericarditis, pleuritis, colitis, or polyserositis [24]. Many of the reported cases were also diagnosed with myocarditis, while others would likely meet the RegiSCAR criteria for probable or definite DRESS based on descriptions. The onset is typically during the early titration (range 8–70 days), although there are some late reports (e.g. 1–9 years) that might relate to other factors [24]. While cases have been described without organ involvement (e.g. isolated pericarditis without myocarditis), rather than considering this as a separate disorder, serositis should be evaluated as a possible manifestation of a DRESS-like syndrome.

Table 12.3 RegisCAR DRESS criteria [18].

Score	−1	0	1	2
1. Fever ≥ 38.5°C	No/Unk	Yes		
2. Enlarged lymph nodes		No/Unk	Yes	
3. Eosinophilia				
– Eosinophil count			700–1499/mm^3	≥ 1500/mm^3
– Eosinophil proportion if leukocytes < 4000/mm^3			10–19.9%	≥ 20%
4. Atypical lymphocytes		No/Unk	Yes	
5. Skin involvement				
– Skin rash extent (% body surface area)			No/Unk	> 50%
– Skin rash suggesting DRESS		No	Unk	Yes
– Biopsy suggesting DRESS		No	Yes/Unk	
6. Organ involvement (after excluding other etiologies)[1]				
– Liver		No/Unk	Yes	
– Renal		No/Unk	Yes	
– Skeletal muscle/heart		No/Unk	Yes	
– Pancreas		No/Unk	Yes	
– Other		No/Unk	Yes	
Final score[2]	_____ points			

Unk, unknown or not recorded.
1. Organ involvement scoring: 1 point = one organ; 2 points = two or more organs.
2. Final score interpretation: < 2: no case; 2–3: possible case; 4–5: probable case; ≥ 5: definite case.

The clinical point to appreciate is that most of these patients report flu-like symptoms, accompanied by fever and complaints related to the organ involved. In general, fever occurring in the first 2 months of clozapine treatment demands evaluation, but the presence of systemic complaints, including vague comments about malaise or flu-like symptoms, should raise red flags concerning more serious immune-mediated reactions. The serosal inflammation resolved in all reported cases after clozapine was discontinued, with two patients experiencing recurrence upon rechallenge [24]. There is one case report of a patient with pericarditis but no other organ involvement that was successfully rechallenged, perhaps suggesting that the other rechallenge failures may have been in patients who met one or more DRESS criteria [12].

 ## Cardiomyopathy

Cardiomyopathy is dissimilar to the other adverse effects described in this chapter, as it is neither an early phenomenon during clozapine treatment, nor does it have an obvious immune-mediated etiology. Although hypotheses previously focused on cardiomyopathy as a consequence of undetected myocarditis, this has been documented in only a few instances. More likely explanations include untreated tachycardia, clozapine-mediated depletion of intracellular selenium, unknown direct myocardial effects of clozapine and contributions from cardiometabolic disorders that predispose to heart disease (e.g. disease, hypertension), and smoking [6]. That clozapine might have a myocardial effect in some is supported by a study of 100 schizophrenia patients with no known prior heart disease history who had been on clozapine > 1 year. While 27% of the clozapine cohort had LVEF values in the impaired range (< 55%) by echocardiography, none of the schizophrenia patients on nonclozapine antipsychotics > 1 year ($n = 21$) and healthy controls ($n = 20$) had impaired LVEF [25]. Supporting the multihit hypothesis, impaired LV function in the clozapine cohort was associated with metabolic syndrome criteria, elevated heart rate, smoking and elevated neutrophil count.

The most common presentation is dilated cardiomyopathy, diagnosed when LVEF is < 50% by echocardiography, or when the patient becomes symptomatic with symptoms of congestive heart failure such as new-onset tiredness, peripheral edema, orthopnea or exertional dyspnea. In the latter instances, LVEF values might be significantly under 40% at the time of clinical presentation [6]. Some cases are only diagnosed at autopsy after the patient has experienced sudden cardiac death

[26]. Less common is hypertrophic cardiomyopathy, in which LVEF is preserved but the thickened ventricle becomes increasingly stiff and noncompliant [6]. The onset is insidious, and the duration of clozapine treatment is typically 1 or more years in most studies, with a range in larger samples from 8 months to 5.5 years. The prevalence ranges from 0% to 12% depending on the sample size and whether patients were identified due to symptomatic disease or through dedicated echocardiographic screening. No study with a sample size ≥ 40 has reported a rate above 5%. The prevalence is low enough that routine echocardiographic screening is not cost-effective based on results of an Australian surveillance program [27]. There is no basis for the use of routine troponin or CRP levels to predict cardiomyopathy, and it is unknown whether certain genetic polymorphisms increase risk.

As routine echocardiograms are not cost-effective, clinicians must be alert to any signs or symptoms suggestive of heart failure so that appropriate diagnostic measures are ordered and treatment can begin. New complaints of tiredness without obvious medication changes, leg swelling, palpitations or shortness of breath should prompt further investigation, particularly when other cardiomyopathy risks are present. Echocardiography is definitive and provides an estimate of LVEF. Given the possible direct effect of clozapine itself in susceptible individuals, tapering off clozapine is recommended along with introduction of standard therapy involving salt restriction, angiotensin-converting enzyme inhibitors or angiotensin II receptor type-1 antagonists, diuretics, beta-adrenergic blockers and neprilysin inhibitors. The degree of improvement after clozapine cessation is widely variable and must be documented by ongoing measurements of LVEF.

Unlike myocarditis, nephritis or DRESS, cardiomyopathy is not an acute emergency requiring abrupt discontinuation of clozapine treatment. This allows time to start standard medical therapy while engaging in discussions with the patient, family and caregivers about the diagnosis and the need to ascertain to what extent LVEF can improve off clozapine and with medical therapy. Psychiatrically stable patients with a history of treatment-resistant schizophrenia might value remaining on clozapine with a degree of mental clarity (despite the foreshortened lifespan) over the prospect of unremitting psychosis irrespective of the improved LVEF. Helpful to this discussion is evidence from three cases in which standard cardiomyopathy treatment was implemented and the patients rechallenged successfully with clozapine. Not only did clozapine not induce further deterioration in cardiac function, there was evidence of gradual improvement in LVEF [6]. A treatment plan can therefore be devised in which clozapine is gradually withdrawn, standard cardiomyopathy treatment provided, and heroic attempts made with nonclozapine antipsychotics to manage the mental illness (e.g. high-dose olanzapine). Should the latter prove fruitless, the patient would be rechallenged with clozapine under close cardiology supervision [12]. An assessment of decision-making capacity and involvement of ethicists can be useful in permitting a patient to remain on clozapine after rechallenge, irrespective of their cardiac status, due to the failure of nonclozapine treatments. Higher functioning schizophrenia patients with excellent psychosocial support might be considered candidates for heart transplantation, the only treatment option with Stage D heart failure (defined as advanced disease requiring hospital-based support, heart transplantation or palliative care). Such decisions require close evaluation, but there are two published cases of successful cardiac transplantation in patients with schizophrenia [28,29].

Box 12.4 Considerations in Cases of Clozapine-Related Cardiomyopathy

1. Suspect when patients complain of feeling tired (without obvious medication changes), leg swelling, palpitations or shortness of breath.

2. All patients should receive standard therapy involving salt restriction, angiotensin-converting enzyme inhibitors or angiotensin II receptor type-1 antagonists, diuretics, beta-adrenergic blockers or neprilysin inhibitors.

3. Clozapine discontinuation is recommended to determine the maximum degree of improvement. Abrupt discontinuation is not necessary, allowing some time for tapering to avoid cholinergic rebound.

4. The possibility of clozapine rechallenge should be part of the treatment plan when psychosis fails to respond to nonclozapine agents. Published cases document lack of deterioration in cardiac parameters and evidence of improved ventricular function (when combined with standard medications for heart failure).

5. Heart transplantation is a viable consideration for stable, high-functioning schizophrenia patients with good psychosocial support who have stage D heart failure.

Summary Points

a. Most cases of fever are benign, but fever occurring in the first 8 weeks of treatment demands work-up for myocarditis, interstitial nephritis, and DRESS, including physical examination and some basic laboratory measures.

b. The addition of routine troponin I or T levels and CRP for the first 6 weeks of treatment is a cost-effective method of screening for myocarditis. Serum creatinine for the first 8 weeks of treatment is a cost-effective method of screening for interstitial nephritis.

c. Routine periodic echocardiography is not a cost-effective method of screening for cardiomyopathy. Clinicians should suspect this adverse effect when patients on stable medication doses complain of feeling tired, or new complaints emerge about leg swelling, palpitations or shortness of breath.

References

1. Citrome, L., McEvoy, J. P. and Saklad, S. R. (2016). Guide to the management of clozapine-related tolerability and safety concerns. *Clinical Schizophrenia & Related Psychoses*, 10, 163–177.

2. Bauer, D. and Gaertner, H. J. (1983). [Effects of neuroleptics on liver function, the hematopoietic system, blood pressure and temperature regulation. Comparison of clozapine, perazine and haloperidol by evaluating medical records]. *Pharmacopsychiatria*, 16, 23–29.

3. Pui-yin Chung, J., Shiu-yin Chong, C., Chung, K. F., et al. (2008). The incidence and characteristics of clozapine-induced fever in a local psychiatric unit in Hong Kong. *Canadian Journal of Psychiatry*, 53, 857–862.

4. Jeong, S. H., Ahn, Y. M., Koo, Y. J., et al. (2002). The characteristics of clozapine-induced fever. *Schizophrenia Research*, 56, 191–193.

5. Tham, J. C. and Dickson, R. A. (2002). Clozapine-induced fevers and 1-year clozapine discontinuation rate. *Journal of Clinical Psychiatry*, 63, 880–884.

6. Ronaldson, K. J. (2017). Cardiovascular disease in clozapine-treated patients: Evidence, mechanisms and management. *CNS Drugs*, 31, 777–795.

7. Vesterby, A., Pedersen, J. H., Kaempe, B., et al. (1980). [Sudden death during treatment with clozapine (Leponex)]. *Ugeskrift for Laeger*, 142, 170–171.

8. Kilian, J. G., Kerr, K., Lawrence, C., et al. (1999). Myocarditis and cardiomyopathy associated with clozapine. *Lancet*, 354, 1841–1845.

9. Legge, S. E., Hamshere, M. L., Ripke, S., et al. (2017). Genome-wide common and rare variant analysis provides novel insights into clozapine-associated neutropenia. *Molecular Psychiatry*, 22, 1502–1508.

10. Ronaldson, K. J., Fitzgerald, P. B., Taylor, A. J., et al. (2012). Rapid clozapine dose titration and concomitant sodium valproate increase the risk of myocarditis with clozapine: A case-control study. *Schizophrenia Research*, 141, 173–178.

11. Ronaldson, K. J., Fitzgerald, P. B., Taylor, A. J., et al. (2012). Observations from 8 cases of clozapine rechallenge after development of myocarditis. *Journal of Clinical Psychiatry*, 73, 252–254.

12. Manu, P., Lapitskaya, Y., Shaikh, A., et al. (2018). Clozapine rechallenge after major adverse effects: Clinical guidelines based on 259 cases. *American Journal of Therapeutics*, 25, e218–e223.

13. Elias, T. J., Bannister, K. M., Clarkson, A. R., et al. (1999). Clozapine-induced acute interstitial nephritis. *Lancet*, 354, 1180–1181.

14. Estebanez, C., Fernandez Reyes, M. J., Sanchez Hernandez, R., et al. (2002). [Acute interstitial nephritis caused by clozapine]. *Nefrologia*, 22, 277–281.

15. Mohan, T., Chua, J., Kartika, J., et al. (2013). Clozapine-induced nephritis and monitoring implications. *Australian & New Zealand Journal of Psychiatry*, 47, 586–587.

16. Fraser, D. and Jibani, M. (2000). An unexpected and serious complication of treatment with the atypical antipsychotic drug clozapine. *Clinical Nephrology*, 54, 78–80.

17. Hunter, R., Gaughan, T., Queirazza, F., et al. (2009). Clozapine-induced interstitial nephritis – A rare but important complication: A case report. *Journal of Medical Case Reports*, 3, 8574.

18. Cacoub, P., Musette, P., Descamps, V., et al. (2011). The DRESS syndrome: A literature review. *American Journal of Medicine*, 124, 588–597.

19. Sanader, B., Grohmann, R., Grotsch, P., et al. (2019). Clozapine-induced DRESS syndrome: A case series from the AMSP Multicenter Drug Safety Surveillance Project. *Pharmacopsychiatry*, 52, 156–159.

20. Ben-Ari, K., Goldberg, I., Shirazi, I., et al. (2008). An unusual case of DRESS syndrome. *Journal of Dermatology Case Reports*, 2, 39–42.

21. Hassine, H., Ouali, U., Ouertani, A., et al. (2017). Clozapine-induced DRESS syndrome with multiple and rare organ involvement. *Asian Journal of Psychiatr*, 28, 146–147.

22. Bommersbach, T. J., Lapid, M. I., Leung, J. G., et al. (2016). Management of psychotropic drug-induced DRESS syndrome: A systematic review. *Mayo Clinic Proceedings*, 91, 787–801.

23. Wang, C. W., Yang, L. Y., Chen, C. B., et al. (2018). Randomized, controlled trial of TNF-alpha antagonist in CTL-mediated severe cutaneous adverse reactions. *Journal of Clinical Investigations*, 128, 985–996.

24. Mouaffak, F., Gaillard, R., Burgess, E., et al. (2009). Clozapine-induced serositis: Review of its clinical features, pathophysiology and management strategies. *Clinical Neuropharmacology*, 32, 219–223.

25. Chow, V., Yeoh, T., Ng, A. C., et al. (2014). Asymptomatic left ventricular dysfunction with long-term clozapine treatment for schizophrenia: A multicentre cross-sectional cohort study. *Open Heart*, 1, e000030.

26. Meyer, J. M., Rao, S. D. and Nielsen, J. R. (2007). Clozapine and dilated cardiomyopathy. *Clinical Schizophrenia & Related Psychoses*, 1, 175–180.

27. Murch, S., Tran, N., Liew, D., et al. (2013). Echocardiographic monitoring for clozapine cardiac toxicity: Lessons from real-world experience. *Australasian Psychiatry*, 21, 258–261.

28. Taborda, J. G., Bordignon, S., Bertolote, J. M., et al. (2003). Heart transplantation and schizophrenia. *Psychosomatics*, 44, 264–265.

29. Le Melle, S. M. and Entelis, C. (2005). Heart transplant in a young man with schizophrenia. *American Journal of Psychiatry*, 162, 453–457.

30. Ronaldson, K. J., Fitzgerald, P. B., Taylor, A. J., et al. (2011). A new monitoring protocol for clozapine-induced myocarditis based on an analysis of 75 cases and 94 controls. *Australian & New Zealand Journal of Psychiatry*, 45, 458–465.

31. Southall, K. E. (2000). A case of interstitial nephritis on clozapine. *Australian & New Zealand Journal of Psychiatry*, 34, 697–698.

32. Au, A. F., Luthra, V. and Stern, R. (2004). Clozapine-induced acute interstitial nephritis. *American Journal of Psychiatry*, 161, 1501.

33. Kanofsky, J. D., Woesner, M. E., Harris, A. Z., et al. (2011). A case of acute renal failure in a patient recently treated with clozapine and a review of previously reported cases. *Primay Care Companion CNS Disorders*, 13, PCC.10br01091.

34. An, N. Y., Lee, J. and Noh, J. S. (2013). A case of clozapine induced acute renal failure. *Psychiatry Investigations*, 10, 92–94.

35. Parekh, R., Fattah, Z., Sahota, D., et al. (2014). Clozapine induced tubulointerstitial nephritis in a patient with paranoid schizophrenia. *BMJ Case Reports*, 2014, bcr2013203502.

36. Chan, S. Y., Cheung, C. Y., Chan, P. T., et al. (2015). Clozapine-induced acute interstitial nephritis. *Hong Kong Medical Journal*, 21, 372–374.

13

Managing Enuresis and Incontinence, Priapism, Venous Thromboembolism, Neuroleptic Malignant Syndrome, Tardive Dyskinesia and Obsessive Compulsive Disorder

QUICK CHECK

INTRODUCTION

Along with metabolic problems, there are a number of other adverse effects not unique to clozapine, but which present unique treatment considerations given the absence of alternatives to clozapine for many patients. An important part of prescribing clozapine is developing patient rapport, and conveying the message that embarrassing adverse effects such as nocturnal enuresis and incontinence can occur in up to 40% of patients, and will be addressed, especially if persistent. Normalizing the experience through education and elucidation of a prior history of such problems is a helpful means of initiating the discussion, and imparting to patients that this is not an unusual issue, and that there are standard approaches to these problems [1]. Nonetheless, direct inquiry is the best method for elucidating complaints about enuresis or incontinence. Large studies of clozapine treatment discontinuation often cite "patient preference" when no specific reason is provided. Given the high prevalence of enuresis early in treatment, and the fact that it may persist in 20% of patients, the absence of this complaint from the literature on clozapine discontinuation suggests a lack of communication with providers [1–3].

- Incontinence and enuresis are more common with clozapine than with other antipsychotics in schizophrenia patients, and can occur in up to 40% of patients early in treatment. Approximately 20% report persistent problems with nocturnal enuresis. This adverse effect must be assessed by direct inquiry – patient embarrassment leads to underreporting and underdiagnosis. Different approaches are needed for patients who only experience nocturnal enuresis vs. those who have daytime incontinence.

- Priapism is related to inherent patient sensitivity and is reported among many medications with potent alpha$_1$-adrenergic antagonism. This is a medical emergency that requires urgent treatment to prevent tissue necrosis and permanent erectile dysfunction.

- Increased risk for venous thromboembolism is not unique to clozapine, and the risk associated with clozapine may not be significantly greater than for other antipsychotics, possibly due to patient factors (e.g. smoking, obesity, inactivity).

- The development of neuroleptic malignant syndrome (NMS) is very rare, and generally related to the concurrent use of another potent dopamine D$_2$ antagonist. Clozapine rechallenge has been successful in seven of seven reported cases.

- Tardive dyskinesia (TD) is also rare with clozapine and not a reason for treatment discontinuation. Use of newer approved agents for TD is the most evidence-based approach.

- New-onset obsessive compulsive symptoms can occur with clozapine. Treatment approach will depend on whether dose reduction is possible, and whether the patient has a prior mania history that precludes use of selective serotonin reuptake inhibitors.

13

Once elicited through patient questioning, nocturnal enuresis and incontinence are generally treatable and should not be causes for treatment discontinuation. Priapism and venous thromboembolism (VTE) represent a more significant challenge, especially as there can be risk of recurrence with significant medical consequences [4,5] The decision to rechallenge patients who have experienced priapism or VTE requires a knowledge of the management options, and a nuanced approach involving assessment of patient decision-making capacity, treatment alternatives for the medical and psychiatric conditions, and the input of caregivers. NMS and TD are much rarer with clozapine than priapism or VTE, and also present less of a management dilemma due to the success with rechallenge in clozapine-related NMS cases [6], and the availability of multiple evidence-based TD treatments in the form of vesicular monoamine transporter type 2 inhibitors [7]. New-onset obsessive compulsive symptoms can occur rarely with other atypical antipsychotics, but is reported more often with clozapine. This also should not be a reason for treatment discontinuation, although the management can require some mental flexibility on the clinician's part when the use of selective serotonin reuptake inhibitor (SSRI) antidepressants is precluded by a prior mania history [8]. As with many of the adverse effects discussed in this volume, the ultimate goal is to maintain patients on clozapine when possible, particularly when there are no acceptable therapeutic options to manage resistant psychosis.

 Nocturnal Enuresis and Incontinence

Nocturnal enuresis is not unique to clozapine, occurs with numerous medications that have central nervous system (CNS) effects, and may be related to schizophrenia itself as noted by Kraepelin [9]. There is a paucity of information on bladder dysfunction among schizophrenia patients, with most studies relying on patient self-report. Nonetheless, one study is available that used detailed questionnaires of inpatients with schizophrenia ($n = 63$) or mood disorders ($n = 45$) to compare rates of enuresis. The prevalence of nocturnal enuresis was twice as high in the psychosis patients: 46% for the schizophrenia cohort vs. 20% for the mood diagnoses [9]. Only one study has reported outcomes from urodynamic testing of incontinence complaints in psychosis patients. Investigators in India found that six of eight antipsychotic-treated patients had abnormal studies, with significant postvoid residual urine volumes in two patients [10]. Numerous hypotheses have been advanced regarding antipsychotic mechanisms that induce nocturnal enuresis, but the authors of the India urodynamic study note: "These hypotheses have been derived indirectly from the various treatments used to treat [urinary incontinence] in this situation; treatments which had limited success only" [10].

What is apparent from the literature is that nocturnal enuresis is more common with clozapine treatment, although it may improve over time. A 2016 review of clozapine adverse effects noted a broad range of published prevalence rates (0.23–42%), and commented on the limitations of the literature, especially for an adverse effect that may be underreported due to patient embarrassment [5]. A retrospective study of 61 Chinese inpatients on clozapine for at least 3 months noted that 41% reported nocturnal incontinence, and 18% had incontinence at night and during the day [11]. Over time, the prevalence of all incontinence symptoms diminished, but persisted in 25% of patients. With systematic inquiry, 39% of a British cohort of 103 clozapine-treated patients reported nocturnal enuresis [12]. A New Zealand study compared nocturnal enuresis rates across multiple antipsychotics by asking providers to directly query patients about "bed-wetting." Among a sample of 606 antipsychotic-treated patients with mean age 40 years, of whom 60% were male, nocturnal enuresis was found in 20.7% of patients on clozapine, compared to 9.6% on olanzapine, 6.7% on quetiapine and 6.2% on risperidone [1]. Significant enuresis risk factors included use of a second antipsychotic (24% vs. 4% for those without enuresis) and a history of childhood bedwetting (43% vs. 20% for those without enuresis).

Clozapine is sedating and has significant affinity for multiple receptors, especially muscarinic cholinergic, so both central and peripheral mechanisms may contribute to the problem. Cholinergic stimulation of muscarinic receptors (M_3 in particular) on the detrusor is necessary for contraction and bladder emptying, hence the use of selective M_3 antagonists for overactive bladder [13]. For those without overactive bladder symptoms, exposure to an M_3 antagonist impairs the contractile action of acetylcholine at the detrusor to the extent that it may induce urinary retention, particularly in males. Urinary retention may be the presenting complaint, but overflow incontinence may also result due to incomplete voiding.

The general approach to incontinence and nocturnal enuresis outlined in Box 13.1 will depend on whether the complaint is solely a nighttime issue, whether the problem persists, and the patient's gender. If a patient sees a provider who is unfamiliar with clozapine's pharmacology, they must be reminded that clozapine is strongly anticholinergic, and that the addition of other anticholinergic medications may double the risk for ileus. Assessment can be aided by the use of noninvasive transabdominal ultrasound. This relatively simple and painless test provides information on postvoid residual urine volume, bladder wall thickness and other parameters [14]. In instances where urodynamic testing is obtained that documents overactive bladder symptoms not due to incomplete voiding, there is a nonanticholinergic option: mirabegron. This agent is an agonist at beta$_3$-adrenergic receptors present in the detrusor, with the net effect being muscle relaxation and increased bladder capacity. Urological consultation may be necessary in persistent

Box 13.1 Approach to Incontinence Complaints

1. **Prior to starting clozapine:** Ask about current symptoms and nocturnal enuresis (past and present).

2. **Nocturnal enuresis developing during titration or after a dose increase:**

   a. Remind the patient that clozapine is sedating and not to be embarrassed. Direct routine inquiry is best.

   b. As tolerance may develop, consider slowing the titration and dividing the dose if administered solely at bedtime. Ask the patient to minimize fluids after 3 pm, avoid the use of diuretics at bedtime, and to empty their bladder before sleep.

   c. If persistent, attempt to taper off other antipsychotics, as their presence increases the risk for nocturnal enuresis sixfold.

   d. One study noted benefit from ephedrine titrated to 150 mg/day in 15/16 patients without adverse effects, but this is often not available due to abuse liability [36]. There is one case report employing pseudoephedrine titrated to 30 mg QID with complete resolution of nocturnal incontinence [37]. There are three case reports for the use of desmopressin, but in one instance severe hyponatremia developed [38].

3. **Daytime incontinence:**

   a. **Inquire:** Ask about symptoms of urgency, incomplete voiding, changes in force of the urinary stream, and the frequency of urination.

   b. **In males:** Assessment can be aided by a simple, noninvasive, transabdominal ultrasound scan that provides information on postvoid residual urine volume, bladder wall thickness and other parameters. Overactive bladder (OAB) can be due to incomplete voiding and overflow incontinence, so consider medications that relax the bladder neck (e.g. tamsulosin) via selective α_{1A}-adrenergic receptor antagonism but have lower orthostasis rates than nonselective α_1-adrenergic receptor antagonists (e.g. prazosin). Anticholinergics for OAB should be avoided for two reasons: they increase risk for ileus; and clozapine is strongly anticholinergic, so additional muscarinic antagonism is unlikely to remedy the problem. If a urodynamic study documents OAB, the β_3-adrenergic receptor agonist mirabegron is the preferred agent.

   c. **In females:** Urinary retention and overflow incontinence is less likely. Consider urological consultation as testing for pelvic floor weakness and other causes may be needed. Anticholinergics for OAB should be avoided for the same reasons as in males. If a urodynamic study is performed that documents OAB, the β_3-adrenergic receptor agonist mirabegron is the preferred agent.

   d. **Urodynamic testing:** This is very helpful when incontinence persists, but is invasive, may be difficult to obtain, and the patient may not be willing or able to cooperate.

cases, particular where initial measures have failed, and when anatomic issues might be suspected (e.g. benign prostatic hypertrophy in males, pelvic floor weakness in females). Urodynamic testing is somewhat invasive as it involves inserting a urinary catheter, but typical tests require only 30 minutes and provide information on urine flow, postvoid volumes, and other parameters if tolerated by the patient [15,16].

B Priapism

Priapism is a medical emergency in which the penis remains erect for 4 or more hours in the absence of stimulation, resulting in ischemia and significant pain. If not promptly treated, complete erectile dysfunction can result due to tissue loss in the corpora cavernosa [17]. Numerous medications are associated with priapism, many of which share the common property of alpha$_1$-adrenergic antagonism, including trazodone, and multiple first- and second-generation antipsychotics [18]. Individual predisposition clearly plays a role as some patients develop priapism on medications with no known adrenergic properties (e.g. SSRIs). For clozapine, the presumed mechanism relates to potent alpha$_1$-adrenergic antagonism, yet there are less than 20 cases reported in the literature [19]. The onset is typically during the titration phase or after a dose increase, although there is one unusual case of onset after 11 years of clozapine treatment [20].

Emergency treatment is performed in a hospital setting, and involves initial aspiration of blood from the engorged corpora cavernosa (at times with saline irrigation), intracavernosal injection of sympathomimetics in certain cases, and, if needed, surgery. The goal of the surgical shunt procedure is to create a fistula that facilitates drainage of deoxygenated blood from the corpora cavernosa [17]. Discontinuation of clozapine is recommended when this is presumed to be the offending agent, and appropriate management of cholinergic rebound and psychosis commenced. (Chapter 4 provides an extensive discussion of strategies for managing cholinergic rebound, and considerations for antipsychotic therapy after clozapine discontinuation.) After resolution, the dilemma facing clinicians is whether to rechallenge the patient with clozapine, especially when there may be little chance of treatment success with other antipsychotics. Even with slow titrations, some patients experience recurrence of priapism upon rechallenge with clozapine [4,19]. These patients likely represent a subgroup of very sensitive individuals, as there are cases of patients experiencing the same problem with multiple antipsychotics [18]. There are, however, three cases in which patients managed to continue with

13

clozapine [4,20,21]. Of note, the patient who developed priapism after 11 years continued clozapine treatment without interruption after surgical shunting [20]. Despite requiring surgical decompression for priapism during his first clozapine trial, one patient with treatment-resistant schizophrenia agreed to be rechallenged due to inadequate response to other antipsychotics. After recurrence of priapism requiring surgical intervention, he agreed to long-term use of the antiandrogen agent goserelin (a gonadotropin-releasing hormone agonist) to prevent future recurrences rather than having clozapine withdrawn and descending again into psychosis [4]. This patient had the decision-making capacity to weigh the risks and benefits of various options, but in other cases involvement of caregivers, urology experts and an ethicist might be needed.

 Venous Thromboembolism

Antipsychotics as a class have been associated with approximately a 1.5-fold increased risk for venous thromboembolism (VTE), but this effect is not seen in all studies [22]. Not only are the putative mechanisms not well understood, certain demographic factors related to the population of interest (e.g. smoking, obesity, sedentary behavior) and possibly biological factors unrelated to medications may play important roles [23]. A comprehensive meta-analysis of 17 published studies noted that the adjusted odds ratio (AOR) for VTE or pulmonary embolism (PE) ranged from 0.9 to 2.0 in the four largest studies comprising millions of antipsychotic-exposed patients [22]. This translates roughly to three cases for every 10,000 antipsychotic users. Due to the small number of events, even the largest studies lack statistical power to differentiate between agents, and for PE specifically, only three studies are of sufficient quality for analysis. Based on this smaller pool of PE studies, exposure to antipsychotics as a class does not appear to significantly increase PE risk, but more data are needed to exclude the possibility of substantial harm [22].

Despite the limited data on individual drugs, compared to antipsychotic nonusers the AOR for clozapine is reported as 1.5–2.7, with values of 1.1–1.9 for olanzapine, and 1.1–2.0 for risperidone [23]. The overlap in these odds ratios and their respective confidence intervals raises questions whether clozapine's VTE risk is significantly different than for other antipsychotics. Even haloperidol has an AOR of 1.2 for PE in a cohort study of 450,951 antipsychotic-exposed patients [24]. This is an important consideration in the risk–benefit decision to rechallenge a patient with clozapine, as switching to other agents may not necessarily lower VTE or PE risk. Prior to the development of VTE, some hospitalized psychiatric patients might merit prophylaxis on the basis of risks scores using a point system (Table 13.1) [25].

Table 13.1 A venous thromboembolism risk assessment tool for hospitalized psychiatric patients [25].

1 point risks	2 point risks	Total score	VTE risk
• Immobilization (including lower extremity paralysis) • Physical restraint ≥ 8 hours, catatonia • Oral contraceptives, hormone replacement therapy • Obesity (BMI ≥ 30 kg/m²) • Age 60–74 years • Varicose veins or venous insufficiency • Dehydration • Thrombophilia • Treatment with antipsychotics	• History of DVT or PE • Malignancy (active/treated) • Age ≥ 75 years • Acute infection (including severe infection/sepsis) or acute respiratory disease (including exacerbation of chronic respiratory disease)		Score 0–3: low Score 4–7: medium* Score ≥ 8: high*

BMI, body mass index; DVT, deep vein thrombosis; PE, pulmonary embolism.

* Risks, benefits and necessity of prophylaxis should be considered for hospitalized inpatients with scores ≥ 4 points.

After an initial episode of VTE (with or without PE) each patient should receive prophylaxis, the length of which depends on a number of clinical factors. Warfarin, factor Xa inhibitors and direct thrombin inhibitors are all treatment options, with the choice of agent relating to the need for dietary adherence and additional monitoring for warfarin, higher cost of newer agents, and proximity of hospital care in the event of bleeding [26]. Given the confluence of medication- and patient-related risks that promote recurrence, including smoking, obesity and the need for antipsychotic treatment, work-up for primary hypercoagulable states may reveal underlying disorders that require extended anticoagulant therapy [27].

A single episode of VTE (even with PE) is not a reason to discontinue clozapine, but is a reason to pursue a risk management strategy to minimize modifiable factors that increase risk, especially smoking, obesity and the use of certain contraceptives in women. If the patient develops a second instance of VTE, the work-up for a primary hypercoagulable state must be pursued. In addition, extensive discussions need to be held with the patient and caregivers about the potential options. Considerations include:

a. Switching from clozapine to an agent that theoretically may have lower VTE/PE risk, but which may be less effective for control of psychotic symptoms, and which may not be entirely free of VTE or PE risk.

b. Lifetime anticoagulant therapy, including the burdens of monitoring, and the bleeding risk.

As with priapism, the wishes of a patient who is a competent decision-maker must be respected. Some may choose the risk of death due to VTE/PE or bleeding rather than be removed from clozapine, while others may wish to try other antipsychotics with the understanding that even haloperidol may impose some risk. When a patient decides to discontinue clozapine, it need not be stopped abruptly, allowing time for appropriate decisions to be made about alternate antipsychotics based on the patient's history (see Chapter 4).

D Neuroleptic Malignant Syndrome

Neuroleptic malignant syndrome (NMS) is a serious medical disorder from exposure to dopamine D_2 antagonists associated with hyperthermia, mental status alteration, sympathetic nervous system lability, muscular rigidity and resultant marked elevation in creatine kinase. While these and associated features have been described for over 40 years, standardized criteria were not arrived at until 2011. Box 13.2 provides the International Consensus Diagnostic Criteria for NMS; moreover, a 2017 validation study found that a cut-off score of 74 had the best agreement with modified DSM-IV-TR criteria for NMS (sensitivity, 69.6%; specificity, 90.7%) based on detailed analysis of 211 cases, and agreed with consultant diagnoses in 85.7% of cases [28,29].

As a weak D_2 antagonist, clozapine is a low-risk agent for inducing NMS and the literature bears this out, yet the risk is not zero. However, there are less than 15 well-documented NMS cases involving clozapine, some of which involve concurrent use of other more potent D_2 antagonists such as haloperidol [30,31]. Whether NMS occurs with clozapine monotherapy, or the more likely scenario of combination antipsychotic treatment, all sources of D_2 antagonism should be withdrawn. Provisions also have to be made for mitigating the cholinergic rebound from abrupt discontinuation of clozapine for two important reasons:

a. Untreated cholinergic rebound may cause delirium, further exacerbating the mental status changes associated with NMS [31].

b. Cholinergic rebound will induce even more extrapyramidal symptoms [32].

The latter is critical in this instance, as NMS patients already have the most extreme form of an extrapyramidal reaction: cholinergic rebound will exacerbate the problem (Chapter 4 provides an extensive discussion of strategies for managing cholinergic rebound, and considerations for antipsychotic therapy after clozapine discontinuation).

That many of the clozapine NMS cases were also receiving other sources of D_2 antagonism may explain why clozapine rechallenge has been successful in seven of seven cases where NMS had occurred during clozapine treatment [6]. The 100% success rate is a strong argument for rechallenge, particularly when there were mitigating factors contributing to the prior episode of NMS.

Table 13.2 International Consensus Diagnostic Criteria for Neuroleptic Malignant Syndrome [28]

Criterion	Priority score
Exposure to dopamine antagonist or dopamine agonist withdrawal within the past 72 hours	20
Hyperthermia (> 100.4°F or > 38.0°C on at least two occasions, measured orally)	18
Rigidity	17
Mental status alteration (reduced or fluctuating level of consciousness)	13
Creatine kinase elevation (at least 4 times the upper limit of normal)	10
Sympathetic nervous system lability, defined by at least two of the following: - Blood pressure elevation (systolic or diastolic ≥ 25% above baseline) - Blood pressure fluctuation (≥ 20 mmHg diastolic change or ≥ 25 mmHg systolic change within 24 hours) - Diaphoresis - Urinary incontinence	10
Hypermetabolism, defined as heart rate increase (≥ 25% above baseline) AND respiratory rate increase (≥ 50% above baseline)	5
Negative work-up for infectious, toxic, metabolic, or neurologic causes	7

Comment: NMS is a clinical diagnosis; however, using the scoring system above, scores of 74 and above agreed with 85.7% of clinical consultant diagnoses during a validation study of 211 NMS cases [29].

Tardive Dyskinesia

Tardive dyskinesia (TD) is a hyperkinetic movement disorder resulting from exposure to dopamine receptor antagonists, primarily antipsychotics and metoclopramide. TD is often irreversible, even when the offending medication is discontinued, with complete remission occurring in < 30% of patients [7]. Older age and higher potency D_2 antagonism are significant risk factors for TD, but cases have been reported for every antipsychotic, including clozapine, although the development of TD on clozapine is often ascribed to prior antipsychotic exposure [33]. Nonetheless, clozapine's low risk for acute movement disorders (parkinsonism, dystonia, akathisia) led to multiple studies exploring its benefit in patients with TD in whom antipsychotic therapy cannot be stopped. The results of these studies were decidedly mixed, and with the availability of three vesicular monoamine transporter type 2 (VMAT2) inhibitors for TD treatment (tetrabenazine, deutetrabenazine, valbenazine), switching to clozapine (or any other antipsychotic with low D_2 affinity) is no longer an evidence-based recommendation for patients who need antipsychotic treatment [7]. For the rare patient who develops TD on clozapine, switching to another antipsychotic is unlikely to impact the movement disorder, but is likely to result in relapse. Thus, clozapine discontinuation is not recommended for patients who develop TD.

A more salient approach is the use of a VMAT2 inhibitor to treat TD while maintaining the patient on clozapine. The two newest VMAT2 inhibitors (deutetrabenazine, valbenazine) have approved indications for TD treatment in the US. The majority of patients in the clinical trials remained on antipsychotic treatment, and with no signal for psychiatric symptom exacerbation. Importantly, the drop-outs due to adverse effects ranged between 10% and 12% for drug and placebo groups alike across studies with deutetrabenazine and valbenazine, speaking to acceptable tolerability even with ongoing psychotropic use [7]. The litany of other medications tried for TD in the past (e.g. vitamin E) had poor evidence for efficacy according to an American Academy of Neurology 2013 review paper [34]. Anticholinergics are effective for parkinsonism and dystonia, but will exacerbate tardive dyskinesia [7].

 Obsessive Compulsive Disorder (OCD)

A 2016 review of atypical antipsychotics and obsessive compulsive symptoms notes an interesting paradox: while atypical antipsychotics are often employed to augment selective serotonin reuptake inhibitors (SSRIs) in treatment-resistant

Box 13.2 Approach to New-Onset Obsessive Compulsive Symptoms

1. Clozapine discontinuation will resolve the problem, but this may be an unacceptable choice for patients with treatment-resistant schizophrenia.

2. There may be a dose or plasma-level relationship with the onset of new obsessive compulsive symptoms (OCS). Check the trough plasma clozapine level, and consider a slow dose reduction (e.g. 5% per month) in stable patients if there is evidence that the current plasma level was achieved after rapid titration. The hypothesis is that the patient's psychosis may respond adequately at lower clozapine levels, and that the OCS will also improve.

3. For schizophrenia patients with no history of mania, the use of SSRI antidepressants is evidence-based. Avoid medications with significant cytochrome P450 interactions with clozapine, including fluvoxamine, fluoxetine and paroxetine. Sertraline is a good choice as it lacks cytochrome P450 interactions, and has no QTc warning as seen with citalopram or escitalopram. There is a small literature about the adjunctive use of aripiprazole, and this can be considered in patients on clozapine as antipsychotic monotherapy. (See Chapter 11 for discussion about concerns when combining aripiprazole with more potent D_2 antipsychotics.)

4. For patients with a history of mania, SSRI antidepressants must be avoided due to the possible exacerbation of the mood disorder, even if treated with mood stabilizers. Adjunctive aripiprazole can be considered in patients on clozapine as antipsychotic monotherapy. (See Chapter 11 for discussion about concerns when combining aripiprazole with more potent D_2 antipsychotics.)

5. Consider use of evidence-based OCD behavioral therapies (exposure and response prevention, stress management training) in lieu of, or in addition to any medication changes.

obsessive compulsive disorder (OCD), atypical antipsychotics have been reported to induce obsessive compulsive symptoms in schizophrenia patients [8]. Clozapine appears to be associated with this adverse effect more than other antipsychotics, possibly related to its higher affinity for $5HT_{2A}$ receptors, although the underlying mechanism is not fully understood. Nonetheless, every year several cases are published in which new-onset OCD symptoms appear after commencing clozapine, and improve abruptly upon discontinuation [35]. The approach to these patients (Box 13.2) depends on whether clozapine can be stopped or the dose (and plasma level) reduced, and whether the patient has a prior history of mania that precludes use of high-dose SSRI treatment needed for OCD management. In general, this should not be a cause of clozapine discontinuation, but management can be complex when the patient requires clozapine for a treatment-resistant schizophrenia spectrum disorder, but also has a history of mania. For more intractable cases, consultation with a local OCD expert may be useful to determine the best combination of behavioral therapies (e.g. exposure and response prevention, stress management training) and other pharmacological approaches.

Summary Points

a. Daytime incontinence is rarely due to overactive bladder (OAB), as clozapine is strongly anticholinergic. Anticholinergics for OAB should be avoided as a routine treatment of daytime incontinence for two reasons: they increase risk for ileus; and clozapine is strongly anticholinergic, so additional muscarinic antagonism is unlikely to remedy the problem.

b. Nocturnal enuresis may wane with time, but persists in approximately 20%. Use of multiple antipsychotics increases risk sixfold.

c. The decision to rechallenge a patient with priapism relates in part to their ability to understand the risks and benefits of rechallenge, and the presence of antipsychotic alternatives with lower priapism risk, as recurrence has been reported in some (but not all) rechallenge cases.

d. As the risk for venous thromboembolism may not be significantly greater for clozapine than for other antipsychotics, the risk–benefit equation may tilt towards ongoing anticoagulant therapy for cases of recurrence instead of clozapine discontinuation.

e. The development of neuroleptic malignant syndrome on clozapine is typically related to the concurrent use of another D_2 antagonist, and not a reason for permanently stopping clozapine. Clozapine rechallenge has been successful in seven of seven reported cases.

f. Tardive dyskinesia (TD) is also rare with clozapine and not a reason for treatment discontinuation. Use of VMAT2 inhibitors for TD is the best approach.

g. New-onset obsessive compulsive symptoms can occur with clozapine. Dose reduction (if possible) and use of selective serotonin reuptake inhibitors are common strategies, although a mania history precludes the latter. Behavioral strategies should always be considered.

References

1. Harrison-Woolrych, M., Skegg, K., Ashton, J., et al. (2011). Nocturnal enuresis in patients taking clozapine, risperidone, olanzapine and quetiapine: Comparative cohort study. *British Journal of Psychiatry*, 199, 140–144.

2. Nielsen, J., Correll, C. U., Manu, P., et al. (2013). Termination of clozapine treatment due to medical reasons: When is it warranted and how can it be avoided? *Journal of Clinical Psychiatry*, 74, 603–613.

3. Legge, S. E., Hamshere, M., Hayes, R. D., et al. (2016). Reasons for discontinuing clozapine: A cohort study of patients commencing treatment. *Schizophrenia Research*, 174, 113–119.

4. Kashyap, G. L., Nayar, J., Bashier, A., et al. (2013). Treatment of clozapine-induced priapism by goserline acetate injection. *Therapeutic Advances in Psychopharmacology*, 3, 298–300.

5. Citrome, L., McEvoy, J. P. and Saklad, S. R. (2016). Guide to the management of clozapine-related tolerability and safety concerns. *Clinical Schizophrenia & Related Psychoses*, 10, 163–177.

6. Manu, P., Lapitskaya, Y., Shaikh, A., et al. (2018). Clozapine rechallenge after major adverse effects: Clinical guidelines based on 259 cases. *American Journal of Therapeutics*, 25, e218–e223.

7. Meyer, J. M. (2016). Forgotten but not gone: New developments in the understanding and treatment of tardive dyskinesia. *CNS Spectrums*, 21, 13–24.

8. Grillault Laroche, D. and Gaillard, A. (2016). Induced obsessive compulsive symptoms (OCS) in schizophrenia patients under atypical antipsychotics (AAPs): Review and hypotheses. *Psychiatry Research*, 246, 119–128.

9. Bonney, W. W., Gupta, S., Hunter, D. R., et al. (1997). Bladder dysfunction in schizophrenia. *Schizophrenia Research*, 25, 243–249.

10. Sinha, P., Gupta, A., Reddi, V. S., et al. (2016). An exploratory study for bladder dysfunction in atypical antipsychotic-emergent urinary incontinence. *Indian Journal of Psychiatry*, 58, 438–442.

11. Lin, C. C., Bai, Y. M., Chen, J. Y., et al. (1999). A retrospective study of clozapine and urinary incontinence in Chinese in-patients. *Acta Psychiatrica Scandinavica*, 100, 158–161.

12. Yusufi, B., Mukherjee, S., Flanagan, R., et al. (2007). Prevalence and nature of side effects during clozapine maintenance treatment and the relationship with clozapine dose and plasma concentration. *International Clinical Psychopharmacology*, 22, 238–243.

13. Callegari, E., Malhotra, B., Bungay, P. J., et al. (2011). A comprehensive non-clinical evaluation of the CNS penetration potential of antimuscarinic agents for the treatment of overactive bladder. *British Journal of Clinical Pharmacology*, 72, 235–246.

14. Foo, K. T. (2010). Decision making in the management of benign prostatic enlargement and the role of transabdominal ultrasound. *International Journal of Urology*, 17, 974–979.

15. Hecht, S. L. and Hedges, J. C. (2016). Diagnostic work-up of lower urinary tract symptoms. *Urology Clinics of North America*, 43, 299–309.

16. Syan, R. and Brucker, B. M. (2016). Guideline of guidelines: Urinary incontinence. *BJU International*, 117, 20–33.

17. Shigehara, K. and Namiki, M. (2016). Clinical management of priapism: A review. *World Journal of Men's Health*, 34, 1–8.

13

18. Doufik, J., Otheman, Y., Khalili, L., et al. (2014). [Antipsychotic-induced priapism and management challenges: a case report]. *Encephale*, 40, 518–521.

19. Donizete da Costa, F., Toledo da Silva Antonialli, K. and Dalgalarrondo, P. (2015). Priapism and clozapine use in a patient with hypochondriacal delusional syndrome. *Oxford Medical Case Reports*, 2015, 229–231.

20. Raja, M. and Azzoni, A. (2006). Tardive priapism associated with clozapine. A case report. *Pharmacopsychiatry*, 39, 199–200.

21. de Nesnera, A. (2003). Successful treatment with clozapine at higher doses after clozapine-induced priapism. *Journal of Clinical Psychiatry*, 64, 1394–1395.

22. Barbui, C., Conti, V. and Cipriani, A. (2014). Antipsychotic drug exposure and risk of venous thromboembolism: A systematic review and meta-analysis of observational studies. *Drug Safety*, 37, 79–90.

23. Jonsson, A. K., Schill, J., Olsson, H., et al. (2018). Venous thromboembolism during treatment with antipsychotics: A review of current evidence thromboembolism during treatment with antipsychotics: a review of current evidence. *CNS Drugs*, 32, 47–64.

24. Allenet, B., Schmidlin, S., Genty, C., et al. (2012). Antipsychotic drugs and risk of pulmonary embolism. *Pharmacoepidemiology and Drug Safety*, 21, 42–48.

25. Maly, R., Masopust, J., Hosak, L., et al. (2008). Assessment of risk of venous thromboembolism and its possible prevention in psychiatric patients. *Psychiatry and Clinical Neurosciences*, 62, 3–8.

26. Khorana, A. A. and Weitz, J. I. (2018). Treatment challenges in venous thromboembolism: an appraisal of rivaroxaban studies. *Thrombosis and Haemostasis*, 118, S23–S33.

27. Hollenhorst, M. A. and Battinelli, E. M. (2016). Thrombosis, hypercoagulable states, and anticoagulants. *Primary Care*, 43, 619–635.

28. Gurrera, R. J., Caroff, S. N., Cohen, A., et al. (2011). An international consensus study of neuroleptic malignant syndrome diagnostic criteria using the Delphi method. *Journal of Clinical Psychiatry*, 72, 1222–1228.

29. Gurrera, R. J., Mortillaro, G., Velamoor, V., et al. (2017). A validation study of the International Consensus Diagnostic Criteria for Neuroleptic Malignant Syndrome. *Journal of Clinical Psychopharmacology*, 37, 67–71.

30. Pope, H. G., Jr., Cole, J. O., Choras, P. T., et al. (1986). Apparent neuroleptic malignant syndrome with clozapine and lithium. *Journal of Nervous and Mental Disorders*, 174, 493–495.

31. Cheng, M., Gu, H., Zheng, L., et al. (2016). Neuroleptic malignant syndrome and subsequent clozapine-withdrawal effects in a patient with refractory schizophrenia. *Neuropsychiatric Disease and Treatment*, 12, 695–697.

32. Simpson, G. M. and Meyer, J. M. (1996). Dystonia while changing from clozapine to risperidone. *Journal of Clinical Psychopharmacology*, 16, 260–261.

33. Ryu, S., Yoo, J. H., Kim, J. H., et al. (2015). Tardive dyskinesia and tardive dystonia with second-generation antipsychotics in non-elderly schizophrenic patients unexposed to first-generation antipsychotics: A cross-sectional and retrospective study. *Journal of Clinical Psychopharmacology*, 35, 13–21.

34. Bhidayasiri, R., Fahn, S., Weiner, W. J., et al. (2013). Evidence-based guideline: Treatment of tardive syndromes: Report of the Guideline Development Subcommittee of the American Academy of Neurology. *Neurology*, 81, 463–469.

35. Dykema, L. R. (2018). Abrupt improvement in obsessive-compulsive symptoms upon discontinuation of clozapine. *Journal of Clinical Psychopharmacology*, 38, 88–89.

36. Fuller, M. A., Borovicka, M. C., Jaskiw, G. E., et al. (1996). Clozapine-induced urinary incontinence: Incidence and treatment with ephedrine. *Journal of Clinical Psychiatry*, 57, 514–518.

37. Hanes, A., Lee Demler, T., Lee, C., et al. (2013). Pseudoephedrine for the treatment of clozapine-induced incontinence. *Innovations in Clinical Neuroscience*, 10, 33–35.

38. Sarma, S., Ward, W., O'Brien, J., et al. (2005). Severe hyponatraemia associated with desmopressin nasal spray to treat clozapine-induced nocturnal enuresis. *Australian and New Zealand Journal of Psychiatry*, 39, 949.

13

14

Eosinophilia, Leukocytosis, Thrombocytopenia, Thrombocytosis, Anemia, Hepatic Function Abnormalities

 QUICK CHECK

 INTRODUCTION

One need not specialize in hematology to prescribe clozapine, but the concern about neutropenia compels all clinicians to develop expertise with concepts such as benign ethnic neutropenia (BEN), and the dose-dependent impact of divalproex/valproate on neutrophil counts and neutropenia risk. The mandatory monitoring has also revealed a propensity for clozapine to induce other hematological abnormalities including eosinophilia, neutrophilia, abnormal platelet counts, and anemia. This spectrum of hematologic abnormalities is not unique to clozapine, but an analysis of 285 antipsychotic-treated patients found that persistent anemia, neutrophilia and eosinophilia occurred at significantly higher rates compared to other antipsychotics during the first 18 weeks of therapy [1]. A retrospective Canadian study of 1-year hematologic outcomes among 101 new clozapine starts found a cumulative incidence of 48.9% for neutrophilia (> 7500/mm^3), 5.9% for eosinophilia (> 1500/mm^3), and 3% each for thrombocytosis (> 500,000/mm^3) and thrombocytopenia (< 100,000/mm^3) [2]. An Italian study of 2404 patients reported a leukocytosis rate of 7.7% using the

- Eosinophilia without evidence of organ involvement is not a reason to permanently discontinue clozapine. When there is no evidence of organ involvement or other systemic reaction to clozapine, eosinophilia is self-limited and resolves without need for treatment interruption, unless dictated by local prescribing guidelines.

- Exposure to divalproex/valproate is associated with neutropenia (see Chapters 6 and 10), but also thrombocytopenia and rarely anemia. Use of alternate agents is necessary to determine whether clozapine (or another etiology) is the offending medication.

- Thrombocytopenia (not due to other causes) and thrombocytosis each occur at rates no higher than 3%. These are usually self-limited processes that resolve without need for treatment interruption unless dictated by local prescribing guidelines. Extremely low ($< 50,000/mm^3$) or high ($> 750,000/mm^3$) platelet counts pose risk for bleeding or thrombosis and will necessitate treatment interruption.

- Anemia can be associated with clozapine treatment (once other causes have been ruled out), but is not a reason for treatment discontinuation.

- Moderate elevations of transaminases (ALT, AST) > 2 times the upper limit of normal (ULN) not part of a systemic reaction do occur early in clozapine treatment in over 30%. When presenting after longer periods (e.g. months or years), nonalcoholic steatohepatitis due to insulin resistance is the likely etiology.

- Patients have been successfully rechallenged after manifesting ALT or AST levels exceeding 3 times ULN but who had no prior evidence of fever or other systemic reaction.

total WBC threshold of $15,000/mm^3$ [3]. Most of the aberrations were self-limited and did not necessitate treatment interruption. Anemia may have multiple causes, and one study of 96 new clozapine starts found that 24.5% developed anemia during the first 2 years of treatment, but it was not a cause of treatment discontinuation [4].

14

While clozapine is prone to a host of unusual adverse effects, in certain instances the problem relates not to clozapine but to other medical conditions, or to the concurrent use of medications, especially divalproex/valproate. Thrombocytopenia rates during the first 24 weeks of divalproex are 18% when defined as a platelet count $< 100,000/mm^3$, with a significant negative correlation found between valproate levels and platelet counts [5]. Divalproex has direct effects on hematopoiesis and is not uncommonly associated with macrocytosis, but anemia and pure red cell aplasia have also been reported [6,7]. The overarching principle is that for each cell line abnormality there are a small number of considerations to evaluate before hematology or other expertise is required. Moreover, these problems typically develop insidiously and do not require urgent action, permitting time for any necessary work-up or concurrent medication changes. Having a comfort level with the expected rates and course of these hematological abnormalities will allow clinicians to focus their energies on more daunting and persistent problems such as weight gain, sialorrhea, and constipation. Eosinophilia and leukocytosis should not be reasons for discontinuing clozapine treatment. Thrombocytosis and thrombocytopenia may necessitate temporary cessation, but are only rarely grounds for permanently stopping clozapine therapy [8].

Abnormalities of hepatic function tests present another source of worry for many clinicians, and may be a more prevalent problem for clozapine compared to other antipsychotics. An early prospective trial found that 37.3% of clozapine-treated patients had alanine aminotransferase (ALT) levels more than 2 times the upper limit of normal (ULN) during the first 18 weeks of treatment compared to 16.6% for a haloperidol-treated cohort [9]. As with certain hematological issues this is typically a transient phenomenon: 61% of patients who exhibited an ALT > 2 times ULN at any point in weeks 1–6 of the 18 week study had ALT levels ≤ 2 times ULN during weeks 13–18 [9]. In a manner analogous to the anemia work-up, the time course and severity will help guide appropriate diagnostic testing to evaluate nonmedication-related reasons for changes in liver function tests. Early increases in ALT or aspartate aminotransferase (AST) beyond 3 times ULN may require a pause in clozapine treatment, but in the absence of systemic illness (e.g. drug reaction with eosinophilia and systemic symptoms syndrome [DRESS]), rechallenge with adjusted titration and careful monitoring often allows patients to be successfully resumed on clozapine [10].

Eosinophilia

Eosinophils are granulocytes akin to neutrophils, but which reside primarily at tissue sites where they mediate a number of allergic responses. The development of eosinophils from myeloid precursors is governed by levels of interleukin-5 (IL-5), and once released, IL-5 and granulocyte colony-stimulating factor (G-CSF) are the most important cytokine signals that govern trafficking and promote survival [11]. Eosinophilia can occur as a reaction to numerous medications including antipsychotics, as well as parasitic diseases, autoimmune disorders and neoplastic syndromes. Due to the association between eosinophilia and serious adverse events occurring in the first 6–8 weeks of treatment (e.g. myocarditis), early clozapine package inserts contained stark warnings about eosinophilia, often including requirements for treatment interruption when counts exceeded 3000/mm³. As noted in Table 14.1, this language persists in many countries, but the accumulated data from the past 30 years of postmarketing experience have led to several insights:

(a) eosinophilia should not be used as a means of diagnosing myocarditis or interstitial nephritis – other tests are more specific and sensitive (see Chapter 12);

(b) eosinophilia is but one of many criteria necessary for the DRESS diagnosis;

(c) eosinophilia in the absence of systemic symptoms is not a reason to discontinue clozapine treatment.

This evolved understanding of eosinophilia led to modified language in the most recent US package insert (Box 14.1) which emphasizes that clozapine can be continued when there is no evidence of organ involvement, and that it may resolve without intervention.

 Table 14.1 UK reference ranges for eosinophils and platelets.

	Value	Action
High eosinophils	> 1000/mm³ - Pretreatment	Initiation/continuation of clozapine treatment is not recommended
		Increase monitoring frequency
	> 3000/mm³ - On-treatment	Clozapine therapy should be started only after blood results have stabilized under 1000/mm³
		Initiation/continuation of clozapine treatment is not recommended
		Increase monitoring frequency
Low platelets	< 50K	Clozapine therapy should be started only after blood results have stabilized at or above 50K.

Eosinophilia, defined as a blood eosinophil count of greater than 700/µl, has occurred with CLOZARIL treatment. In clinical trials, approximately 1% of patients developed eosinophilia. Clozapine-related eosinophilia usually occurs during the first month of treatment. In some patients, it has been associated with myocarditis, pancreatitis, hepatitis, colitis, and nephritis. Such organ involvement could be consistent with a drug reaction with eosinophilia and systemic symptoms syndrome (DRESS), also known as drug-induced hypersensitivity syndrome (DIHS). If eosinophilia develops during CLOZARIL treatment, evaluate promptly for signs and symptoms of systemic reactions, such as rash or other allergic symptoms, myocarditis, or other organ-specific disease associated with eosinophilia. If CLOZARIL-related systemic disease is suspected, discontinue CLOZARIL immediately.

If a cause of eosinophilia unrelated to CLOZARIL is identified (e.g., asthma, allergies, collagen vascular disease, parasitic infections, and specific neoplasms), treat the underlying cause and continue CLOZARIL.

Clozapine-related eosinophilia has also occurred in the absence of organ involvement and can resolve without intervention. There are reports of successful rechallenge after discontinuation of clozapine, without recurrence of eosinophilia. In the absence of organ involvement, continue CLOZARIL under careful monitoring. If the total eosinophil count continues to increase over several weeks in the absence of systemic disease, the decision to interrupt CLOZARIL therapy and rechallenge after the eosinophil count decreases should be based on the overall clinical assessment, in consultation with an internist or hematologist.

There are varying thresholds used to define eosinophilia (400/mm³, 500/mm³, 700/mm³) so prevalence estimates in the literature display a range of values. The US package insert states that 1% experienced counts > 700/mm³ in early clinical trials, while the rate was 2.2% in a large Italian study ($n = 2404$) with a threshold of 400/mm³ after excluding those with other pathologies [3]. The Italian paper comments that none of the eosinophilia cases required the interruption of clozapine administration, and all spontaneously resolved 3–4 weeks after onset. Lastly, using a threshold of 1500/mm³ a 1-year study of 101 new clozapine starts found a cumulative incidence of 5.9% for eosinophilia [2].

Mandatory treatment interruption is required in many countries when eosinophil counts exceed a predefined threshold (typically 3000/mm³), so clinicians in those regions will have no option but to follow local guidelines. If clozapine must be held, there are multiple reports in the literature of successful rechallenge where organ involvement did not occur [12,13]. A slower titration during the rechallenge and more frequent CBC assessments for the first month (e.g. biweekly) might help alleviate anxiety from other providers, but the expectation is that eosinophilia will spontaneously resolve if no prior evidence of a systemic reaction. When there is no mandated threshold for pausing clozapine treatment, it is still reasonable to consult with an internist or hematologist if eosinophil counts continue to climb despite lack of evidence for a systemic reaction or organ involvement (as recommended in the US package insert). This expertise can help a clinician decide whether another medication might be the offending agent, or if further work-up for parasitic or other illness is needed. Once the 6–8-week risk period has passed for myocarditis, interstitial nephritis and DRESS, the absence of systemic symptoms in a seemingly healthy individual narrows down the differential diagnosis of eosinophilia considerably, with self-limited drug reaction of no clinical consequence being the leading candidate. Figure 14.1 provides an illustration of longitudinal eosinophil counts depicting the self-limited nature of the problem in an otherwise asymptomatic patient continued on clozapine therapy [14]. The underlying mechanism is unknown, but almost certainly

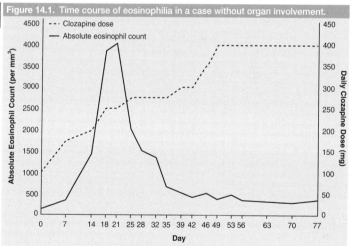

Figure 14.1. Time course of eosinophilia in a case without organ involvement.

(Adapted from: Ho, Y. C. and Lin, H. L. (2017). Continuation with clozapine after eosinophilia: a case report. *Annals of General Psychiatry*, 16, 46 [14].)

involves cytokine activation. In particular, clozapine treatment has been associated with increases in G-CSF levels, and this cytokine promotes eosinophil survival [15].

 ## Leukocytosis

To prescribe clozapine is to be intimately familiar with neutropenia, but there is a significant rate of the opposite problem, neutrophilia. As with eosinophilia, the underlying mechanism may relate to increases in G-CSF levels seen in some patients, but this remains speculative [15]. The literature in this area is sparse, and consists of a number of case reports, and aggregate data from three surveillance papers. Some papers only report increases in total WBC, although the presumed effect is solely on neutrophils. In the Italian study of 2404 patients, the prevalence of leukocytosis was 7.7% using the WBC threshold of 15,500/mm^3 [3]. While much smaller, a 1-year Canadian study of 101 clozapine starts found a cumulative incidence of 48.9% for neutrophilia (absolute neutrophil count > 7500/mm^3)[2]. As with eosinophilia, the appearance of leukocytosis is both early and self-limited in the vast majority of cases, with rare exceptions. A 1994 study of 68 new clozapine starts indicated that 40.9% met criteria for leukocytosis (WBC > 10,000/mm^3), but this lasted only 1–3 weeks in all patients but one individual whose WBC counts varied from 11,100 to 15,600/mm^3 over the ensuing 2 years [16]. A series of seven persistent leukocytosis cases with no known cause (aside from clozapine) was subsequently reported in 2007 (peak WBC 19,800/mm^3) and another in 2010 (peak WBC 27,700/mm^3) [17,18].

Before concluding that clozapine is the underlying etiology, two important causes of neutrophilia must be excluded: infection (or other acute insults such as trauma, burns), and the use of lithium. Lithium possesses G-CSF agonist properties that stimulate neutrophil production, and at therapeutic serum levels can increase neutrophil counts as much as 88% [19]. In one case of long-term clozapine-induced leukocytosis, the patient remained on lithium, so the association with clozapine is unclear [20]. While clozapine-induced chronic leukocytosis is decidedly rare, it must be included in the differential diagnosis to obviate an expensive work-up for occult sources of infection in an apparently healthy individual. In one case report, a patient underwent HIV testing, Lyme antibody IgG/IgM testing, a sinus CT scan, pulmonary and abdominal CT scans and a dental examination before it was concluded that clozapine was the cause [18]. Consultation with a hematologist knowledgeable about drug-related leukocytosis may help confine the evaluation to likely sources of infection. Once these have been ruled out, leukocytosis should never be a reason to stop clozapine treatment, even temporarily [8].

Box 14.2 General Approach to Leukocytosis, Thrombocytopenia, Thrombocytosis and Anemia

1. Leukocytosis:

   a. Eliminate lithium use and infections as possible contributors.

   b. Leukocytosis is almost always time-limited. In rare circumstances it may persist in the absence of other etiologies. Expensive work-ups are not necessary in otherwise healthy-appearing patients.

   c. Leukocytosis is not a reason to hold or discontinue clozapine.

2. Thrombocytopenia:

   a. Eliminate divalproex/valproate use as a possible contributor.

   b. When not due to divalproex, thrombocytopenia is almost always time-limited. In rare circumstances it may persist in the absence of other etiologies.

   c. Thrombocytopenia is not a reason to hold or discontinue clozapine unless mandated by local prescribing guidelines or counts approach 50,000/mm³ after ruling out other etiologies.

3. Thrombocytosis:

   a. Thrombocytosis is time-limited in all reported cases.

   b. Thrombocytosis is not a reason to hold or discontinue clozapine, unless the platelet count is extremely high (> 750,000/mm³).

4. Anemia:

   a. Eliminate other causes including blood loss (e.g. gastrointestinal), iron deficiency and divalproex/valproate use as possible etiologies.

   b. When not due to another etiology or divalproex, anemia is not a reason to hold or discontinue clozapine.

   c. Long-term data indicate that almost 25% of clozapine-treated patients will meet anemia criteria over 2 years of follow-up. Attention should be given to hemoglobin and red blood cell indices provided with routine hematological monitoring.

Thrombocytopenia and Thrombocytosis

Platelet adhesion and aggregation are the first steps in hemostasis, so platelet dysfunction can lead to bleeding or abnormal thrombosis when counts are significantly below or above normal physiologic ranges. The normal platelet count is 150,000–450,000/mm³, so technically any value below 150,000/mm³ is considered thrombocytopenia; however, there are racial/ethnic variations in platelet counts, with values from 100,000 to 150,00/mm³ not uncommon in certain non-Western

14

groups, and there is also a benign phenomenon known as pregnancy-related thrombocytopenia [21,22]. As chronic platelet counts of 100,000–150,000/mm^3 in these groups appear to pose no risk (in a manner analogous to low neutrophil counts in benign ethnic neutropenia), a working definition of thrombocytopenia as a platelet count < 100,000/mm^3 is commonly used [21]. Mild bleeding can occur when the count is less than 50,000/mm^3, but the risk for serious bleeding does not appear until the count is less than 20,000/mm^3, and especially when under 10,000/mm^3.

The best estimate of thrombocytopenia prevalence in a large sample ($n = 6316$) comes from clozapine registry data amassed in the UK and Ireland January 1990–July 1994. Only six cases of thrombocytopenia were found (rate 0.095%) using the definition of platelet count < 50,000/mm^3 [23]. Using a threshold of 100,000/mm^3 the Italian cohort ($n = 2404$) reported a rate of 0.083% [3], and the Canadian 1-year data on 101 new clozapine starts cited a value of 3.0% [2]. When not due to other causes this appears as a self-limited phenomenon, and resolution in most cases requires no intervention [24]. As further evidence for the limited impact of clozapine on long-term platelet indices, the Canadian sample of new starts reported no change in mean platelet volume (MPV) for the 65 patients who had MPV data at baseline and after one year of treatment [25].

Comparable to the focus on lithium exposure in cases of clozapine-related leukocytosis, the primary consideration in thrombocytopenia is the concurrent use of divalproex/valproate. Divalproex is known to induce thrombocytopenia in a serum level-dependent manner, with rates as high as 17.7% reported in a 24-week epilepsy monotherapy study ($n = 265$) using the threshold of 100,000/mm^3, although psychiatric samples have documented somewhat lower incidences [5]. Cross-sectional data on 264 valproate-treated psychiatric patients in Pittsburgh found that 9.5% had mild thrombocytopenia (101,000–150,000/mm^3) and 2.3% moderate thrombocytopenia (40,000–100,000/mm^3) for a total rate of 11.8% [26]. British data on 126 individuals found a 5% rate using the threshold of 150,000/mm^3 [27]. Higher serum valproate levels in both of these studies were associated with lower platelet counts.

When not due to the effects of divalproex, all of the available literature suggests that thrombocytopenia is transient, and not a reason to hold clozapine treatment in the majority of patients unless treatment interruption is dictated by prescribing guidelines (see Table 14.1). The latest US package insert contains no comments about platelet counts, and lists thrombocytopenia among a group of adverse effects noted in postmarketing experience. Nonetheless, there are two case reports of persistent thrombocytopenia without leukopenia or other concurrent medication-related etiologies [23,28]. The first case involved a 43-year-old male with chronic hepatitis and cirrhosis, both of which may have contributed, but the second case was a healthy 22-year-old woman with schizophrenia who developed platelet counts under 100,000/mm^3 after 17 weeks of clozapine treatment, and whose counts dropped to 60,000/mm^3 over the next 4 months without leukopenia or anemia, and no other possible etiologies. It was assumed that clozapine was the cause and was tapered off. Within a week of stopping clozapine the platelet count improved, and after 6 weeks it was 180,000/mm^3 [23].

A small number of thrombocytosis cases not due to the use of colony-stimulating factors have appeared in the literature, but only two studies provide incidence rates. Seven of 43 patients (17.9%) had at least one platelet count > 400,000/mm^3 in one study, and 3% of a sample ($n = 101$) followed for 1 year had at least one count > 500,000/mm^3 [2,24]. In the 1-year study the mean time to thrombocytosis was 12 weeks (range 4–22 weeks), with all cases resolving. High platelet counts (> 750,000/mm^3) present a risk for thrombosis, but this has been reported with clozapine in only one case, and was directly related to the use of the G-CSF agonist filgrastim for severe neutropenia [23]. There are no reported cases of persistent thrombocytosis, so clinicians should monitor platelet counts under the assumption that it is a self-limited process and should resolve without intervention.

D Anemia

Anemia presenting insidiously has many causes, with iron deficiency and blood loss being leading etiologies. Autoimmune processes are also a consideration when a new medication has been introduced. Based on hemoglobin values, red cell indices (e.g. mean corpuscular volume (MCV), mean corpuscular hemoglobin content), and the presence of reticulocytes (immature red blood cells), hypotheses can be formed regarding the leading candidates, and further diagnostic work-up pursued.

Despite the abundance of CBC data from decades of clozapine prescribing, there was no systematic study documenting clozapine's impact on red blood cell or hemoglobin indices until recent years. In 2015 a retrospective analysis was published from data gathered during the first 2 years of treatment in 94 Canadian patients. Using a hemoglobin threshold for anemia of < 12.0 g/dl for women and < 13.0 g/dl for men, 24.5% of the sample developed anemia over the 2 years of clozapine, although no patient discontinued treatment for this reason [4]. Among those who developed anemia, in 87% it was recurrent or persistent. The majority of all anemia cases (78%) were normochromic (normal mean corpuscular hemoglobin) and normocytic (normal MCV), and anemia tended to occur more often in those with lower baseline hemoglobin values and in nonsmokers. Smoking was protective of clozapine's effect due to the chronic carbon monoxide exposure and resultant higher hemoglobin and mean corpuscular hemoglobin concentrations in these individuals [29]. Of note, cases continued to develop throughout the 2 years of monitoring.

The underlying mechanism for the insidious development of anemia is unclear. *In vitro* studies have indicated that the metabolite norclozapine may impact erythrocyte development, but neither clozapine dose, nor plasma clozapine or norclozapine levels were associated with anemia risk in the Canadian study [4]. There are two case reports of pure red cell aplasia resulting from clozapine use, suggesting that rare individuals might be uniquely susceptible. Because the predominant form of anemia for the Canadian cohort was normochromic and normocytic, iron deficiency is ruled out, as these patients would be microcytic (low MCV) in addition to having abnormal iron studies. Renal failure, hypothyroidism, and pituitary failure are other causes of normochromic, normocytic anemia, but were not seen, and toxic effects of other medications were deemed unlikely.

The implications of these 2-year data are summarized in Box 14.2. Fortunately, every patient on clozapine is monitored for anemia due to the routine complete blood count obtained. Consultation with an internist can be helpful when anemia appears, iron studies are normal, and additional hypotheses need to be considered before concluding that the anemia is clozapine-related. Anemia is an adverse effect of a number of other medications including divalproex, and a hematologist can be helpful in evaluating the likelihood of other offending agents being present. Aside from the extremely rare cases of red cell aplasia, anemia should never be a reason to stop clozapine treatment.

 Hepatic Function Abnormalities

A number of medications and medical conditions commonly seen in schizophrenia patients can induce abnormal liver function tests. Alcohol abuse, other antipsychotics, anticonvulsants, and chronic hepatitis C are leading etiologies for abnormal liver function tests in schizophrenia patients, but increasingly nonalcoholic fatty liver disease (NAFLD) is recognized as a source of persistent hepatic disease. In a sample of 180 treatment-naive German schizophrenia patients followed for 3 years, 25.1% manifested high scores on the fatty liver index, indicative of steatosis (i.e. fatty liver) [30]. Given the range of possibilities and the high NAFLD prevalence among schizophrenia patients, the etiology of abnormal liver function tests must be determined before initiating clozapine, and appropriate treatment started including discontinuing offending medications. This is especially true for patients diagnosed with NAFLD, as clozapine-associated weight gain and worsening insulin resistance will exacerbate this problem.

That antipsychotics can induce liver function abnormalities has been known since early experience with chlorpromazine. Interestingly, chlorpromazine tended to induce changes indicating inflammation or "toxicity" in only 20% of cases with abnormal liver function, while in 80% the pattern was one of cholestasis, with increases in alkaline phosphatase and total bilirubin [9]. This cholestatic picture is not typically seen with newer antipsychotics, so evidence of hepatotoxicity (inflammation) is tracked using changes in the level of two enzymes: ALT and AST. Treatment decisions for most medications are often based on whether AST or ALT levels exceed certain thresholds such as 2 or 3 times the upper limit of normal (ULN). A early German study of 215 patients found that ALT or AST exceeded 2 times ULN in 31% of patients on clozapine monotherapy [31]. A retrospective analysis of naturalistic data from the initial 18 weeks of treatment in an affiliated group of Austrian hospitals found that 37.3% of clozapine-treated patients ($n = 167$) experienced ALT levels > 2 times ULN compared to 16.6% for the haloperidol group ($n = 71$) [9]. There was lesser impact on AST, with 11.7% of clozapine patients and 0% of haloperidol patients having values > 2 times ULN. There were no significant differences in rates of abnormalities for bilirubin or alkaline phosphatase. Importantly, 61% of clozapine patients whose ALT exceeded 2 times ULN during the first 6 weeks of treatment had lower levels by weeks 13–18. Surveillance data on drug-induced liver injury amassed from Berlin hospitals 2002–2011 did not find significantly different rates between clozapine (five cases) and olanzapine (six cases), with the 95% confidence intervals for the odds of developing liver injury (compared to a control group) overlapping for the two antipsychotics [32].

There are limited additional data on this topic aside from a number of case reports. In many instances these cases are labeled as examples of hepatotoxicity, but the patient manifested fever and other systemic symptoms strongly suggestive of DRESS [33]. As with the hematological issues discussed earlier in this chapter, the time

14

course, severity and associated features are very instructive in determining a course of action. Significant ALT/AST abnormalities presenting early in treatment with fever and other somatic complaints will point towards systemic reactions such as DRESS syndrome, while insidious and later onset indicates other possibilities (e.g. NAFLD, chronic hepatitis C, other medications).

Box 14.3 General Approach to Abnormal Liver Function Tests

1. Monitoring:
   a. After starting treatment: there is no consensus, but liver function tests must be included as part of the chemistry panel obtained during any work-up of fever or systemic symptoms occurring during the first 60 days of treatment (the risk period for DRESS and other systemic reactions).
   b. Routine: yearly as part of routine annual history and physical examination.

2. Response to abnormal ALT/AST with early onset (days to 8 weeks):
   a. Systemic signs or fever present: discontinue clozapine while the work-up for DRESS or other systemic reactions is proceeding.
   b. No systemic signs or fever present: may continue clozapine while values remain ≤ 3 times ULN. Evaluate for other causes including effects of other medications (e.g. divalproex), or possibility of NAFLD, especially in those who have gained significant weight and show signs of insulin resistance (e.g. elevated serum triglycerides, elevated fasting glucose). Consider a trial of dose reduction before ALT or AST exceed 3 times ULN if no other cause is found. Clozapine will need to be paused when ALT or AST exceed 3 times ULN, but rechallenge should be considered (see below).

2. Late insidious onset (> 90 days):
   a. Evaluate for other causes including effects of other medications (e.g. divalproex), or possibility of NAFLD, especially in those who have gained significant weight and show signs of insulin resistance (e.g. elevated serum triglycerides, elevated fasting glucose).
   b. If ALT/AST ≤ 3 × ULN there is no reason to hold or discontinue clozapine. Consider a trial of dose reduction before ALT or AST exceed 3 times ULN if no other cause is found. Clozapine will need to be paused when ALT or AST exceed 3 times ULN, but rechallenge should be considered (see below).

3. Rechallenge: should be considered in patients where no systemic symptoms or fever accompanied the increase in ALT or AST and work-up revealed no evidence of DRESS. Use slower titration, and check liver function tests 2–3 times weekly for the first 4 weeks. The monitoring frequency can be adjusted over time if results return to normal.

As with many of clozapine's adverse effects, the underlying cause of hepatotoxicity when not associated with an obvious systemic allergic response is unknown [10]. When other etiologies have been excluded, management of elevated ALT or AST often involves watchful waiting, as many early cases will spontaneously resolve over time. When AST or ALT exceed 3 times ULN, pausing treatment is necessary. In cases where no other cause is found, the liver function tests will normalize over 1–4 weeks [10,34]. There are two well-documented cases in which a patient was successfully rechallenged after manifesting ALT or AST levels exceeding 3 times ULN but who had no prior evidence of fever or other systemic reaction. In the second case, the patient underwent numerous tests to exclude other etiologies including: serology for hepatitis A, B, and C, and for HIV; serology for acute infection with Cytomegalovirus, herpes simplex, and Epstein–Barr viruses; antinuclear antibody, liver–kidney microsomal antibody; antimitochondrial antibody; smooth muscle antibody; perinuclear antineutrophil cytoplasmic antibody; abdominal ultrasound [10]. All of the testing was normal, the patient was rechallenged with thrice-weekly liver function tests, and the course is illustrated in Figure 14.2. Upon rechallenge the AST and ALT climbed again over the next 3 weeks as the dose was advanced to 500 mg/day. When the ALT exceeded 200 IU/l a liver biopsy was performed that showed mild inflammatory changes. The dose was reduced slightly to 400 mg/day, and the ALT and AST normalized over the next week. The patient was discharged on 400 mg/day and his liver function tests remained normal over the ensuing 9 months of outpatient treatment. In the first case sporadic elevations of AST and ALT were noted after rechallenge, but no intervention was performed when the patient again showed no fever or systemic symptoms, and clozapine treatment continued. The liver function tests normalized, and remained normal 1 year later on 600 mg/day [34]. These cases provide a compelling argument that, with careful monitoring, patients can be safely rechallenged with clozapine who have isolated AST or ALT elevations without systemic symptoms during the prior trial. Although peak transaminase levels may be higher than those seen in other patients, the time course and complete resolution suggests that these patients are no different than many others who experience elevated transaminases during early clozapine treatment.

14

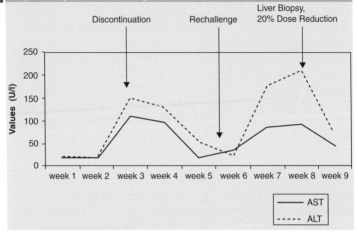

Figure 14.2. Time course of liver function test changes in a patient without fever or systemic symptoms rechallenged with clozapine.

(Adapted from: Erdogan, A., Kocabasoglu, N., Yalug, I., et al. (2004). Management of marked liver enzyme increase during clozapine treatment: A case report and review of the literature. *International Journal of Psychiatry in Medicine*, 34, 83–89 [10].)

Summary Points

a. Eosinophilia without evidence of organ involvement is not a reason to permanently discontinue clozapine. It is self-limited and resolves without need for treatment interruption.

b. Thrombocytopenia (not due to valproate or other causes) and thrombocytosis are usually self-limited processes that resolve without need for treatment interruption.

c. Anemia can be associated with clozapine treatment, but is not a reason for treatment discontinuation.

d. Moderate elevations of ALT or AST > 2 times ULN occur in over 30% of clozapine patients, usually early in the treatment course. When presenting after longer periods (e.g. months or years), NAFLD due to insulin resistance is the likely etiology.

e. Patients who had no prior evidence of fever or other systemic reaction from clozapine have been successfully rechallenged after manifesting ALT or AST levels exceeding 3 times ULN during the prior clozapine trial.

References

1. Fabrazzo, M., Prisco, V., Sampogna, G., et al. (2017). Clozapine versus other antipsychotics during the first 18 weeks of treatment: A retrospective study on risk factor increase of blood dyscrasias. *Psychiatry Research*, 256, 275–282.

2. Lee, J., Takeuchi, H., Fervaha, G., et al. (2015). The effect of clozapine on hematological indices: A 1-year follow-up study. *Journal of Clinical Psychopharmacology*, 35, 510–516.

3. Lambertenghi Deliliers, G. (2000). Blood dyscrasias in clozapine-treated patients in Italy. *Haematologica*, 85, 233–237.

4. Lee, J., Bies, R., Bhaloo, A., et al. (2015). Clozapine and anemia: A 2-year follow-up study. *Journal of Clinical Psychiatry*, 76, 1642–1647.

5. Nasreddine, W. and Beydoun, A. (2008). Valproate-induced thrombocytopenia: A prospective monotherapy study. *Epilepsia*, 49, 438–445.

6. Acharya, S. and Bussel, J. B. (2000). Hematologic toxicity of sodium valproate. *Journal of Pediatric Hematology and Oncology*, 22, 62–65.

7. Chateauvieux, S., Eifes, S., Morceau, F., et al. (2011). Valproic acid perturbs hematopoietic homeostasis by inhibition of erythroid differentiation and activation of the myelo-monocytic pathway. *Biochemical Pharmacology*, 81, 498–509.

8. Nielsen, J., Correll, C. U., Manu, P., et al. (2013). Termination of clozapine treatment due to medical reasons: When is it warranted and how can it be avoided? *Journal of Clinical Psychiatry*, 74, 603–613.

9. Hummer, M., Kurz, M., Kurzthaler, I., et al. (1997). Hepatotoxicity of clozapine. *Journal of Clinical Psychopharmacology*, 17, 314–317.

10. Erdogan, A., Kocabasoglu, N., Yalug, I., et al. (2004). Management of marked liver enzyme increase during clozapine treatment: A case report and review of the literature. *International Journal of Psychiatry in Medicine*, 34, 83–89.

11. Akuthota, P. and Weller, P. F. (2012). Eosinophils and disease pathogenesis. *Seminars in Hematology*, 49, 113–119.

12. McArdle, P. A., Siskind, D. J., Kolur, U., et al. (2016). Successful rechallenge with clozapine after treatment associated eosinophilia. *Australasian Psychiatry*, 24, 365–367.

13. Manu, P., Lapitskaya, Y., Shaikh, A., et al. (2018). Clozapine rechallenge after major adverse effects: Clinical guidelines based on 259 cases. *American Journal of Therapeutics*, 25, e218–e223.

14. Ho, Y. C. and Lin, H. L. (2017). Continuation with clozapine after eosinophilia: A case report. *Annals of General Psychiatry*, 16, 46.

15. Pollmacher, T., Fenzel, T., Mullington, J., et al. (1997). The influence of clozapine treatment on plasma granulocyte colony-stimulating (G-CSF) levels. *Pharmacopsychiatry*, 30, 118–121.

16. Hummer, M., Kurz, M., Barnas, C., et al. (1994). Clozapine-induced transient white blood count disorders. *Journal of Clinical Psychiatry*, 55, 429–432.

17. Madhusoodanan, S., Cuni, L., Brenner, R., et al. (2007). Chronic leukocytosis associated with clozapine: A case series. *Journal of Clinical Psychiatry*, 68, 484–488.

18. Sopko, M. A. and Caley, C. F. (2010). Chronic leukocytosis associated with clozapine treatment. *Clinical Schizophrenia & Related Psychoses*, 4, 141–144.

14

19. Focosi, D., Azzara, A., Kast, R. E., et al. (2009). Lithium and hematology: Established and proposed uses. *Journal of Leukocyte Biology*, 85, 20–28.

20. Trinidad, E. D., Potti, A. and Mehdi, S. A. (2000). Clozapine-induced blood dyscrasias. *Haematologica*, 85, E02.

21. Rodeghiero, F., Stasi, R., Gernsheimer, T., et al. (2009). Standardization of terminology, definitions and outcome criteria in immune thrombocytopenic purpura of adults and children: Report from an international working group. *Blood*, 113, 2386–2393.

22. Kadir, R. A. and McLintock, C. (2011). Thrombocytopenia and disorders of platelet function in pregnancy. *Seminars in Thrombosis and Hemostasis*, 37, 640–652.

23. Kate, N., Grover, S., Aggarwal, M., et al. (2013). Clozapine associated thrombocytopenia. *Journal of Pharmacology and Pharmacotherapy*, 4, 149–151.

24. Atmaca, M., Kilic, F., Temizkan, A., et al. (2013). What about platelet counts in clozapine users? *Reviews of Recent Clinical Trials*, 8, 74–77.

25. Lee, J., Powell, V. and Remington, G. (2014). Mean platelet volume in schizophrenia unaltered after 1 year of clozapine exposure. *Schizophrenia Research*, 157, 134–136.

26. Conley, E. L., Coley, K. C., Pollock, B. G., et al. (2001). Prevalence and risk of thrombocytopenia with valproic acid: Experience at a psychiatric teaching hospital. *Pharmacotherapy*, 21, 1325–1330.

27. Vasudev, K., Keown, P., Gibb, I., et al. (2010). Hematological effects of valproate in psychiatric patients: What are the risk factors? *Journal of Clinical Psychopharmacology*, 30, 282–285.

28. Gonzales, M. F., Elmore, J. and Luebbert, C. (2000). Evidence for immune etiology in clozapine-induced thrombocytopenia of 40 months' duration: A case report. *CNS Spectrums*, 5, 17–18.

29. Malenica, M., Prnjavorac, B., Bego, T., et al. (2017). Effect of cigarette smoking on haematological parameters in a healthy population. *Medical Archives*, 71, 132–136.

30. Morlan-Coarasa, M. J., Arias-Loste, M. T., Ortiz-Garcia de la Foz, V., et al. (2016). Incidence of non-alcoholic fatty liver disease and metabolic dysfunction in first episode schizophrenia and related psychotic disorders: A 3-year prospective randomized interventional study. *Psychopharmacology (Berlin)*, 233, 3947–3952.

31. Gaertner, H. J., Fischer, E. and Hoss, J. (1989). Side effects of clozapine. *Psychopharmacology (Berlin)*, 99(Suppl), S97–100.

32. Douros, A., Bronder, E., Andersohn, F., et al. (2015). Drug-induced liver injury: Results from the hospital-based Berlin Case-Control Surveillance Study. *British Journal of Clinical Pharmacology*, 79, 988–999.

33. Wu Chou, A. I., Lu, M. L. and Shen, W. W. (2014). Hepatotoxicity induced by clozapine: A case report and review of literature. *Neuropsychiatric Disease and Treatment*, 10, 1585–1587.

34. Eggert, A. E., Crismon, M. L., Dorson, P. G., et al. (1994). Clozapine rechallenge after marked liver enzyme elevation. *Journal of Clinical Psychopharmacology*, 14, 425–426.

15

Special Topics: Child and Adolescent Patients, Elderly Patients, Patients With Intellectual Disability, Pregnancy and Risk for Major Congenital Malformation, Lactation, Overdose, Postmortem Redistribution

QUICK CHECK

INTRODUCTION

Clozapine's effectiveness for treatment-resistant schizophrenia and mania, and its anti-aggressive properties, has led to trials for younger and older patients with severe mental disorders, and for those with intellectual disability (ID) who have treatment-resistant psychosis or nonpsychotic behavioral disorders. There is a paucity of double-blind data supporting some of these

PRINCIPLES

- Clozapine is effective for treatment-resistant adolescent and childhood onset schizophrenia. Schizophrenia patients under age 18 may respond to plasma levels below the response thresholds defined for adults (i.e. < 350 ng/ml or < 1070 nmol/l). Lack of efficacy at these lower plasma levels should prompt further titration, assuming no dose-limiting adverse effects.

- Initial titration for children and young adolescents is based on body weight and tolerability. Patients under age 18 are more sensitive to weight gain, so prophylactic metformin should be started along with clozapine. Very young patients (age 8–13) started on clozapine may also develop akathisia in a manner not seen with older adolescents or adults.

- Clozapine has been used successfully in older schizophrenia patients from ages 65 to 100 years. Slower titrations must be used to minimize the risk of sedation and orthostasis, both of which can result in falls. Older age is not a reason to withdraw clozapine or refuse to commence clozapine in a treatment-resistant schizophrenia patient. With advancing age (i.e. ≥ 70 years of age), patients may require lower doses and maintain psychiatric stability even with plasma clozapine levels below the response threshold of 350 ng/ml or 1070 nmol/l.

- For intellectually disabled (ID) adults with treatment-resistant psychosis, clozapine remains the antipsychotic of choice. There are limited data to support use of clozapine to manage aggression and self-injurious behavior in nonpsychotic adult ID patients, mostly derived from case reports. Careful monitoring for adverse effects, especially constipation, is crucial in ID patients, many of whom may lack communication abilities to adequately describe somatic complaints.

- According to the latest research, atypical antipsychotics as a class do not increase risk for major congenital malformations. For treatment-resistant patients requiring clozapine, it should be continued throughout pregnancy, but breastfeeding is precluded due to the risk of neutropenia in the infant.

- Clozapine shows a biphasic elimination process after overdose. Supportive measures in a monitored hospital setting are needed to manage sedation, orthostasis, tachycardia, myoclonus or seizure issues until plasma

15

continued overleaf

Principles continued

> levels return to the patient's therapeutic baseline. Clozapine remains
> the antipsychotic of choice for schizophrenia patients with a history of
> suicidality. Overdose is not a reason to discontinue clozapine treatment,
> but to institute measures (e.g. restricted medication supply) to minimize its
> recurrence.
>
> • Clozapine is highly lipophilic and undergoes extensive postmortem
>   redistribution. Interpretation of postmortem drug levels requires knowledge
>   of the sample source (i.e. central or peripheral), and whether appropriate
>   measures were taken to isolate the peripheral blood vessel from central
>   sources.

uses, but a compelling picture of efficacy based on case series and a small
number of clinical trials. The common theme for these patient groups is
managing tolerability concerns through adjustment of initial titration, use of
plasma clozapine levels, and careful tracking of adverse effects. Pregnant
women represent a patient population with a different set of issues; however,
recent developments in the literature on major congenital malformations and
first-trimester antipsychotic exposure support the conclusion that *atypical
antipsychotics as a class* are not associated with increased risk [1]. This
finding is consistent with the available clozapine case data, and thereby
allows clinicians to focus their energies on monitoring for maternal gestational
diabetes, and minimization of postnatal exposure to avoid excessive sedation
in the newborn [2]. Clinicians should be familiar with the risk nomenclature
and data on psychotropics during breastfeeding as a matter of routine clinical
competence; however, due to risk of neutropenia, clozapine is the only
antipsychotic that is absolutely contraindicated in breastfeeding women [3].

Lastly, clozapine is associated with lower rates of self-harm in schizophrenia
spectrum patients compared to other antipsychotics, but intentional and unintentional
overdose do occur, and at times can lead to fatal outcomes [4]. Kinetic data provide useful
guidelines for monitoring patients shortly after the overdose. When clozapine-treated
patients expire due to natural or unnatural causes, the accuracy of postmortem drug
levels depends on a number of factors including time to postmortem examination and
implementation of procedures that minimize "contamination" from central blood sources

[4]. An appreciation of the literature on postmortem redistribution of lipophilic molecules such as clozapine, and the preferred methods for obtaining postmortem drug levels, is crucial to anyone involved in such cases as the treating clinician, or as an expert witness.

A Children and Adolescents

Childhood-onset schizophrenia (COS), defined as symptom presentation before the age of 13, is exceedingly rare, but many patients with schizophrenia will present as teenagers, and a significant proportion of both groups will be identified as treatment-resistant (see Table 15.1). In particular, COS is a model for treatment resistance because most COS patients respond inadequately to nonclozapine antipsychotics [5]. Unfortunately COS is so rare that a dedicated group at the US National Institute of Mental Health (NIMH) managed to amass only 131 cases from 1990 to 2015 of patients started on clozapine therapy. Nonetheless, there are three double-blind studies of treatment-resistant COS patients that point to clinically meaningful efficacy differences compared to haloperidol or olanzapine, with the largest effect size seen for negative symptom improvement. Although clozapine treatment carries the same hematological monitoring burdens for children as for adults, 72.5% of COS patients started on clozapine at NIMH or shortly thereafter adhered to long-term clozapine therapy ($\geq$ 2 years of treatment) with median dosage

Table 15.1 Summary of randomized, double-blind studies for childhood-onset schizophrenia.

Study	N	Duration (weeks)	Mean age (years)	Mean clozapine dose (mg)	Mean dose of comparator (mg)	Effect size for outcomes
Kumra, 1996 [58]	21	6	14.0 ± 2.3	176 ± 149	Haloperidol 16 ± 8	BPRS 0.26 SANS 1.16 CGAS 1.37
Shaw, 2006 [59]	25	8	12.3 ± 2.3	327 ± 113	Olanzapine 18.1 ± 4.3	BPRS 1.0 SANS 0.7 CGI-S 0.6
Kumra, 2008 [60]	39	12	15.6 ± 2.1	403 ± 202	Olanzapine 26.2 ± 6.5	BPRS 0.29 SANS 0.92 CGI-S 0.4

BPRS, Brief Psychiatric Rating Scale; SANS, Scale for the Assessment of Negative Symptoms; CGAS, Children's Global Assessment Scale; CGI-S, Clinical Global Impression – Severity.

at follow-up of 500 mg/day (interquartile range: 275–500 mg/day) [5]. Despite the early age at which clozapine was initiated, this retention rate significantly exceeds that in adult patients, and speaks both to the long-term tolerability and comparative efficacy of clozapine in COS. Children starting clozapine are also more sensitive to akathisia, an uncommon adverse effect among adult clozapine patients [6]. The NIMH group found akathisia in approximately 20% of their COS patients and recommends vigilance for this adverse effect, as children often cannot describe the experience adequately, and it can result in symptomatic worsening (see Box 15.1) [7]. The NIMH group also found higher-than-expected rates of neutropenia, although this result may be distorted by the large proportion of African Americans in the treatment cohort, many of whom developed neutropenia (47%) using older ANC thresholds [8]. It is thus unclear whether children are at higher neutropenia risk using the lower ANC thresholds and BEN adjustments now present in the US. Without question children are more sensitive to weight gain and lipid abnormalities, although these were comparable to olanzapine in the double-blind trials [7]. All of the other common adverse effects experienced in adults (e.g. constipation, orthostasis, sialorrhea, tachycardia, enuresis) are also experienced by children, but without any pattern of unusual sensitivity [7].

Unless working in a tertiary referral center, many clinicians can spend their entire lives treating schizophrenia patients without encountering COS. Conversely, adolescent-onset schizophrenia is quite common, with many programs dedicated to early identification of treatment resistance in order to prevent unnecessary delays in starting clozapine. As discussed in Chapter 1, a delay in commencing clozapine after treatment resistance is recognized diminishes chances of response [9]. Despite the association with earlier onset and treatment resistance, records of 112 adolescents (mean age 15.2 years) at a German tertiary referral center found that 34% received three or more antipsychotics before their first clozapine prescription, and 40% received antipsychotic polypharmacy [10]. Although this prescribing pattern is concerning, the mean time from first psychiatric hospitalization to clozapine initiation was 1.1 ± 1.0 years, which compares favorably to general population data on clozapine initiation. Using the Danish healthcare registry data from 1995 to 2006, 662 schizophrenia patients with onset before age 18 were located of whom only 17.6% had started clozapine by December 31, 2008 [11]. There were three antipsychotic trials on average prior to clozapine, and the mean time between first antipsychotic

Box 15.1 Principles for Clozapine Use in Children and Adolescents

1. Clozapine is effective for childhood-onset schizophrenia (onset under age 13) and for treatment-resistant adolescent schizophrenia.

2. As younger age is associated with greater weight gain, prophylactic metformin must be started at the outset. Metformin should be started at 500 mg with a meal once daily for 1 week, increased to 500 mg BID with meals at week 2, and then slowly advanced by no more than 500 mg/week. A metformin dose of 850 mg BID was well tolerated in children of mean age 13.1 years [61]. If gastrointestinal adverse effects develop, try extended-release preparations.

3. Titration should proceed based on tolerability (see Table 15.2), but a reasonable starting dose is approximately 0.3 mg/kg rounded to the nearest multiple of 6.25 mg (one-fourth of a 25-mg tablet). Thus, a 36-kg 11-year-old girl would receive 12.5 mg QHS as the initial dose, while an adult-sized 16-year-old boy weighing 70 kg would start at 25 mg QHS. The starting dose should never exceed 25 mg QHS due to concerns about orthostasis and sedation.

4. Therapeutic levels seen in adults also achieve efficacy in children and adolescents. These levels typically correspond to doses between 3.0 and 6.0 mg/kg, but many children and adolescents require higher doses and plasma levels for sufficient efficacy. Management of adverse effects will permit pursuit of higher plasma levels. As with adults there is generally limited benefit for clozapine levels > 1000 ng/ml or > 3057 nmol/l.

5. The clozapine:norclozapine metabolic ratio (MR) of 1.32 seen in adult nonsmokers is slightly higher in adolescents (1.60) [19]. The ratio may be < 1.00 in children under 10.

6. Adverse effects: aside from weight gain, the only adverse effect that is unusually common in COS and younger adolescents is akathisia, occurring in approximately 20% [7]. The distress of akathisia not uncommonly exacerbates underlying psychotic symptoms. Children may not be able to describe akathisia symptoms clearly, so akathisia may be unrecognized in a patient with worsening psychosis, prompting an unnecessary increase in the clozapine dose. A high index of suspicion must be maintained when worsening occurs *during early titration or shortly after a clozapine dose increase in a COS patient*. Dose reduction may prove diagnostic for akathisia as the cause of increased psychotic symptoms. Propranolol starting in small doses (e.g. 5 mg TID) and titrated as blood pressure tolerates is also effective in 50% of patients [7]. *Other adverse effects (e.g. constipation, sialorrhea, tachycardia, seizures, etc.) are managed in the same manner as in adults, but doses of medications may need to be adjusted for younger patients.*

15

treatment and clozapine initiation was 3.2 ± 2.9 years [11]. Underuse of clozapine in adolescents remains a worldwide problem, with only 58.8% of patients deemed eligible for a clozapine trial in an Australian first-episode psychosis program actually starting clozapine [12].

The ability to recognize treatment resistance earlier in adolescent schizophrenia patients is highlighted by the fact that onset before age 20 is associated with 2.5 times greater likelihood of treatment resistance, and for males threefold higher risk [13]. Although onset in adolescence carries a better prognosis than COS, 10-year follow-up data from 323 first-episode schizophrenia patients followed at the South London and Maudsley NHS Trust showed that 23% were treatment-resistant. Importantly, among those who were identified as treatment-resistant, 84% were treatment-resistant from the onset of their illness [14]. For adolescents who are not treatment-resistant, Cochrane meta-analyses published in 2013 and 2017 concluded that there are few demonstrable efficacy differences between agents but significant tolerability differences, especially with respect to weight gain [15,16].

Once an adolescent is identified as having schizophrenia, the possible need for clozapine should be gently introduced as part of the concept that earlier onset is associated with greater odds of treatment resistance. If the patient has failed two antipsychotic trials (ideally with plasma levels to verify adequate exposure), clozapine should be commenced as soon as possible, particularly when there has been minimal response to prior treatment. Whether due to parent/guardian cooperation, or patient recognition that other agents have offered little benefit, retention on clozapine remains high in naturalistic settings, at rates very similar to those seen with the COS patients started at NIMH. The Danish registry study found that 88.8% of patients prescribed clozapine continued on it as evidenced by prescription refills [11]. A 2018 report from a Melbourne first-episode program (mean age 19.5 years) also noted that 75.6% of treatment-resistant patients started on clozapine remained on treatment [12]. In addition, 76.6% of those who were commenced on clozapine achieved symptomatic remission of positive psychotic symptoms by the time of discharge from the program or transfer to adult mental health services.

● Levels

The data in COS and adolescent schizophrenia patients indicate that these younger patients tend to respond at plasma clozapine levels slightly below the thresholds used for adults, with response seen at times with levels < 300 ng/ml or

< 917 nmol/l [7,17]. Nonetheless, as with adults, failure to respond after several weeks at a particular plasma level is a reason to pursue further titration. In addition to nonadherence and cytochrome P450 polymorphisms, age, gender and smoking status will influence plasma clozapine levels. Data analyzed from 1408 samples obtained in 484 UK and Irish patients 8–17 years of age found that clozapine levels did correlate with prescribed dose, and were 34% higher in females than in males, and 41% higher in nonsmokers than in smokers. The mean metabolic ratio (MR), defined as the ratio of clozapine to the metabolite norclozapine, is typically 1.32 in adults [18], but was 1.6 in this large sample [19]. In young children aged 8–9 the plasma norclozapine level was higher than that for clozapine, a finding noted in another small sample ($n = 6$) with mean age of 13.3 years [17], but over time the MR assumes ratios closer to that seen with adults as shown in Figure 15.1 [19].

Figure 15.1. Median clozapine and norclozapine plasma levels and median clozapine dose by age in 1408 samples from 454 patients under age 18.

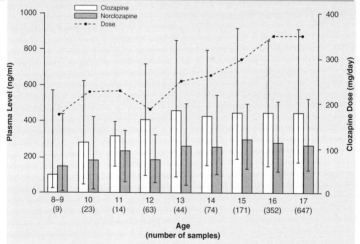

(Adapted from: Couchman, L., Bowskill, S. V., Handley, S., et al. (2013). Plasma clozapine and norclozapine in relation to prescribed dose and other factors in patients aged <18 years: Data from a therapeutic drug monitoring service, 1994–2010. *Early Interventions in Psychiatry*, 7, 122–130 [19].)

● **Adverse Effects**

No unusual patterns of tolerability have been observed in children or adolescents starting on clozapine with the one exception noted previously: COS and young adolescent patients appear prone to developing akathisia in a manner rarely seen with adult patients commencing clozapine [6]. While uncommon adverse events such as myocarditis have been reported, there is no evidence of increased rates in younger patients [12,20]. Tachycardia and orthostasis must be managed aggressively as these appeared to be disproportionate causes of treatment discontinuation in a large case series from an early psychosis service in Melbourne [12]. Adverse effects are managed in the same manner as for adults, although doses of adjunctive medications need to be adjusted in much younger patients. Consultation with a pediatrician can be helpful to decide on initial doses and titration schedule of beta-adrenergic antagonists for tachycardia, medications for constipation, and other agents.

● **Use in Mania**

Some bipolar patients present early in life, and may experience mania that is resistant to treatment with usual combinations of mood stabilizers and antipsychotics. Although there are no controlled data for adolescent mania, there is one large case series describing the benefit of clozapine in 10 adolescent

Table 15.2. Child/adolescent clozapine titration.

Day	Slower titration (mg QHS)	Day	Faster titration (mg QHS)
1	12.5	1	12.5
3	25	3	25
6	50	5	50
9	75	7	75
12	100	9	100
15	125	11	125
18	150	13	150
21	175	15	175
24	200	17	200

QHS, at bedtime.

Comments:

1. All titrations must be adjusted based on tolerability, with sedation, orthostasis and tachycardia being important limiting adverse effects. In childhood-onset schizophrenia, akathisia with clozapine is also reported in a manner not seen with adults (see Box 15.1). As with adults, a faster titration may be possible in inpatient settings where vital signs can be monitored daily.

2. Unlike adults, the use of divided doses early in treatment may be necessary; however, the bulk of the clozapine dose should be administered at bedtime.

3. A plasma clozapine level should be obtained at 100 mg/day, ideally after 4–5 days on that dose.

inpatients (age range 12–17) with severe treatment-resistant acute manic or mixed episodes [21]. All patients were successfully discharged after 15–28 days of clozapine treatment, and changes in mood rating scales and in the Clinical Global Impression – Severity scale were significant ($p < 0.001$). The mean clozapine dose at time of discharge was 142.5 ± 73.6 mg/day (range 75–300 mg/day). Although adverse effects did occur (sedation, enuresis, sialorrhea, increased appetite), these were not severe enough to warrant dosage reduction. Long-term follow-up (12–24 months) revealed a mean 10.7% weight gain, but no episodes of seizures or neutropenia [21].

B Elderly

Treatment of older patients (i.e. those ≥ 60 years of age) creates concerns related to increased intolerance of certain adverse effects, combined with reduced drug clearance [22]. Aside from the double-blind studies for Parkinson's disease psychosis (see Chapter 1), there are no prospective studies specifically targeting the use of clozapine for older severely mentally ill patients; however, there are a number of papers that have retrospectively examined outcomes in nondemented patients with schizophrenia spectrum disorders. While many of these papers include data on older patients who had been started on clozapine when younger, one group provided outcomes data on 43 Israeli schizophrenia patients of mean age 69.4 ± 8.7 years, all of whom were new starts to clozapine [23]. These patients had been ill on average 39 years and had all failed at least three first- and second-generation antipsychotics. Clozapine was well tolerated with no patients having to stop treatment due to adverse effects. Plasma levels were not provided, but the mean clozapine dose was 264 ± 110 mg/day (range 25–700 mg/day). Over the next 5 years, psychiatric hospitalization rates were significantly lower than for the 5-year period prior to clozapine therapy (0.41 vs. 3.8; $p < 0.001$). The authors also noted that the mortality rate in the clozapine-treated cohort was equal to that for other older schizophrenia patients treated at the same clinic with nonclozapine antipsychotics [23].

The titration used in older patients is limited by tolerability, especially those adverse effects that can contribute to fall risk [24]. As with younger adults, failure to respond after several weeks at a particular plasma level without dose-limiting

15

285

adverse effects is a reason to pursue further titration. The mean dose at which older schizophrenia patients respond may be lower than that used with younger patients even after controlling for differences in smoking behavior. Consistent with the Israeli data noted above, dosing records from 778 UK and Irish elderly schizophrenia patients (363 males, median age 67, range 65–100 years; 415 females, median age 68, range 65–90 years) yielded a median dose of 300 mg/day in those aged 65–70 years, and 200 mg/day in those aged 75 and older (see Figure 15.2) [25]. An important contributor to tolerability issues is decreased drug metabolism with advanced age, along with decreased body mass. More than 1900 plasma level samples were obtained from this UK/Irish cohort, and the metabolic ratio (MR) was 1.8 in this older patient sample, higher than the value of 1.32 in younger adults [25]. Importantly, the plasma clozapine level was estimated to

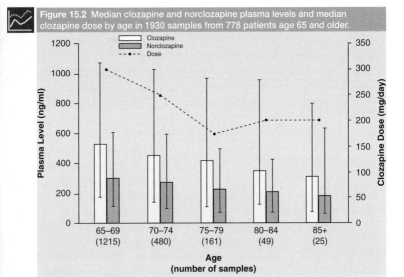

Figure 15.2 Median clozapine and norclozapine plasma levels and median clozapine dose by age in 1930 samples from 778 patients age 65 and older.

(Adapted from: Bowskill, S., Couchman, L., MacCabe, J. H., et al. (2012). Plasma clozapine and norclozapine in relation to prescribed dose and other factors in patients aged 65 years and over: Data from a therapeutic drug monitoring service, 1996–2010. *Human Psychopharmacology*, 27, 277–283 [25].)

Table 15.3 Clozapine titration for nonsmoking schizophrenia patients age 65 and above not receiving cytochrome P450 inhibitors.

Day	Dose (mg QHS)
1	12.5
3	25
6	50
9	75
12	100
15	125
18	150
21	175
24	200

QHS, at bedtime.

Comments

1. All titrations must be adjusted based on tolerability, with sedation, orthostasis and tachycardia being important limiting adverse effects as they contribute to fall risk. As with younger adults, a slightly faster titration may be possible in inpatient settings where vital signs can be monitored daily. Clozapine levels in nonsmokers are 32% higher than for smokers, so the titration in smokers can be increased by 33% (i.e. advancing the dose every 2 days instead of every 3 days).

2. A plasma clozapine level should be obtained at 150 mg/day. A greater proportion of older schizophrenia patients may respond at plasma levels below the response threshold seen with younger adults (< 350 ng/ml or < 1070 nmol/l). In large naturalistic samples, the median dose was 300 mg/day in those aged 65–70 years, and 200 mg/day in those aged 75 and older.

increase by 3% for each 10 kg decrease in body weight from 74 kg (the cohort mean weight). Thus, as people advance beyond the age of 65, tracking plasma clozapine levels is key to minimizing level creep that can be associated with aging. Not only might patients require lower daily doses to maintain equivalent plasma levels, they may remain psychiatrically stable at plasma levels below those needed in prior decades, at times even below the response threshold of 350 ng/ml or 1070 nmol/l [25].

● **Adverse Effects**

There are a small number of adverse effects to which older patients are more prone including the central nervous system (CNS) impact of histamine H_1 antagonism and cholinergic antagonism, orthostasis from peripheral $alpha_1$-adrenergic blockade, and anticholinergic impact on gastrointestinal motility and urination (in males) [24]. Mitigation of early problems with orthostasis or sedation is crucial because even mild problems with alertness or dizziness can result in a fall that itself can have catastrophic consequences. Although early analyses

15

1. Plasma clozapine levels may be higher for a given dose due to age-related decreases in cytochrome P450 activity, and possibly lower serum albumin levels. The clozapine:norclozapine metabolic ratio (MR) of 1.32 seen in younger adults is higher in those age 65 and older (MR = 1.8) [25].

2. Older patients will be more sensitive to orthostasis and sedation, with the net effect being higher fall rates than in younger patients. The starting dose should be no higher than 12.5 mg QHS, and a slower titration must be used in this age group along with careful monitoring of orthostatic vital signs, and prompt action for complaints of dizziness or gait instability (see Table 15.3).

3. Patients aged 65 and older will often require plasma clozapine levels above the response threshold of 350 ng/ml or 1070 nmol/l; however, there will be a substantial proportion of these older patients who achieve therapeutic benefit with plasma levels below this threshold.

4. In established patients on clozapine, doses may need to be reduced as the patient reaches age 65 due to tolerability reasons, or due to higher plasma levels from reduced rates of drug metabolism. Possibly due to reduced absorptive capacity, plasma levels decline in patients starting at age 80 despite remaining on the same dose.

5. Adverse effects: older patients are more sensitive to developing orthostasis (as noted above). They are also more sensitive to the sedating effects of histamine H_1 antagonism, and to anticholinergic effects including CNS issues (sedation, confusion or delirium) and peripheral adverse effects (constipation, urinary retention [in males]) [24]. The management of adverse effects is similar to that for younger patients but with greater diligence during the titration phase, and the possible need for expert consultation due to comorbid medical problems, or complex nonpsychiatric medication regimens that pose risk for drug–drug interactions.

indicated an association between older age and neutropenia risk [26], this is not consistently seen in later literature. Older patients need not be subjected to hematological monitoring that differs from that in younger individuals. Once on established therapy, attentiveness to peripheral anticholinergic issues including constipation and urinary retention (in males) is important due to the higher age-related prevalence of these problems independent of clozapine treatment. Treatment of adverse effects is the same as for younger patients, bearing in mind the complexity of nonpsychiatric medical conditions and medications. Consultation with a geriatrician can prove useful in circumstances where there is uncertainty about a course of action due to underlying medical disorders or possible interactions with other medications. With these caveats in mind, the data sets from Israel and UK/Ireland indicate that clozapine has been used in patients up to age 100. The conclusions from this research are twofold: (a) schizophrenia spectrum patients can be maintained on clozapine throughout their lifetime; and (b) patients 65 years of age and older need not be deprived of a clozapine trial solely on the basis of age.

C Intellectual Disability

Intellectual disability (ID) patients represent a heterogeneous cohort of individuals, some of whom manifest identifiable psychosis symptoms, while others present problematic behaviors (e.g. self-injury, aggression) that do not respond to behavioral interventions. Certain atypical antipsychotics have been approved in the US and elsewhere for treatment of irritability associated with autistic disorder in children and adolescents aged 5–16 years [27], but there are very few double-blind, placebo-controlled studies of antipsychotic use in ID adults, with clozapine being no exception. Although psychosis afflicts no more than 3% of the ID population, antipsychotics are widely prescribed for behavioral disturbances despite limited controlled studies supporting efficacy, tolerability, or improved quality of life [28,29]. One significant problem for pharmacological trials in ID adults relates to recruitment of a vulnerable population for medication studies. A 2010 paper summarizes these challenges in describing the hurdles to recruiting aggressive adult ID patients in Queensland, Australia to participate in a double-blind trial comparing risperidone, haloperidol and placebo. The authors note that clinician concerns over the efficacy of antipsychotics in these patients, ethical concerns over medication trials in the ID population, and practical issues with engaging treatment teams were all impediments [30]. The investigators did manage to recruit 86 subjects out of the intended sample of 120, and found that aggression declined dramatically in all groups by 4 weeks, with placebo showing a 79% reduction in aggressive events, compared to 57% reduction for the combined antipsychotic cohort ($p = 0.06$) [31].

● Use of Clozapine in Nonpsychotic Adult ID Patients

With the paucity of controlled data supporting obvious efficacy advantages for nonclozapine antipsychotics in adult ID patients without psychosis, widespread use of antipsychotics to manage challenging behavior is not the standard of care. Nonetheless, there are instances where antipsychotics may prove useful, and clinicians must develop expertise in managing their safe use in this patient group. A leading expert on psychotropic use in the adult ID population, Professor Jose De Leon MD (University of Kentucky Mental Health Research Center, Lexington, KY) published a comprehensive guideline on the use of nonclozapine atypical antipsychotics in ID adults, including information on: initiation, dosing, drug–drug interactions, adverse drug reactions, and discontinuation syndromes [32]. (Note: this review also provides drug utilization review forms for nonclozapine antipsychotics to facilitate implementation of the guidelines.) In a manner analogous to the use of clozapine for treatment-resistant mania, the application of clozapine for behavioral disturbances in nonpsychotic adult ID patients has largely been motivated by lack of response to traditional treatment, in this instance to the combination of behavioral interventions and other psychotropics. Supporting this logic is the literature noting that clozapine has unique benefits for suicidality and aggression, benefits that are independent of its antipsychotic effects [33]. (See Chapter 1 for additional discussion of clozapine's anti-aggressive properties.) The literature on use of clozapine for behavioral disturbances in nonpsychotic ID patients extends back to a 1974 publication describing 40 adolescents (mean age 16.4 years) with mild to profound ID treated with clozapine in 1971–1972 [34]. Of note, 80% of those in the higher IQ range (36–59) had good or very good improvement compared to only 20% of those with more profound ID. Since that publication there have been several dozen case reports and series published covering clozapine use in adult ID cohorts, but no controlled studies and few papers mention use of any rating scales beyond a general global impression [35]. When global impressions are reported, 14/14 papers noted improvement. The doses employed ranged from 25 to 900 mg/day, but the dose ranges cited most often are 200–500 mg/day, somewhat lower than those used for treatment-resistant schizophrenia. The reasons for this are twofold: (a) the majority of these patients are nonsmokers; (b) the anti-aggression effect of clozapine is seen at lower plasma levels than that required for resistant schizophrenia [36]. As the majority of reports cite doses $\geq$ 200 mg/day, this is a reasonable target for the initial titration, assuming tolerability. As will be discussed below in the section on Adverse Effects, vigilance has to be maintained for all adverse effects but particularly constipation and orthostasis, as patients may not be able to adequately verbalize these complaints. Before proceeding to higher dosages and plasma clozapine levels, it is reasonable to allow at least 2–3 weeks to observe changes in behavior patterns, bearing in mind the results of the Queensland study that indicate a natural fluctuation in the frequency of aggression in adult ID patients. Longer observation periods might be required before deciding that a particular dose/plasma level is ineffective, especially when the problematic behavior is infrequent. When problematic behaviors go into remission for extended periods, it is not unreasonable to gradually taper down clozapine to ascertain whether there is ongoing need for this medication, especially when environmental or behavioral interventions have been implemented that may address precipitating circumstances for the behaviors.

● Use of Clozapine in Psychotic Adult ID Patients

For ID patients with treatment-resistant schizophrenia clozapine remains the medication of choice, but this conclusion is not based on controlled trials, of which there are none. This statement is derived solely from the absence of viable therapeutic options, and the 31 publications (case reports or series, retrospective chart reviews) that document improved psychiatric outcomes in psychotic adults with ID that inadequately respond to nonclozapine antipsychotics [37]. Among the largest case series in the past 20 years is a sample of 33 treatment-resistant ID patients (17 male, 16 female) managed at an academic hospital in North Carolina, 88% diagnosed with psychotic disorders, and 12% diagnosed as bipolar I [38]. The patients were of mean age 40 years, and were titrated using standard adult dosing starting at 25 mg/day. All 33 patients were successfully discharged on clozapine after a mean hospital stay of 39.9 ± 16.6 days, and 26 remained on clozapine as outpatients through a mean 25 months of follow-up at a median dose of 400 mg/day. Among the seven who stopped clozapine as outpatients, two were due to poor adherence, four due to perceived lack of efficacy, and one was lost to follow-up. Side effects were described as "mild and transient," with constipation being the most prevalent (30%). There were no significant cardiovascular side effects, no seizures, and no treatment discontinuation due to severe neutropenia [38]. A 2004 paper described outcomes in 24 treatment-resistant adult ID patients managed at a London, UK treatment center [39]. The cohort was 83% schizophrenia spectrum disorders, 8% bipolar disorder, and 8% with no diagnosis other than ID. The patients were of mean age 38 years, and had four antipsychotic trials on average prior to clozapine. The mean maximum dose of clozapine was 488 mg/day, and 71% were deemed much improved or very much improved. Importantly, 53% of those from the medium secure unit were discharged to homes in the community. Only four patients discontinued treatment, three of which were due to neutropenia and one due to worsening diabetes mellitus [39].

Box 15.3 Principles for Clozapine Use in Adult Patients with Intellectual Disability

1. For adult ID patients with treatment-resistant schizophrenia spectrum or bipolar I disorders, target doses are generally comparable to those for non-ID patients.

2. For nonpsychotic adult ID patients with behavioral disturbances, effective doses may be lower than those often required for treatment-resistant schizophrenia.

3. The starting dose should be no higher than 25 mg QHS, and a slower titration is recommended to minimize issues with orthostasis and sedation. Daily monitoring of orthostatic blood pressure is important during the first 2 weeks of treatment and for several days after dose increases. A daily temperature should be obtained during the first 8 weeks of treatment, as this is the risk period for developing myocarditis, interstitial nephritis and other systemic drug reactions. Moreover, this patient group may be unable to verbalize complaints of malaise or systemic symptoms that suggest a serious drug reaction during the first 8 weeks of treatment.

4. Adverse effects: there is no unusual pattern of sensitivity, but vigilance must be observed for any sign of constipation, as patients may be unable to report issues until they become catastrophic. It may be preferable to be aggressive with laxative use to the point of causing loose stools than risk a patient developing ileus. A similar logic applies to the management of sialorrhea: patients may not complain of nocturnal sialorrhea and thus remain at risk for aspiration pneumonia unless aggressively managed. Prophylactic metformin should also be started at the onset of clozapine therapy to minimize weight gain. The general management of other adverse effects is similar to that for non-ID patients.

● **Adverse Effects**

There is no unusual pattern of sensitivity to adverse effects in the adult ID population, but constipation looms as the most easily overlooked and potentially life-threatening problem in a group that may have limited verbal abilities or underreport somatic complaints. Aggressive management of weight gain with prophylactic metformin, sialorrhea with orally applied agents and constipation with use of multiple agents should start early in treatment, as outlined in Box 15.3. Protocols must be in place to act promptly when initiatives to address adverse effects, especially constipation, do not meet with results in a timely manner. For constipation, this is set at 48 hours (see Chapter 7). For outpatients, appropriate education of caregivers is a crucial part of the management process, as they will be the ones to note adverse effects, implement measures to manage adverse effects, and quickly report the success (or lack thereof) of new treatments.

D Pregnancy and Lactation

Antipsychotics have been available for 60 years without compelling evidence of increased risk for major congenital malformations following first-trimester exposure [40]. Nonetheless, the earlier literature was comprised primarily of case reports and other nonsystematic collections of case data. Moreover, attempts to perform comparative analyses with control groups were complicated by the problem of confounding bias: those who received antipsychotics prior to 2000 were primarily schizophrenia spectrum patients, and thus had all of the associated risks (e.g. smoking, substance use) and care access issues not seen in a control group. Thus, any differential pregnancy outcome might be more related to the cohort of women who received antipsychotic therapy, and not to the medication itself [1].

With the broader use of antipsychotics for mood and other disorders, an opportunity arose to examine a more diverse population of exposed women. In 2016, Krista Huybrechts, PhD and her group in the Division of Pharmacoepidemiology and Pharmacoeconomics at Harvard Medical School published a study that overcame many of the limitations of the prior literature [1]. Using US data from 1,341,715 pregnancies in women enrolled in a Medicaid program from 3 months before their last menstrual period through at least 1 month after delivery, the investigators identified 9258 pregnancies with a prescription for an atypical antipsychotic and 733 with prescriptions for a typical antipsychotic that were filled during the first trimester (total $n = 9991$). In addition to matching this sample with a control group for covariates associated with increased risk of adverse birth outcomes, the two cohorts were also matched on the basis of *propensity scores.* One important source of bias in pregnancy outcome studies may depend more on characteristics that influence whether a woman received antipsychotic therapy (e.g. diagnosis age, geographic location, race, etc.). This issue can be managed in randomized studies because the likelihood of

15

treatment exposure is equal. For naturalistic data sets, the assignment of treatment is not random. Propensity score matching addresses the unevenness in real-world drug prescribing by matching the antipsychotic-exposed and unexposed women on the basis of empirically derived factors that influenced the likelihood (or propensity) of getting an antipsychotic among the 1,341,715 pregnancies in this data set. The groups can then be balanced for important covariates that relate to the outcome, major congenital malformations.

As a point of comparison, data from the US put the rate of major congenital malformations at 2–4% of live births, or 20–40 per 1000. In the Huybrechts study, the absolute risks for major congenital malformations per 1000 live-born infants was 38.2 (95% CI 26.6–54.7) for those treated with typical antipsychotics and 44.5 (95% CI 40.5–48.9) for those treated with atypical antipsychotics compared to 32.7 (95% CI 32.4–33.0) for untreated women [1]. However, in the fully adjusted analysis, there was no increased relative risk (RR) in the atypical antipsychotic exposed infants for malformations overall (RR 1.05; 95% CI 0.96–1.16) or for cardiac malformations (RR 1.06; 95% CI 0.90–1.24). In contrast, the risk remained elevated for risperidone, especially among those who filled ≥ 2 prescriptions or had ≥ 1-day supply in the first trimester (RR for any malformation 1.46 [95% CI 1.01–2.10]; RR for cardiac malformations, 1.87 [95% CI 1.09–3.19]) [1]. Unfortunately, there were no clozapine-exposed women in this large sample. Nonetheless, the important conclusion from this study is that atypical antipsychotics as a class do not appear to be associated with increased risk for major congenital malformations, although statements about individual agents cannot be made due to lack of large samples. Risperidone is possibly an exception, but the finding in this study requires replication from another data source.

● Review of Clozapine and Pregnancy Outcomes

In 2017, the British Association for Psychopharmacology published a consensus guidance paper on the use of psychotropic medication during preconception, pregnancy and the postpartum period [3]. Using data from the Huybrechts study and numerous other sources, the British Association for Psychopharmacology concluded that if a woman is established on clozapine prior to conception, she should continue with clozapine if the benefits are likely to outweigh the risks. This conclusion is bolstered by a comprehensive review of clozapine safety during pregnancy and lactation also published in 2017 [2]. The authors found four case-control or cohort studies ($n = 61$), one summary paper ($n = 102$), individual case reports or case series

($n = 18$), and information located in the Novartis database ($n = 523$) [2]. With respect to maternal risk, the only adverse effects noted were weight gain and a higher rate of gestational diabetes mellitus (DM). The latter is based on a case-control analysis of 11 clozapine-treated women that found a 2.4-fold increased risk of gestational DM compared to controls without mental illness and receiving no antipsychotic treatment [2]. Disentangling the specific impact of clozapine on risk of major congenital malformations in a group of women with serious mental illness, some of whom are taking multiple psychotropic medications or have behaviors associated with adverse fetal outcomes (e.g. smoking, substance use, etc.), is fraught with many of the issues noted at the beginning of this section. Nonetheless, the large data set from Novartis noted 22 major congenital malformations among 523 cases (42.1 per 1000 live births), a rate very similar to the crude rate of 44.5 per 1000 live births for those treated with the class of atypical antipsychotics in the Huybrechts study. The limited data on miscarriages also do not point to increased risk. Due to clozapine's sedating properties and impact on seizure threshold, there are multiple case reports of floppy infant syndrome at delivery and neonatal seizures. As noted in Box 15.4, decreasing clozapine exposure in the 48 hours prior to delivery may help minimize risk of seizures or poor infant tone. The dose reduction should be modest (i.e. ≤ 50%), as discontinuing clozapine abruptly will induce cholinergic rebound or psychiatric decompensation.

● Lactation

Breastfeeding provides enormous benefits for mother and baby by strengthening the maternal bond and providing the infant with secretory antibodies and nutrients important to short-term and long-term health [41]. Given the modern efforts to encourage breastfeeding, a leading expert in the field (Thomas W. Hale, PhD, Department of Pediatrics, Texas Tech University School of Medicine) has created a risk classification scheme to help clinicians advise women taking a variety of medications about the benefits and risks of breastfeeding [41]. The Hale classification uses empirical observations combined with relative infant dose estimates (a method to calculate infant drug exposure) to rank medications on a scale from L1 to L5 based on the degree of compatibility with breastfeeding. L1 is defined as compatible, meaning that this is a widely used medication with supporting controlled trials showing no adverse effects. The other categories are: L2, probably compatible; L3, possibly compatible; L4, possibly hazardous; and L5, hazardous. Although the quality of studies and accuracy of relative infant dose calculations for antipsychotics

15

Box 15.4 Use of Clozapine during Pregnancy

1. As a class, atypical antipsychotics do not increase risk for major congenital malformations following first-trimester fetal exposure [1]. On the basis of the accumulated data, the British Association for Psychopharmacology concluded that if a woman is established on clozapine prior to conception, she should continue with clozapine if the benefits are likely to outweigh the risks.

2. For treatment-resistant schizophrenia or mania patients, the lack of viable treatment options tilts the risk–benefit equation towards remaining on clozapine. Poorly managed or relapsed severe mental disorders are associated with worse pregnancy outcomes.

3. Use of clozapine during pregnancy is associated with 2.4-fold increased risk for gestational diabetes mellitus (DM) compared to mothers not taking antipsychotics [2]. How much of this risk can be separately attributed to factors associated with the mental illness or clozapine is unclear, but increased monitoring for gestational DM is recommended.

4. If possible, consideration can be given to modestly reducing the clozapine dose in the 48 hours prior to delivery to minimize the risk of floppy infant syndrome at delivery and neonatal seizures. The dose reduction should be modest (no greater than 50%) to lessen risk of psychiatric destabilization and cholinergic rebound symptoms. The full clozapine dose must be resumed immediately following delivery.

5. Clozapine is highly lipophilic and accumulates in breast milk. Due to the risk of severe neutropenia in the infant, breastfeeding is contraindicated.

is weak, nonclozapine antipsychotics are L2 or L3 level risk, meaning probably or possibly compatible [41,42]. Were the antipsychotic any agent other than clozapine, one could parse through the data to understand the extent of infant exposure and possible adverse effects. The relative infant dose exposure for clozapine is quite low (1.4%), but unfortunately clozapine presents a unique source of infant risk that is not dose-dependent – severe neutropenia. For this reason, the British Association for Psychopharmacology 2017 guidance paper advises that breastfeeding while on clozapine is not recommended due to the risk of neutropenia in the infant [3]. The subsequent 2017 review on the safety of clozapine during pregnancy and lactation also noted that in a case series of four breastfed infants, one developed severe neutropenia [2]. The true incidence of severe neutropenia in breastfed infants may never be known, but at the present time the risk of this potentially fatal complication appears to outweigh the multiple benefits of breastfeeding.

E Overdose

In colloquial usage overdose most commonly refers to intentional acts, but clinicians must be mindful that iatrogenic causes of excessive drug exposure (e.g. unrecognized drug–drug interactions) or other kinetic issues (e.g. smoking cessation) are all possible etiologies [4,43,44]. In most instances the need for supportive care will be obvious; however, the decision to refer a patient for hospital evaluation and monitoring should be based on the clinical scenario and not just the plasma clozapine level (see Chapter 5, Response to Levels Markedly Above or Below Expected Values, and Suspected Nonadherence). Spurious plasma clozapine levels that appear inconsistent with the clinical presentation are a reason to repeat the plasma level. For example, the laboratory returns a plasma clozapine level of 1400 ng/ml or 4280 nmol/l in a patient on a stable clozapine dose whose baseline plasma level is 700 ng/ml or 2140 nmol/l. If the patient shows no evidence of sedation, orthostasis, tachycardia or other plasma level-related adverse effects, and there is no viable explanation for the sudden jump (e.g. smoking cessation), suspicion of laboratory error should be high.

The presentation in intentional clozapine overdose cases relates in part to the dosage consumed, the presence of other medications or substances, and whether the patient has been adherent with clozapine treatment and thus tolerant to some degree to its adverse effects [45]. The leading expert on clozapine overdose (Dr. Robert Flanagan, Medical Toxicology Unit, Guy's and St Thomas' NHS Foundation Trust, London) notes that a dose of 300 mg in a clozapine-naive adult can cause unconsciousness, while 400 mg may be life-threatening [45]. Conversely, a 19-year-old female on clozapine 400 mg/day who ingested 5000 mg intentionally was reported to suffer only from somnolence, intermittent agitation, tachycardia and slight hypotension despite a plasma clozapine level 2.5 hours after ingestion of 3800 ng/ml or 11,600 nmol/l [46]. Adults have survived ingestions as high as 10,000 mg, but the degree to which an overdose is survivable primarily depends on the rapidity of supportive care, with case reports in clozapine-naive toddlers, children and teenagers describing complete recovery after receipt of prompt hospital interventions [47–50]. In addition to profound CNS depression, hypotension, tachycardia, generalized seizure activity and myoclonus are not uncommon, and QT prolongation may also occur [48, 51–53]. The presence of rhabdomyolysis has been reported and is hypothesized to be an epiphenomenon of myoclonic jerking. Significant elevations of creatine kinase ($\gg$ 5000 U/l) require appropriate intravenous hydration to minimize risk of acute renal tubular necrosis from myoglobin deposition [48]. Thromboembolic events have

15

also been reported, so patients with prolonged hospital stays may require prophylaxis [53]. Other complications related to aspiration of gastric contents, gastrointestinal hypomotility, and circulatory collapse can occur and require specific management.

The 12-hour trough metabolic ratio (MR) (defined as the ratio of clozapine:norclozapine) is typically 1.32 in adult nonsmokers, but shortly after an overdose this will be increased markedly, with median MR values of 7.6 (range 5.3–18) noted among samples obtained soon after hospital admission [45]. The high MR values are related to two processes: (a) the time since drug consumption may be relatively short (e.g. several hours) so insufficient time has elapsed for conversion of clozapine to norclozapine; (b) the metabolism of clozapine is primarily dependent on cytochrome P450 (CYP) 1A2, and this mechanism becomes saturated at high plasma clozapine levels [43]. As a result of these kinetic processes and delayed absorption, clozapine and norclozapine clearance demonstrate a biphasic elimination curve (Figure 15.3). Although single overdose cases and small series report a clozapine half-life estimate in these circumstances < 20 hours, pharmacokinetic modeling software using a larger Chinese cohort ($n = 21$) with mean overdose of 3740 mg (range 1250–10,000 mg) calculated a clozapine elimination half-life of 26.9 hours [50]. This extended half-life may explain cases of prolonged tachycardia that persist up to 10 days after the overdose event [48]. Based on serial monitoring of plasma clozapine levels, a time can be chosen to resume clozapine treatment when plasma levels are at or expected to be slightly below the patient's baseline. Withholding clozapine for prolonged periods risks symptoms of cholinergic rebound as well as psychiatric destabilization, all of which may complicate ongoing medical treatment.

For treatment-resistant schizophrenia or schizophrenia patients with a history of suicidality, intentional overdose is not a reason to discontinue clozapine therapy, as there are no viable therapeutic alternatives. Moreover, circumstances leading to the overdose must be investigated to determine whether the precipitant was related to undertreatment (e.g. subtherapeutic plasma clozapine levels) or clozapine nonadherence, because both will be associated with increased suicide risk [45]. When recent plasma levels and other clinical data (e.g. medication refill records, observed medication adherence) point to consistent medication adherence, other stressors, borderline personality disorder or substance use may underlie the overdose. In all instances of an intentional overdose, measures should be taken to limit medication access. For suboptimally treated or poorly adherent patients, routine monitoring of plasma clozapine levels is crucial to insuring that clozapine

Figure 15.3. The time course of plasma clozapine and norclozapine levels in an overdose case.

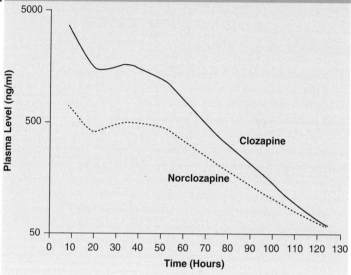

(Adapted from: Renwick, A. C., Renwick, A. G., Flanagan, R. J., et al. (2000). Monitoring of clozapine and norclozapine plasma concentration-time curves in acute overdose. *Journal of Toxicology and Clinical Toxicology*, 38, 325–328 [43].)

levels remain at the therapeutic threshold *for that patient.* For adherent patients with personality disorder or substance use diagnoses, appropriate evidence-based therapies must be provided including dialectical behavior therapy for borderline personality disorder patients [54].

 Postmortem Redistribution

Fatal overdoses on clozapine are relatively less common than deaths from other causes in clozapine-treated patients, but the contribution of clozapine to the patient's demise can become an issue when postmortem drug levels appear markedly elevated [45]. When extensive time may have elapsed after death and before blood samples are obtained, postmortem redistribution of lipophilic antipsychotics occurs resulting in distorted levels and inappropriate conclusions about the cause of death. This is especially true when samples are not obtained from femoral veins but central sources such as heart, vena cava or liver where postmortem redistribution effects are most pronounced [55]. The first report discussing postmortem redistribution of clozapine did not appear until 2003, and was based on the doubtful validity of an intracardiac clozapine blood level of 4500 ng/ml (13,750 nmol/l) obtained from a deceased patient who had been on a stable clozapine dose of 350 mg/day and who had refused clozapine for 24 hours before her death [56]. The expected trough plasma level in a female nonsmoker on 350 mg/day would be less than 500 ng/ml or 1500 nmol/l, and presumably even lower due to medication refusal prior to death [18]. To explore the correlation between antemortem and postmortem drug levels and MR values in patients whose death was not due to clozapine overdose, Flanagan examined cases from the UK/Ireland Clozaril Registry 1992–2003 [45]. In 38 cases where postmortem drug levels were obtained the median MR was 1.5, very similar to the value of 1.32 expected in the general population, and markedly lower than that seen in fatal and nonfatal overdose cases (4.4 and 7.6, respectively) [45]. Of these 38 cases, 21 also had plasma levels obtained within 30 days of death (median 14 days), with no clozapine dose changes in 19/21 since the last level was obtained. The median increase in postmortem levels was substantial: clozapine +489% and norclozapine +371%; however, the median MR increased only from 1.03 to 1.56 [45]. Subsequent data from animal studies and human cases have defined a number of considerations in interpreting postmortem levels in clozapine-related deaths [45,55] (see Box 15.5). The two most important principles are: (a) central postmortem clozapine levels are unreliable and differ by 10-fold or more from those obtained in a peripheral vein; (b) under ideal circumstances samples obtained from femoral veins may rise as much as 1.5-fold after death even when the vein is ligated proximally to minimize central contamination prior to the blood draw [57].

The use of plasma clozapine levels is crucial to effective management of patients, but these data are useful when the question is raised of overdose vs. postmortem redistribution of clozapine, and where a clinician may be accused of patient mismanagement on the basis of elevated postmortem levels. The availability of antemortem levels establishes the baseline MR and the baseline clozapine and norclozapine levels for the prescribed dose, all of which are needed to interpret postmortem levels. For anyone testifying in proceedings involving such issues, the extensive list of concerns elaborated by Flanagan in 2012 are listed in Box 15.5 [55]. While pathologists are increasingly aware of the problem of postmortem distribution, improper withdrawal of femoral vein samples without proximal ligation still occurs, as does reliance on central drug levels in determining a cause of death. The knowledge to challenge such procedural errors or errant conclusions may spare families, caregivers and colleagues from unfounded accusations, guilt or blame in certain cases of clozapine-associated death.

Box 15.5 List of Issues to Address When Investigating a Clozapine-Related Death [55]

1. Is there circumstantial or pathological evidence of self-poisoning?
2. Is there evidence of prior recent exposure to clozapine (i.e. is the patient likely to have been tolerant of the hypotensive effects of the drug)?
3. Was blood collected postmortem by venipuncture from a peripheral vein before opening the body?
4. Was the patient prescribed any other drugs and were other drugs looked for on toxicological analysis?
5. What was the clozapine dose and dosage regimen?
6. Were tablets or suspension dispensed?
7. Did smoking habit or clozapine dosage change recently?
8. Was there a history of substance abuse?
9. Was the blood norclozapine level measured?
10. Are antemortem plasma or whole blood clozapine/norclozapine results available?
11. Was histology performed, especially heart and liver?
12. Was there evidence of pneumonia?
13. Was there clinical or postmortem evidence of vomiting, aspiration of vomit, or other GI tract problem?

Summary Points

a. Clozapine is effective for treatment-resistant adolescent and childhood-onset schizophrenia, and younger patients may respond to plasma levels below the response thresholds defined for adults.

b. Clozapine has been used successfully in older schizophrenia patients from ages 65 to 100 years of age. Older age is not a reason to withdraw clozapine or refuse to commence clozapine in a treatment-resistant schizophrenia patient.

c. Clozapine is the antipsychotic of choice for intellectually disabled adults with treatment-resistant psychosis. There are some limited data to support use of clozapine to manage aggression and self-injurious behavior in adult ID patients, and its use in those circumstances must be balanced by careful monitoring for somatic adverse effects.

d. Treatment-resistant patients requiring clozapine should continue the medication throughout pregnancy with increased monitoring for weight gain and gestational diabetes. Breastfeeding is contraindicated due to the risk of neutropenia in the infant.

e. Supportive measures in a monitored hospital setting are needed after an overdose to manage sedation, orthostasis, tachycardia, and seizures until plasma levels return to the patient's therapeutic baseline. Overdose is not a reason to discontinue clozapine treatment, but to institute measures (e.g. restricted medication supply) to minimize its recurrence.

f. Clozapine is highly lipophilic and undergoes extensive postmortem redistribution. Interpretation of postmortem drug levels requires knowledge of the sample source (i.e. central or peripheral), and whether appropriate measures were taken to isolate the peripheral blood vessel from central sources.

References

1. Huybrechts, K. F., Hernandez-Diaz, S., Patorno, E., et al. (2016). Antipsychotic use in pregnancy and the risk for congenital malformations. *JAMA Psychiatry*, 73, 938–946.

2. Mehta, T. M. and Van Lieshout, R. J. (2017). A review of the safety of clozapine during pregnancy and lactation. *Archives of Women's Mental Health*, 20, 1–9.

3. McAllister-Williams, R. H., Baldwin, D. S., Cantwell, R., et al. (2017). British Association for Psychopharmacology consensus guidance on the use of psychotropic medication preconception, in pregnancy and postpartum 2017. *Journal of Psychopharmacology*, 31, 519–552.

4. Meyer, J. M., Proctor, G., Cummings, M., et al. (2016). Ciprofloxacin and clozapine – A potentially fatal but underappreciated interaction. *Case Reports in Psychiatry*, 2016, 5606098.

5. Kasoff, L. I., Ahn, K., Gochman, P., et al. (2016). Strong treatment response and high maintenance rates of clozapine in childhood-onset schizophrenia. *Journal of Child and Adolescent Psychopharmacology*, 26, 428–435.

6. Gogtay, N., Sporn, A., Alfaro, C. L., et al. (2002). Clozapine-induced akathisia in children with schizophrenia. *Journal of Child and Adolescent Psychopharmacology*, 12, 347–349.

7. Gogtay, N. and Rapoport, J. (2008). Clozapine use in children and adolescents. *Expert Opinion in Pharmacotherapy*, 9, 459–465.

8. Maher, K. N., Tan, M., Tossell, J. W., et al. (2013). Risk factors for neutropenia in clozapine-treated children and adolescents with childhood-onset schizophrenia. *Journal of Child and Adolescent Psychopharmacology*, 23, 110–116.

9. Yoshimura, B., Yada, Y., So, R., et al. (2017). The critical treatment window of clozapine in treatment-resistant schizophrenia: Secondary analysis of an observational study. *Psychiatry Research*, 250, 65–70.

10. Trinczek, E., Heinzel-Gutenbrunner, M., Haberhausen, M., et al. (2016). Time to initiation of clozapine treatment in children and adolescents with early-onset schizophrenia. *Pharmacopsychiatry*, 49, 254–259.

11. Schneider, C., Papachristou, E., Wimberley, T., et al. (2015). Clozapine use in childhood and adolescent schizophrenia: A nationwide population-based study. *European Neuropsychopharmacology*, 25, 857–863.

12. Thien, K., Bowtell, M., Eaton, S., et al. (2018). Clozapine use in early psychosis. *Schizophrenia Research*, 199, 374–379.

13. Lally, J., Ajnakina, O., Di Forti, M., et al. (2016). Two distinct patterns of treatment resistance: Clinical predictors of treatment resistance in first-episode schizophrenia spectrum psychoses. *Psychological Medicine*, 46, 3231–3240.

14. Demjaha, A., Lappin, J. M., Stahl, D., et al. (2017). Antipsychotic treatment resistance in first-episode psychosis: Prevalence, subtypes and predictors. *Psychological Medicine*, 47, 1981–1989.

15. Kumar, A., Datta, S. S., Wright, S. D., et al. (2013). Atypical antipsychotics for psychosis in adolescents. *Cochrane Database of Systematic Reviews*, 10, Cd009582.

16. Pagsberg, A. K., Tarp, S., Glintborg, D., et al. (2017). Acute antipsychotic treatment of children and adolescents with schizophrenia-spectrum disorders: A systematic review and network meta-analysis. *Journal of the American Academy of Child and Adolescent Psychiatry*, 56, 191–202.

15

17. Frazier, J. A., Cohen, L. G., Jacobsen, L., et al. (2003). Clozapine pharmacokinetics in children and adolescents with childhood-onset schizophrenia. *Journal of Clinical Psychopharmacology*, 23, 87–91.

18. Rostami-Hodjegan, A., Amin, A. M., Spencer, E. P., et al. (2004). Influence of dose, cigarette smoking, age, sex, and metabolic activity on plasma clozapine concentrations: A predictive model and nomograms to aid clozapine dose adjustment and to assess compliance in individual patients. *Journal of Clinical Psychopharmacology*, 24, 70–78.

19. Couchman, L., Bowskill, S. V., Handley, S., et al. (2013). Plasma clozapine and norclozapine in relation to prescribed dose and other factors in patients aged < 18 years: Data from a therapeutic drug monitoring service, 1994–2010. *Early Interventions in Psychiatry*, 7, 122–130.

20. Wehmeier, P. M., Schuler-Springorum, M., Heiser, P., et al. (2004). Chart review for potential features of myocarditis, pericarditis, and cardiomyopathy in children and adolescents treated with clozapine. *Journal of Child and Adolescent Psychopharmacology*, 14, 267–271.

21. Masi, G., Mucci, M. and Millepiedi, S. (2002). Clozapine in adolescent inpatients with acute mania. *Journal of Child and Adolescent Psychopharmacology*, 12, 93–99.

22. Mukku, S. S. R., Sivakumar, P. T. and Varghese, M. (2018). Clozapine use in geriatric patients – Challenges. *Asian Journal of Psychiatry*, 33, 63–67.

23. Pridan, S., Swartz, M., Baruch, Y., et al. (2015). Effectiveness and safety of clozapine in elderly patients with chronic resistant schizophrenia. *International Psychogeriatrics*, 27, 131–134.

24. Bishara, D. and Taylor, D. (2014). Adverse effects of clozapine in older patients: Epidemiology, prevention and management. *Drugs & Aging*, 31, 11–20.

25. Bowskill, S., Couchman, L., MacCabe, J. H., et al. (2012). Plasma clozapine and norclozapine in relation to prescribed dose and other factors in patients aged 65 years and over: Data from a therapeutic drug monitoring service, 1996–2010. *Human Psychopharmacology*, 27, 277–283.

26. Alvir, J. M., Lieberman, J. A., Safferman, A. Z., et al. (1993). Clozapine-induced agranulocytosis. Incidence and risk factors in the United States. *New England Journal of Medicine*, 329, 162–167.

27. Unwin, G. L. and Deb, S. (2011). Efficacy of atypical antipsychotic medication in the management of behaviour problems in children with intellectual disabilities and borderline intelligence: A systematic review. *Research in Developmental Disabilities*, 32, 2121–2133.

28. La Malfa, G., Lassi, S., Bertelli, M., et al. (2006). Reviewing the use of antipsychotic drugs in people with intellectual disability. *Human Psychopharmacology*, 21, 73–89.

29. Romeo, R., Knapp, M., Tyrer, P., et al. (2009). The treatment of challenging behaviour in intellectual disabilities: Cost-effectiveness analysis. *Journal of Intellectual Disability Research*, 53, 633–643.

30. Oliver-Africano, P., Dickens, S., Ahmed, Z., et al. (2010). Overcoming the barriers experienced in conducting a medication trial in adults with aggressive challenging behaviour and intellectual disabilities. *Journal of Intellectual Disability Research*, 54, 17–25.

31. Tyrer, P., Oliver-Africano, P., Romeo, R., et al. (2009). Neuroleptics in the treatment of aggressive challenging behaviour for people with intellectual disabilities: A randomised controlled trial (NACHBID). *Health Technolopgy Assessments*, 13, iii–iv, ix–xi, 1–54.

32. de Leon, J., Greenlee, B., Barber, J., et al. (2009). Practical guidelines for the use of new generation antipsychotic drugs (except clozapine) in adult individuals with intellectual disabilities. *Research in Developmental Disabilities*, 30, 613–669.

33. Frogley, C., Taylor, D., Dickens, G., et al. (2012). A systematic review of the evidence of clozapine's anti-aggressive effects. *International Journal of Neuropsychopharmacology*, 15, 1351–1371.

34. Vyncke, J. (1974). The treatment of behavior disorders in idiocy and imbecility with clozapine. *Pharmakopsychiatrie, Neuropsychopharmakologie*, 7, 225–229.

35. Singh, A. N., Matson, J. L., Hill, B. D., et al. (2010). The use of clozapine among individuals with intellectual disability: A review. *Research in Developmental Disabilities*, 31, 1135–1141.

36. Brown, D., Larkin, F., Sengupta, S., et al. (2014). Clozapine: An effective treatment for seriously violent and psychopathic men with antisocial personality disorder in a UK high-security hospital. *CNS Spectrums*, 19, 391–402.

37. Ayub, M., Saeed, K., Munshi, T. A., et al. (2015). Clozapine for psychotic disorders in adults with intellectual disabilities. *Cochrane Database of Systematic Reviews*, 9, Cd010625.

38. Antonacci, D. J. and de Groot, C. M. (2000). Clozapine treatment in a population of adults with mental retardation. *Journal of Clinical Psychiatry*, 61, 22–25.

39. Thalayasingam, S., Alexander, R. T. and Singh, I. (2004). The use of clozapine in adults with intellectual disability. *Journal of Intellectual Disability Research*, 48, 572–579.

40. Cohen, L. S., Viguera, A. C., McInerney, K. A., et al. (2016). Reproductive safety of second-generation antipsychotics: Current data from the Massachusetts General Hospital National Pregnancy Registry for Atypical Antipsychotics. *American Journal of Psychiatry*, 73, 263–270.

41. Newton, E. R. and Hale, T. W. (2015). Drugs in breast milk. *Clinical Obstetrics and Gynecology*, 58, 868–884.

42. Hummels, H., Bertholee, D., van der Meer, D., et al. (2016). The quality of lactation studies including antipsychotics. *European Journal of Clinical Pharmacology*, 72, 1417–1425.

43. Renwick, A. C., Renwick, A. G., Flanagan, R. J., et al. (2000). Monitoring of clozapine and norclozapine plasma concentration–time curves in acute overdose. *Journal of Toxicology and Clinical Toxicology*, 38, 325–328.

44. Meyer, J. M. (2001). Individual changes in clozapine levels after smoking cessation: Results and a predictive model. *Journal of Clinical Psychopharmacology*, 21, 569–574.

45. Flanagan, R. J., Spencer, E. P., Morgan, P. E., et al. (2005). Suspected clozapine poisoning in the UK/Eire, 1992–2003. *Forensic Science International*, 155, 91–99.

46. Broich, K., Heinrich, S. and Marneros, A. (1998). Acute clozapine overdose: Plasma concentration and outcome. *Pharmacopsychiatry*, 31, 149–151.

47. Borzutzky, A., Avello, E., Rumie, H., et al. (2003). Accidental clozapine intoxication in a ten-year-old child. *Veterinary and Human Toxicology*, 45, 309–310.

48. Gupta, G. B. and Sahu, M. K. (2006). Myotoxicity in acute clozapine overdose. *International Journal of Psychiatry and Clinical Practice*, 10, 303–304.

49. Toepfner, N., Wohlfarth, A., Naue, J., et al. (2013). Accidental clozapine intoxication in a toddler: Clinical and pharmacokinetic lessons learnt. *Journal of Clinical Pharmacy and Therapeutics*, 38, 165–168.

50. Li, A. N., Dong, F., He, J. L., et al. (2015). The elimination rate after clozapine overdose in Chinese schizophrenia patients: A population pharmacokinetics model study. *Pharmacopsychiatry*, 48, 150–155.

15

51. Rotella, J. A., Zarei, F., Frauman, A. G., et al. (2014). Refractory hypotension treated with vasopressin after intentional clozapine overdose. *European Journal of Emergency Medicine*, 21, 319–320.

52. Jansman, F. G., Crommelin, H. A., van Hout, F. J., et al. (2015). Rhabdomyolysis in clozapine overdose. *Drug Safety Case Reports*, 2, 9.

53. Sackey, B., Miller, L. J. and Davis, M. C. (2018). Possible clozapine overdose-associated thromboembolic event. *Journal of Clinical Psychopharmacology*, 37, 364–366.

54. Rohde, C., Polcwiartek, C., Correll, C. U., et al. (2018). Real-world effectiveness of clozapine for borderline personality disorder: Results from a 2-year mirror-image study. *Journal of Personality Disorders*, 32, 823–837 .

55. Flanagan, R. J. (2012). Was it poisoning? *Transactions of the Medical Society of London*, 129, 40–61.

56. Kerswill, R. M. and Vicente, M. R. (2003). Clozapine and postmortem redistribution. *American Journal of Psychiatry*, 160, 184.

57. Stark, A. and Scott, J. (2012). A review of the use of clozapine levels to guide treatment and determine cause of death. *Australian & New Zealand Journal of Psychiatry*, 46, 816–825.

58. Kumra, S., Frazier, J. A., Jacobsen, L. K., et al. (1996). Childhood-onset schizophrenia. A double-blind clozapine–haloperidol comparison. *Archives of General Psychiatry*, 53, 1090–1097.

59. Shaw, P., Sporn, A., Gogtay, N., et al. (2006). Childhood-onset schizophrenia: A double-blind, randomized clozapine–olanzapine comparison. *Archives of General Psychiatry*, 63, 721–730.

60. Kumra, S., Kranzler, H., Gerbino-Rosen, G., et al. (2008). Clozapine and "high-dose" olanzapine in refractory early-onset schizophrenia: A 12-week randomized and double-blind comparison. *Biological Psychiatry*, 63, 524–529.

61. Klein, D. J., Cottingham, E. M., Sorter, M., et al. (2006). A randomized, double-blind, placebo-controlled trial of metformin treatment of weight gain associated with initiation of atypical antipsychotic therapy in children and adolescents. *American Journal of Psychiatry*, 163, 2072–2079.

Index